Essays in Cell Metabolism

Essays
in
Cell Metabolism

Hans Krebs Dedicatory Volume

W. Bartley
Professor of Biochemistry, University of Sheffield

H. L. Kornberg
Professor of Biochemistry, University of Leicester

J. R. Quayle
Professor of Microbiology, University of Sheffield

WILEY—INTERSCIENCE

a division of John Wiley & Sons Ltd.

LONDON   NEW YORK   SYDNEY   TORONTO

1970

Library of Congress catalog card number
75–128168

ISBN 0 471 05480 1

PRINTED BY Unwin Brothers Limited,
The Gresham Press, Old Woking, Surrey, England
a member of the Staples Printing Group

DEDICATION

When Hans Krebs in 1925 appeared at Berlin-Dahlem in the Kaiser-wilhelminstitute of Biology, he was a modest thoughtful youth, very intelligent and already wise in spite of his youth. At the beginning of his four years' visit you could not see who he was. But at the end you could.

Nearly 40 years later I met him in Dublin at an important meeting. He was now Sir Hans and the chairman of the meeting. Few scientists were more famous. How civilized he is, I thought, if I compared him, even with myself.

What had he achieved since 1925? He had discovered the essential chemical reactions of the energy-transformations in life; and he had calculated the amount of energy that is transformed by each of these reactions and had therefore explained thermodynamically why these reactions occur. Compare this to the state of bioenergetics in 1925!

Yet there are still dark areas in the field of bioenergetics, for example the oxidative phosphorylation or—perhaps related to it—the activation of carbon dioxide in photosynthesis. It is the hope of his friends that Sir Hans, now freed from administrative duties, will finally solve these very important problems too.

OTTO WARBURG

PREFACE

There are two themes that unite these essays. All their authors are or were close colleagues or students of Professor Sir Hans Krebs, F.R.S.; most were members of the Medical Research Council's Unit that he directed for over twenty years. The researches of that Unit ranged as widely as implied by its permissive title: it was a Unit for Research in Cell Metabolism. We feel it peculiarly appropriate to reflect this title also in the title of this volume. We have resisted the temptation to impose any artificial uniformity of subject-matter or style on these essays: they are printed as submitted, unedited and unvarnished, because we know that Sir Hans would wish to hear unmuted the voices of his friends.

The other common factor in these essays is their intention. On 24th August, 1970, Sir Hans will reach his seventieth birthday, and his friends wish to give him particular pleasure on that occasion. They know that he sets but little store on gifts, on ceremonies and on public honours, and that he rejoices chiefly in the advancement of that field of human endeavour which is the mainspring of his life and to which he himself has so richly contributed. It is for that reason that his friends offer their work to him, in the hope that he will accept it as tangible evidence of their gratitude, their good wishes, and their warm affection.

W. BARTLEY
H. L. KORNBERG
J. R. QUAYLE

CONTRIBUTING AUTHORS

Bacon, J. S. D.   *Department of Biochemistry, Macaulay Institute for Soil Research, Craigiebuckler, Aberdeen, Scotland.*

Bartley, W.   *Department of Biochemistry, University of Sheffield, Sheffield, England.*

Birt, L. M.   *Department of Biochemistry, School of General Studies, Australian National University, Canberra, Australia.*

Brosnan, J. T.   *The Banting and Best Department of Medical Research, The Charles H. Best Institute, University of Toronto, Canada.*

Burton, K.   *Department of Biochemistry, University of Newcastle upon Tyne, Newcastle upon Tyne, England.*

Davies, R. E.   *University of Pennsylvania School of Veterinary Medicine, Department of Animal Biology, Laboratories of Biochemistry, Pennsylvania, U.S.A.*

Eggleston, L. V.   *Metabolic Research Laboratory, Nuffield Department of Clinical Medicine, Radcliffe Infirmary, Oxford, England.*

Hems, R.   *Metabolic Research Laboratory, Nuffield Department of Clinical Medicine, Radcliffe Infirmary, Oxford, England.*

Hughes, D. E.   *Microbiology Department, University College, Cardiff, Wales.*

Kornberg, H. L.   *Department of Biochemistry, University of Leicester, Leicester, England.*

Lowenstein, J. M.   *Graduate Department of Biochemistry, Brandeis University, Waltham, Massachusetts 02154, U.S.A.*

Lund, Patricia   *Metabolic Research Laboratory, Nuffield Department of Clinical Medicine, Radcliffe Infirmary, Oxford, England.*

Newsholme, E. A.   *Agricultural Research Council Unit of Muscle Mechanisms and Insect Physiology, Department of Zoology, University of Oxford, Oxford, England.*

Quayle, J. R.   *Department of Microbiology, University of Sheffield, Sheffield, England.*

Terner, C.   *Department of Biology, Biological Science Center, Boston University, Boston, Massachusetts, U.S.A.*

Whittam, R.   *Department of Physiology, University of Leicester, Leicester, England.*

Williamson, D. H. *Metabolic Research Laboratory, Nuffield Department of Clinical Medicine, Radcliffe Infirmary, Oxford, England.*

CONTENTS

ASPECTS OF THE TURNOVER OF MITOCHONDRIAL CONSTITUENTS

W. Bartley

Department of Biochemistry, University of Sheffield

L. M. Birt

Department of Biochemistry, School of General Studies, Australian National University

H.A.K. as a supervisor

My interest in mitochondria stems from the research I carried out for my Ph.D. in Sheffield under the supervision of Dr. Krebs. The title of the thesis *Studies on the Metabolism of Mitochondria* would never be accepted now but in those days (early 1950's) it expressed the situation that almost any experiments with mitochondria were meaningful. Thus I was able to make progress by the straightforward use of manometers, paper chromatography and conventional chemical analyses of substrates, although later isotopes were also used. The elaborate armoury of electronic devices, such as recording spectrophotometers, recording polarographs and electron microscopes, that are used by modern mitochondriacs were undreamed of. H.A.K.'s attitude was that you made use of the apparatus available to the limit but you did not use lack of apparatus as an excuse for not doing experiments. I am convinced he could have devised meaningful experiments using jamjars only. As a supervisor H.A.K.'s main disadvantage was having so many ideas for experiments that only a tiny fraction could actually be tested. The other difficulty was that he believed that we students could carry out experiments about twice as fast as humanly possible and his cry of 'have you mixed?' at a time when we were only halfway through the pipetting of the Warburg vessels used to produce rebellious rumblings. The other cry of 'are you in the bath?' often provoked comment, particularly when preceded by the christian name of one of the female technicians. Apart from this, H.A.K. was an ideal supervisor. In between the stirrings up he allowed time for his students to think and develop their own lines of experimental approach and he was a great believer in serendipity. Thus there was complete freedom to develop any promising line of work even if the connection between the original problem

1

was extremely tenuous. The most harrowing times were when written-up papers were first presented for his scrutiny. He was merciless in his criticism and sometimes one would emerge exhausted after an hour's discussion, having dealt with only about half a page of the typescript which was now covered with crossings out, interjections and marginal notes to such an extent that nothing remained of the original. Sometimes three or four drafts were necessary before the paper was allowed to be sent to the Journal. The maddening thing was that he was always right, or nearly always. I remember on one occasion having a page cut to ribbons and after modifying it so that it was pure Krebs it received the same drastic treatment on re-submitting it to H.A.K. Thinking I could now point out the error of his ways I told him what he was criticizing was his own modification. His reply was 'yes, but I am my most severe critic' which completely deflated me. He meted out to his own papers the same treatment as he did to others and was in fact 'his most severe critic'.

On looking back one realizes that here was a Master teaching his apprentice the craft of scientific communication and I shall always be grateful that he was willing to spend so much time on my education. I hope I have not given an impression of H.A.K. as an intolerant slave driver. This would be far from the truth. He is the most kindly of men to whom one can turn with any personal difficulty and be assured of receiving sympathy and help. I shall always be grateful to him for the training he gave me in biochemistry, but I am even more grateful to have been accepted as his apprentice with the opportunity of learning from him his attitude to research, scientific integrity and human relationships.

W. BARTLEY

In a discussion of 'scientific family trees' Sir Hans has remarked that direct personal contact between the great innovators of scientific thought and those colleagues fortunate enough to work with them is an extremely potent factor in the process of scientific education.

For my own part, and speaking as a second generation member of Krebs' own 'scientific family', a striking illustration of the accuracy of this proposition is my recollection of the extent to which his concern with scientific integrity and persistence had become part-and-parcel of the mental climate of his entire laboratory. Conversations with those who had worked with him for long periods brought to light again and again the attributes described by Professor Bartley; my own work with him—both at the bench and the writing desk—quickly provided personal confirmation of the strength and value of Sir Hans' approach to research and scientific training and of his ability to transmit this approach to his colleagues. His first two sentences to me on my arrival in Oxford provided a succinct illustration of the fundamental concerns mentioned by Professor Bartley— for personal relations, for a sense of compelling urgency in getting on with the job and for clarity and brevity in communication. 'Have you found yourself satisfactory digs?' was the first enquiry. When I said 'Yes', Prof. replied, 'Well then you will start work this afternoon?'—and that was that! The time that has elapsed since that first meeting has deepened my gratitude for the opportunity of learning in his laboratory and my respect and admiration for a great man and a great scientist.

L. M. BIRT

INTRODUCTION

Although it is generally accepted that the macromolecules of the cell have a finite life and that the amount found at any one time is the result of the balance of synthesis and breakdown, there appears to be a general feeling that there may be some special factors to be taken into consideration when the macromolecules form part of a visible cell structure. Studies on the induction and repression of enzymes tend to be concentrated on 'soluble enzymes', with the implicit suggestion that enzymes in cell structures are stable throughout the life of the cell organelle and that the destruction of such enzymes is a consequence of the complete dissolution of the organelle itself. The accumulating evidence for positional organization of even the 'soluble enzymes' within the cell seems to leave no rational reason for believing that structurally-associated enzymes are controlled in any fundamentally different way from any other enzymes. In the work to be described we shall be concerned with some variations in the biochemical composition of the mitochondria from a variety of species and tissues which throw light on the question of the turnover of their component enzymes.

Mitochondrial morphogenesis

Apart from bacteria, cells actively consuming oxygen have structures called mitochondria that are responsible for catalysing the oxidation of hydrogen to water. In most studies of mitochondrial morphogenesis differentiating tissue or rapidly growing tissue is used because the increase in the mass of the tissue is matched by an increase in that of the mito-chondria. It appears that only in those fungi (in particular yeast) which are able to grow under anaerobic conditions (at which stage mitochondria may be absent) can the *de novo* appearance of mitochondria be studied. In what follows mitochondrial changes will be described in the developing flight muscle of an insect, in regenerating rat liver, in tissues from animals under metabolic stress and in *Saccharomyces cerivisae* that has been transferred from anaerobic to aerobic conditions. Subsequently, experiments on the turnover of mitochondrial constituents will be discussed and lastly the degradation of mitochondria and the selective removal of mitochondrial enzymes will be described.

THE DEVELOPMENT OF MITOCHONDRIA IN RAT LIVER, INSECT FLIGHT MUSCLE AND AEROBICALLY ADAPTING YEAST

Changes in physical properties and structure

Mitochondrial development in muscle, liver and yeast is characterized by an increasing structural elaboration, resulting from increases in the number of cristae and also, in flight muscle (Plate 1) in the complexity of their alignment (Lennie, Gregory and Birt, 1967; Gregory, Lennie and Birt, 1968). At the same time, both flight muscle and liver mitochondria increase in size and specific gravity ($1 \cdot 193$–$1 \cdot 198$ in the regenerating rat liver (Gear, 1965) and $1 \cdot 180$–$1 \cdot 200$ in the developing insect (Walker and Birt, 1968)). These changes reflect the pattern of incorporation of phospholipid and protein into the mitochondrial structure as shown, for example, by the analyses of the developing insect particles (Table 1). There was a 6-fold increase in the amount of mitochondrial lipid phosphorus per insect and a parallel incorporation of protein. The proportions of the various phospholipids changed during development; phosphatidylethanolamine became twice as concentrated, phosphatidylcholine was almost unchanged. Polyglycerophosphatide was most concentrated in the pharate adult; at the time of emergence its concentration fell to the level in the mature adult (12% of the total mitochondrial lipid phosphorus). In the blowfly, it is possible to distinguish a particular period centred about adult emergence, in which the rate of 'structural' development, i.e. the incorporation of 'non-dehydrogenase' or 'structural' protein accelerates, until it greatly exceeds that of other proteins like the extremely active glycerol-l-phosphate dehydrogenase (Figure 1) and the group of respiratory enzymes which change synchronously with this dehydrogenase. This conclusion, based on changes in the specific activities of dehydrogenase and oxidase at different stages of adult development, can be correlated with the changes occurring in mitochondrial DNA (increasing 2–3-fold in amount at the beginning of the period (Table 2) and in the frequency of occurrence of the cristae (which increases 2–3-fold during the same period (Lennie, Gregory and Birt, 1967)).

Table 1. The phospholipids of sarcosomes isolated from thoraces of developing adult flies

Stage of life cycle	μg lipid P per mg protein	Calculated mμg atoms lipid P in thoracic sarcosomes	Calculated mμg atoms sarcosomal lipid P per thorax as				
			Phosphatidylethanolamine	Phosphatidylcholine	Phosphatidylserine	Lysophosphatides	Polyglycerophosphatides
Pharate Adult (2 days before emergence)	10·4	35	11	7	1	4	11
Flies (at emergence)	13·2	128	60	35	16	1	15
Flies (5 days)	11·9	230	143	48	5	7	28

Lipid extracts of sarcosomes from 20 thoraces were fractionated on silicic acid columns to yield the total phospholipid fraction, which was further fractionated by thin-layer chromatography

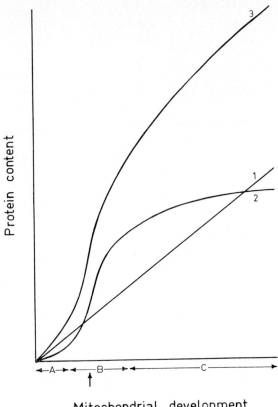

Mitochondrial development

Figure 1. Sarcosomal development. Schematic representation of the asynchronous incorporation of dehydrogenase and non-dehydrogenase protein into developing blowfly sarcosomes. The 'respiratory' protein (curve 1) includes the primary dehydrogenases and redox proteins of the respiratory chain, and the 'non-respiratory' protein (curve 2) the structural proteins together with enzymes not directly concerned with primary redox reactions. Curve 3 represents the total protein of the mitochondria. The developmental period is divided into three stages, the limits of which are determined by the rate of incorporation of the 'non-respiratory' protein. In Stage A, there is a preferential accumulation of the dehydrogenase protein; mitochondria enlarge (but do not exceed 1 μ in diameter) and increase in specific gravity (from less than $1 \cdot 185$ to $1 \cdot 185$–$1 \cdot 195$). In Stage B there is a preferential accumulation of non-dehydrogenase protein; mitochondria continue to increase in size (diameter greater than 1 μ) and in specific gravity (to greater than $1 \cdot 195$). In Stage C both types of protein are accumulated and the mitochondria continue to increase in size and specific gravity. The point at which an individual particle reaches a diameter of 1 μ during its development is indicated by the arrow

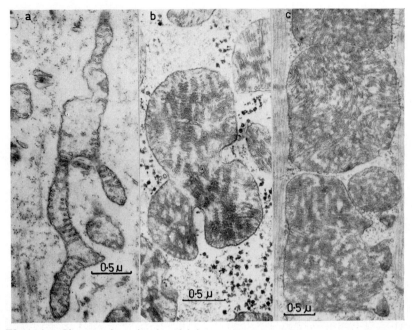

Plate 1. Changes in mitochondrial structure at different stages of adult development in the blowfly *Lucilia*. Mitochondria were isolated from the longitudinal dorsal indirect flight muscle of the fly and were fixed with osmium (see Gregory, Lennie and Birt, 1968). The ages of the insects were: (a) three days before adult emergence; (b) one day after emergence; (c) five days after emergence. Note the increase in the frequency of cristae, which is most rapid during the period of adult emergence; and the development of channels or fenestrations during maturation

Some features of the enzymic changes are summarized in Table 3 and Figure 1. During Stage A (Figure 1 and Table 3) the amount of non-dehydrogenase protein decreases as a proportion of the total protein of the mitochondria, because dehydrogenases are accumulated preferentially; thus increasing specific gravity from less than $1 \cdot 185$ to $1 \cdot 185$–$1 \cdot 195$ produces mitochondria of greater specific activity (Walker and Birt, 1969; Table 3). Two days before emergence, only a small group of mitochondria (16% of the total mitochondrial protein) have undergone this change; at this stage of development these denser mitochondria have sufficient internal structure to 'express' the accumulated dehydrogenase as oxidase. In Stage B (which for most of the mitochondrial population is reached about the time of emergence) there is a rapid incorporation of non-dehydrogenase protein, so that a denser fraction (specific gravity greater

Table 2. Changes in blowfly mitochondrial nucleic acids with age

	Age											
Mitochondrial diameter	1 day before emergence			At emergence			1 day after emergence			7 days after emergence		
	$<1\mu$	$>1\mu$	Total	$<1\mu$	$>1\mu$	Total	$<1\mu$	$>1\mu$	Total	$<1\mu$	$>1\mu$	Total
(a) μg DNA/mg protein	1·0	4·3	2·6[a]	4·0	5·3	4·7[a]	2·7	3·1	2·9[a]	1·6	1·4	1·4[a]
(b) μg RNA/mg protein	48	36	42[a]	35	29	32[a]	21	16	18a	11	4	5[a]
(c) μg Protein/insect (calc)	100	100	200	140	160	300	190	190	380	140	520	660
(d) μg DNA/insect (calc)	0·10	0·43	0·53	0·56	0·85	1·41	0·51	0·59	1·10	0·22	0·73	0·95
(e) μg RNA/insect (calc)	4·8	3·6	8·4	4·9	4·6	9·5	4·0	3·0	7·0	1·5	2·1	3·6
RNA/DNA	48	8·4	16·0[a]	8·8	5·5	6·7[a]	7·8	5·2	6·4[a]	6·9	2·9	3·8

The values for the concentrations of nucleic acids in the mitochondrial fractions were determined experimentally (lines (a) and (b)). The amount of mitochondrial protein (line (c)) in the fractions was derived from Figure 3 of Lennie and Birt (1967). The values for the amount (μg) of nucleic acids/insect (lines (d) and (e)) were determined from the values in lines (a), (b) and (c)

[a] Values were calculated from the total amount (μg) of mitochondrial nucleic acid/insect (lines (d) and (e)) and the total amount (mg) of mitochondrial protein/insect (line (c)) and therefore represent the average values for the whole mitochondrial population

Table 3. Enzymic and structural changes during the development of blowfly mitochondria

Age of insect	α-glycerophosphate dehydrogenase activity [a] in mitochondria of specific gravity			α-glycerophosphate oxidase activity [a] in mitochondria of specific gravity			Respiratory Control Ratio [b]	Stimulation by Ca^{2+} [c]	No. of cristae per μ of mitochondrial profile
	<1·185	1·185–1·195	>1·195	<1·185	1·185–1·195	>1·195			
2 days before emergence	780	1,400	–	300	1,650	–	∞ (∞)	+	Approximately 14
At emergence	850	1,450	800	600	650	650	5–10 (∞)	++	29
5–7 day fly	850	1,550	850	200	750	400	1·2 (10)	+++	34
Stage (see Figure 1)	←–A→	←––B––→	←–C–	←–A→	←––B––→	←–C–			

[a] Activities expressed as $\mu1O_2$/mg/protein/hour.

[b] The ratio is respiratory rate with ADP/respiratory rate before addition of ADP. Values in parenthesis are for the oxidation of pyruvate.

[c] Stimulation by Ca^{2+} was estimated in the absence of ADP in a medium containing 2mM EGTA and 3mM α-glycerophosphate (see Handsford and Chappell, 1967)

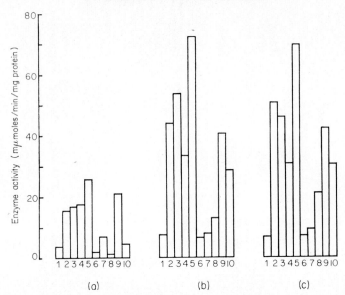

Figure 2. Pattern of 'mitochondrial' enzymes in yeast grown on a synthetic medium with 0.9% glucose as the carbon source initially. The three blocks of columns represent (reading from left to right): (a) after 12 hours of growth when roughly one-half the glucose is consumed; (b) after 15 hours of growth when all glucose has been consumed; and (c) after 30 hours of growth. (1) Pyruvate oxidase; (2) Condensing enzyme; (3) Aconitase; (4) Isocitrate dehydrogenase (NAD linked); (5) Isocitrate dehydrogenase (NADP linked); (6) α-oxoglutarate oxidase; (7) Succinyl CoA synthetase; (8) Succinate-cytochrome c reductase; (9) Fumarase; (10) Malate DH = Malate dehydrogenase

than 1.195) appears; consequently the specific activity of the dehydrogenase falls (by about 45%) while that of the oxidase remains almost constant. A small group of mitochondria are still undergoing the Stage A transition. Continuing growth of the mitochondria involves the further accumulation of both dehydrogenase and non-dehydrogenase protein so that there is little further change in the specific activities of either oxidase or dehydrogenase in the specific gravity range above 1.185 (at emergence, 5–7 day fly; Stage C). These studies emphasize the extent to which an independent accumulation of different protein fractions occurs during mitochondrial development. Similar conclusions have been reached by investigations of changes in enzyme activities in mitochondria of different size in developing insects (Lennie and Birt, 1967). All these data are consistent with the accumulating evidence for separate and independently controlled formation of mitochondrial structure and enzymes.

The incorporation of enzymes

(a) In yeast

It is well known that yeast cells are capable of considerable adaptation, varying their enzyme content in changing environmental conditions.

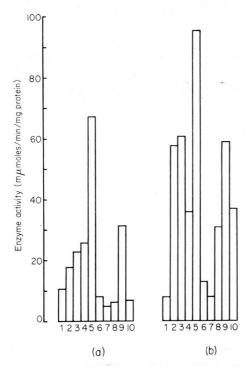

Figure 3. Pattern of mitochondrial enzymes in yeast grown on a synthetic medium with 0·9% galactose as the carbon source initially. The two blocks of columns represent: (a) after 14 hours of growth when roughly half the galactose is consumed; (b) after 27 hours when all the galactose had been consumed. Enzymes indicated as in Figure 2

Yeast grown aerobically with glucose as the carbon source degrade it continually until it has been converted firstly to ethanol (Stage 1) and, subsequently, to acetate (Stage 2). Initially, the cells lack well-developed mitochondria and the relatively feeble TCA-cycle activity is probably located in simple vesicles. During Stage 1 (glucose to ethanol), TCA cycle activity increases somewhat, especially that of the enzymes metabolizing citrate, isocitrate and malate. The components of the electron transport chain also appear to be present in the vesicles, but in low concentration.

Table 4. Ratios of enzyme activities in yeast growing on different substrates

Main substrate for growth	Pyr / α-oxo	Con / Mal	Acon / Fum	Iso NAD / Iso NADP	Succ syn / succ ox	cyt ox / NADH ox
Glucose	1·9	0·35	0·8	0·69	5·2	2·3
Ethanol	1·1	0·15	1·3	0·45	0·6	3·8
Acetate	1·0	0·19	1·1	0·44	0·42	5·5
Galactose	1·3	0·25	0·7	0·39	0·77	3·1
Acetate	0·6	0·15	1·0	0·37	0·26	5·3
Pyruvate	0·6	0·06	1·0	0·35	0·50	1·1

Pyr	= Pyruvate oxidase
α-oxo	= α-oxoglutarate oxidase
Con	= Condensing enzyme
Mal	= Malate dehydrogenase
Acon	= Aconitase
Fum	= Fumarase
Iso NAD	= Isocitrate dehydrogenase (NAD linked)
Iso NADP	= Isocitrate dehydrogenase (NADP linked)
Succ syn	= Succinyl CoA synthetase
Succ ox	= Succinic oxidase
Cyt ox	= Cytochrome oxidase
NADH ox	= NADH oxidase

As the cells can obtain almost all the ATP they require from glycolysis, respiratory activity is probably only 'loosely coupled' to phosphorylation; hence the respiratory vesicles do not contain the structural elements (cristae) required for the efficient coupling of oxidation and phosphorylation. Figure 2 illustrates the enzyme patterns in yeast under these conditions. In contrast, where galactose is the original carbon source (Figure 3) and the glycolytic generation of ATP is much slower, the cells must meet some of their demand for ATP from oxidative phosphorylation. Relatively complex mitochondrial structures are then visible and the concentration of respiratory enzymes is greater. Figure 4 illustrates the cytochrome oxidase and NADH oxidase activities in glucose and galactose grown yeast at the same stages as in Figures 2 and 3.

During the second stage (ethanol to acetate) both the number of mitochondria per cell and of cristae per mitochondrion increase. TCA cycle enzymes become more concentrated. Since the glyoxylate cycle also becomes more active at this time, these changes are probably required for the entry of acetate into the TCA cycle. The cells are now entirely dependent on these processes for the provision of all biosynthetic inter-

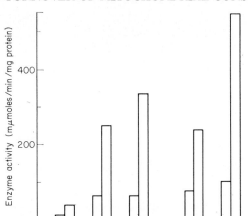

Figure 4. NADH oxidase and cytochrome oxidase in yeast grown on glucose or galactose

mediates and, in conjunction with the respiratory chain and its associated ATP synthetase, for the generation of ATP. Hence, there are striking increases in the concentrations of the components of the respiratory chain and in the structural complexity of the particles. Table 4 shows the changes in ratios of some enzymes of the mitochondria brought about by growth on different substrates.

In summarizing the significance of these observations, it should be stressed that in yeast, individual enzymes of the TCA cycle, redox components of the respiratory chain and the components responsible for coupling oxidation and phosphorylation, can all vary independently in response to different environmental conditions. It seems that a 'constant proportion group' hypothesis of the type proposed by Bucher and his colleagues (Brosemer and coworkers 1963; Bucher, 1965) cannot be applied to the enzymes of these mitochondria.

(b) In regenerating rat liver

The biogenesis of mitochondria in regenerating rat liver has been examined by Gear (1965) who has studied the appearance of various enzyme activities in light (smaller) and heavy (larger) mitochondrial fractions. He interprets his results as indicating independent incorporation of related components, for example of cytochrome c, cytochrome oxidase and various dehydrogenases. Thus, if in the normal animal the activities of cytochrome oxidase and succinic dehydrogenase are designated 100%, the ratio cytochrome oxidase/succinic dehydrogenase may increase during

Table 5. Changes in proportions of membrane bound mitochondrial enzymes under different conditions
The enzyme activity before the experimental procedure is given the arbitrary value of 100. Thus all ratios start as 1

Tissue	Experimental condition	Growth of Tissue + or −	Cytochrome oxidase NADH-cyt c reductase	Cytochrome oxidase Succ-cyt c reductase	Cytochrome oxidase Succinic dehydrogenase
Mouse liver	Hypoxia 24 hours	−	1·2	—	4·2
	48 hours	−	1·05	—	0·6
	1 week	−	0·75	—	0·73
Chick liver	Normal growth from day 10 after hatching to day... (daily injection of vehicle) 13	+	0·52	0·33	—
	16	+	1·17	0·28	—
	19	+	0·66	0·22	—
	21	+	0·38	0·16	—
	25	+	0·42	0·33	—
	Extra growth induced by daily cortisol injections (2 mg/100 g body wt) from day 10 to day... 13	+	0·30	0·16	—
	16	+	1·53	0·65	—
	19	+	0·52	0·30	—
	21	+	0·39	0·23	—
	25	+	0·47	0·38	—
Mouse kidney	Hypoxia 24 hours	0	1·14	—	2·3
	48 hours	0	0·94	—	1·24
	1 week	0	0·48	—	0·71
Rat kidney	21 days after removal of 1 kidney and DOCA implant in neck + high salt diet	+ ?	—	1·13	—
Mouse heart	Hypoxia 24 hours	?	2·2	—	0·67
	48 hours	?	1·9	—	1·9
	1 week	?	1·6	—	1·9
Rat heart	21 days after removal of heart and DOCA implant in neck + high salt diet	+ ?	—	1·5	—
Mouse skeletal	Hypoxia 24 hours	?	—	—	0·53
	48 hours	?	—	—	0·56

regeneration to a value of $1 \cdot 85$ in about three weeks. Although the range of differences in the rates of enzyme incorporation is much smaller than that used to detect significant deviations from a 'constant proportion group' by Bucher, Gear has concluded that such an hypothesis probably does not apply to these mitochondria.

Support for the non-constancy of proportions of enzymes in rat liver mitochondria is given also by the work of Swick, Stange, Nance and Thomson (1967) who found that the ratio of one mitochondrial enzyme to another was not constant when mitochondria were separated in a linear density gradient. The less dense mitochondria had a higher proportion of cytochrome oxidase but it appeared that the total membrane-bound enzyme composition of a mitochondrion was constant with the heavier mitochondria having a larger matrix and more of the enzymes localized in this matrix. Bearing in mind the experimental evidence (see later) that soluble protein such as cytochrome c (Haldar, Freeman and Work, 1966) is synthesized outside the mitochondria and transported into the particles, it might be expected that the variation would be in the non-structural enzymes of the mitochondria. Constant proportions of enzymes might then be expected in specialized mitochondria in which the membrane component is a relatively higher proportion of the total protein, as, for example, in sarcosomes of mature blowflies (see later).

Changes in membrane-bound enzymes of the mitochondria under different conditions

A somewhat similar situation to the regeneration of rat liver is the natural increase in size which occurs as the young animal grows towards maturity. The rate of cell division slows as the maximum adult size of the organ is approached. In the chick the rate of liver growth can be accelerated by the injection of cortisol (Bellamy and Leonard, 1965) and the proportion of body weight represented by the liver is very much increased under these conditions. In Table 5 are shown changes in the proportions of some membrane-bound mitochondrial enzymes during normal growth of the chick liver and during the accelerated growth induced by cortisol. At the start of the experiment the enzyme activities are given the arbitrary values of 100, and thus the ratio of one enzyme to another starts as 1. The percentage change of one enzyme is then compared with that of another enzyme over the experimental period and expressed as a ratio. Thus, a ratio greater than 1 (e.g. for cytochrome oxidase/NADH cytochrome c reductase) means that the relative proportions of the enzymes have changed (e.g. in favour of cytochrome oxidase) but it does not indicate whether the change is brought about by increase or decrease of either or both of the enzymes. Substantial changes in enzyme proportions occur in both normal and cortisol-induced growth and the pattern of change varies under the two conditions.

Changes in the membrane-bound enzymes of the mitochondria of several tissues may be induced by placing the animal in a condition of metabolic stress. For example, keeping mice under conditions of hypoxia corresponding to an altitude of about 18,000 feet changes the proportions of cytochrome oxidase to NADH cytochrome c reductase and of cytochrome oxidase to succinic dehydrogenase, but the extent of the changes varies with the tissues and with the time of exposure to hypoxia (Table 5). In the liver these changes are associated with a decrease in organ size and suggest that selective removal of enzymes as well as selective induction may play a part in adjusting the membrane-bound mitochondrial enzymes to the required proportions for the new metabolic situation. Similar types of change may be shown in the heart and kidneys of animals made artificially hypertensive by removal of one kidney and the implantation of DOCA. Exposure of these animals to a high salt diet results in hypertension and in the growth of the remaining kidney and the heart. Table 5 shows the change in the ratio of cytochrome oxidase to succinic cytochrome c reductase that occurs under these conditions. It is clear that even if the enzyme is membrane-bound, this localization does not prevent its individual induction and removal if the metabolic situation requires such a change.

Enzyme proportions in developing flight muscle

There are, however, tissues where the proportions of one enzyme to another do remain almost constant throughout a change in net mitochondrial quantity. The appearance of glycerol-l-phosphate dehydrogenase in blowfly sarcosomes has already been mentioned. Other studies (Lennie and Birt, 1967) show that a number of dehydrogenases and cytochrome oxidase increase at the same relative rate as the mitochondria enlarge; at the same time, variations in the activity of two non-mitochondrial enzymes (soluble malic dehydrogenase and NADP-isocitric dehydrogenase) are somewhat greater. It has been concluded that there are 'constant proportion groupings' of related enzymes in these mitochondria. This is in contrast to the situation in liver and yeast, as is the state of the tissue during the period studied. In the insect, there is a very limited range of variations in the internal environment within the enclosed puparium, so that the bulk of mitochondrial development takes place in a precisely regulated system.

However, as has been pointed out already, not all the proteins of the blowfly sarcosomes are incorporated synchronously. Immature mitochondria can accumulate dehydrogenase in excess of their oxidase capacity, but at all stages such oxidase activity as is present appears to be coupled to the phosphorylation system (Table 3). During adult development, the increasing *total* capacity for carrying out oxidative phosphorylation

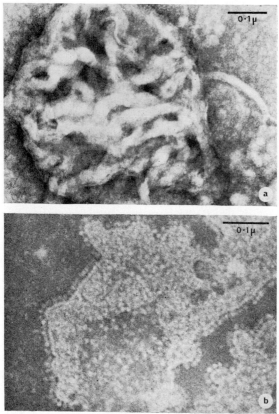

Plate 2.   (a) Part of a mitochondrion isolated from *Lucilia* flight muscle two days before adult emergence and negatively stained with potassium phosphotungstate. There is a clearly-defined outer membrane and relatively few cristae, apparently free from elementary particles; (b) Cristal membrane isolated from tissue 3 days after adult emergence and negatively stained with potassium phosphotungstate. The membrane is lined with elementary particles

accompanies an increasing internal complexity of the mitochondria, most notably an appearance of 'elementary particles' (Kagawa and Racker, 1966) on the cristal membranes (Plate 2, Walker, Gregory and Birt, 1969). The development of new physical structures in the membranes may be responsible for the changing proportions of the component phospholipids in the mitochondria (Table 1) during development. The chemical changes may also be important in determining the physiological behaviour of the mitochondria as shown by the shift in the pattern of respiratory control by ADP and calcium. During development there was a gradual increase in the stimulatory effect of calcium in the absence of ADP, parallel to the decline in respiratory control (Walker and Birt, 1969; Table 3). This may be a reflection of the onset of the extraordinary high activity of the insect flight muscle after emergence (in *Lucilia* this muscle contracts some 20 times faster than vertebrate muscle). In the emerged adult, which begins to fly a few hours after eclosion, it is possible that the process requiring ATP (muscular contraction) and the process generating ATP, are controlled by the release of the same component, calcium. In contrast, the respiratory activity of the pharate adult, in which the muscles are not engaged in locomotion, is more directly linked to energy transformations producing ADP.

All the data on the flight muscle sarcosomes are consistent with a pattern of development in which the immature particles accumulate groups of enzymes, but have a relatively poorly developed structural framework in which to assemble them. This develops independently (synthesis of its protein presumably being controlled by mitochondrial nucleic acids) over the period of adult emergence, producing denser, larger particles of considerable structural complexity, capable of oxidizing TCA cycle intermediates and glycerol-l-phosphate to provide the ATP necessary for flight. It is also clear that not all the dehydrogenase systems of these mitochondria develop synchronously. Thus, early in adult life, fatty acids can be oxidized by a carnitine-dependent pathway which reaches maximum activity at about emergence and then, although other enzymes are still increasing in activity, declines in both specific and absolute activities, until it is virtually absent in mature flies (D'Costa and Birt, 1967; Figure 5). These changes and the loss of fat from the tissues indicate that thoracic development is energized by the oxidation of fatty acids which cannot be utilized for flight; conversely, the relatively small carbohydrate reserves of the insect (Crompton and Birt, 1967) are conserved and can support the initial flights undertaken by the newly emerged insect.

Thus, in the three different situations considered there are three different patterns of mitochondrial development. Yeast cells capable of considerable adaptation can apparently vary the proportions of individual enzymes and the elaboration of mitochondrial structure to provide pathways for carbon transformation, hydrogen transfer and oxidative phosphorylation in relative independence. Mammalian and avian mitochondria, somewhat

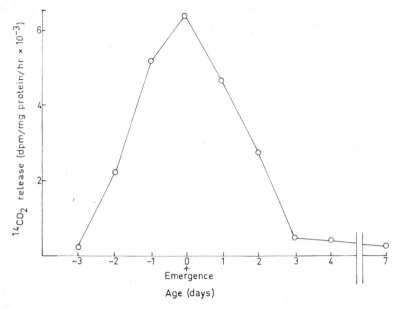

Figure 5. Changes in the activity of fatty acid oxidase in thoracic mitochondria from the developing blowfly. Mitochondria were isolated from the thoracic muscles of insects in the developmental period from three days before adult emergence till seven days after emergence. They were incubated for one hour in a buffered isotonic medium containing coenzyme-A (0·2 mM), carnitine (0·5 mM) and palmitate (2 mM potassium salt, pH 7·5; 0·8 μC ^{14}C per flask). The CO_2 released was collected and its content of ^{14}C determined

more specialized, show less variability, while blowfly sarcosomes, which are highly specialized (being designed to produce ATP in the adult insect from a limited range of substrates) clearly show synchronous incorporation and removal of groups of related enzymes.

The turnover of mitochondrial constituents

Besides enzymic components the mitochondria contain protein ('structural protein'; Criddle, Bock, Green and Tisdale, 1962) which has no apparent enzymic activity, phospholipids and some nucleic acid. In a study of the turnover of insoluble protein, soluble protein, lipid and cytochrome c by measuring the decay of radioactivity that had been incorporated into these components, Fletcher and Sanadi (1961) came to the conclusion that the mitochondrion turned over as a whole with a half-life of 10·3 days. The flexibility shown in the enzymic composition of some mitochondria suggested that a similar flexibility might also exist in some of the non-enzymic components. This possibility was explored using mature rats injected with ^{35}S methionine, ^{32}P and ^{14}C acetate (Bailey, Taylor and Bartley, 1967; Taylor, Bailey and Bartley, 1967). In a manner similar to that in which the enzyme composition of the mitochondria is altered by metabolic stress, the fatty acid composition of the phospholipids of the mitochondria can also be altered. In the experiments to be described some of the rats were kept on a diet deficient in essential fatty acids. Since the proportion of essential fatty acids in the phospholipids of the mito-chondria (in particular those in the cardiolipin fraction) is substantial it might be expected that differences in the turnover of the mitochondria might ensue.

Turnover of phospholipids

Figure 6 gives the decay curve of ^{32}P in the mitochondrial phospholipids of the normal and essential fatty acid deficient rats. It is clear that there

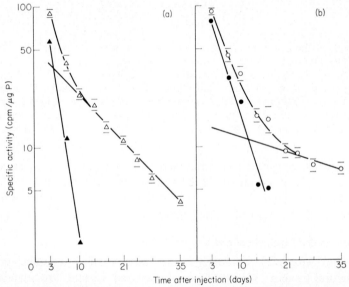

Figure 6. Change in logarithm of mitochondrial [^{32}P] phospholipid specific activity with time. Each point is the mean result for three animals. The horizontal bars represent the range of results. The points for the fast components were obtained by subtracting the values deduced from the extrapolation of the linear 'tail' of the experimental graph from the initial experimental points. (a) control rats; △, experimental results; ▲, calculated fast component; (b) EFA-deficient rats; ○, experimental results; ● calculated fast component

are fast and slow components of the curves and that these are different in the two cases. The turnover of both components is slower in the EFA deficient animals. If the change in specific activity in the individual phospholipids of the mitochondria is followed after a single injection of labelled phosphate into the animal it can be shown that the phospholipid becomes labelled at very different rates (Figure 7).

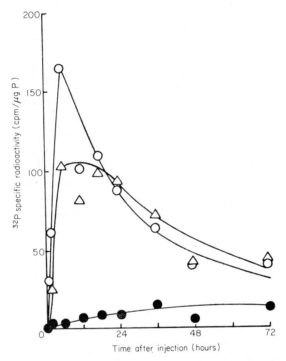

Figure 7. Changes in ^{32}P specific radioactivity of mitochondrial phospholipid with time. Each point is the mean of the results from four animals. △, Lecithin; ○, phosphatidylethanolamine; ●, cardiolipin

[32]P was incorporated most rapidly into phosphatidyl ethanolamine (maximum in 6 hours) and phosphatidyl choline (maximum in 6–12 hours); labelling of cardiolipin was much slower, the activity increasing up to 24 hours. (These values are calculated from the percentage of ^{32}P in the different lipid classes and the percentage composition of the total phospholipid, assuming that no change occurs in this composition during the experimental period.) Thus the bulk phospholipid is labelled maximally about 6 hours after injection as it consists mainly of phosphatidyl choline (56%) and phosphatidyl ethanolamine (28%).

B

The decay of the ^{32}P in the bulk phospholipid indicates a half-life of 1·9 days. The curve also suggests the presence of a component of much longer half-life—about 10 days; this is probably a reflection of the cardiolipin content of this protein.

The data are consistent with either a mitochondrial synthesis of phospholipid or with the rapid transfer of phospholipid from extra mitochondrial pools to the mitochondria. The first possibility appears more likely, as recent evidence (Bygrave, 1969) on the turnover of cephalin and lecithin of liver mitochondria, labelled by the injection of ^{14}C-acetate and choline, indicates that there is a transfer of phospholipid from the outer to the inner membrane, but not from microsomes to mitochondria. These studies have also shown that the label turns over more rapidly in the lecithin and cephalin of the inner membrane than in that of the outer membrane. The relatively slow turnover of cardiolipin in whole mitochondria suggests that it is less concerned with 'metabolic changes' in the mitochondria than the other components; there is other evidence that it may be concentrated in the inner mitochondrial membrane (Parsons, Williams, Thompson, Wilson and Chance, 1966) and there is some proportionality between cardiolipin content and cytochrome c (Getz and Bartley and coworkers, 1968). Thus the molar ratio of cardiolipin to cytochrome is about 800 or a weight ratio of about 10. It has also been suggested (McGivan and Chappell, 1968) that cardiolipin determines the special permeability properties of the mitochondria.

Despite the differences in the rates of turnover of lipid phosphorus, changes in the specific activities of ^{14}C-labelled phospholipids after the injection of ^{14}C-acetate were similar for all three components. Thus it appears that the acyl groups of lecithin, cephalin and cardiolipin all turn over at about the same rate—maximum incorporation had occurred after about 6 hours and the half-lives were all about 4 hours: there is also evidence for a ^{14}C-labelled component with a half-life of about 100 days or more but this may be a reflection of the turnover of the pool of precursor fatty acids, which probably has a long half-life (e.g. 163–187 days).

Turnover of protein

Mitochondrial protein was subdivided into soluble (in ice-cold 0·15 M NaCl) and insoluble fractions. Incorporation of ^{35}S into both fractions occurred without any lag phase. In contrast to the results of Beattie and coworkers (1966) (using ^{14}C-labelled amino acids), the soluble protein was labelled more rapidly than the insoluble; however, the specific activities are expressed as dpm/mg benzidine sulphate and will, therefore, depend on the relative *amounts* of S in the two fractions. After incorporation the isotope was lost from the insoluble protein with a half-life of about 9 days. The decline in the radioactivity of the soluble protein was not linear, suggesting the loss of a number of components at different rates; only between 14 and 28 days after injection was the half-life also 9–10 days (i.e. about the same as for the insoluble protein). Thus it is clear that there are a number of separate components in this soluble fraction, each with a characteristic half-life—a conclusion consistent with those reached from the studies of enzymic incorporation discussed previously. Recently Brunner and Neupert (1968) have shown that the protein of the outer mitochondrial membrane differs in its turnover time from that of the inner mitochondrial membrane (half-life of $4 \cdot 2$ days for the outer membrane compared with $12 \cdot 6$ days for the inner membrane) and the mitochondrial soluble protein turns over at a rate which is intermediate between that of the two membranes.

The data for the turnover of proteins and lipids make it clear that different mitochondrial constituents are incorporated and turn over independently of one another; and that in a particular class of compounds, or even within one compound, individual components may turn over in isolation (e.g., cardiolipin in phospholipid, acyl and phosphoryl groups in cardiolipin).

The loss of mitochondrial enzymes

In the previous sections consideration has been given largely to the control of the enzyme composition of mitochondria by the accretion of specific enzymes. Since the total enzymic protein of the fully developed mitochondrion is likely to remain constant, the selective synthesis of one particular enzyme must be accompanied by a cessation or slackening in the synthesis of another. It is also possible to visualize circumstances where the bulk of adjustment of the enzyme pattern is brought about by the active removal of one of the enzymes as well as by a diminution in its rate of synthesis. In the mammal, it is clear from turnover studies that the amount of an enzyme at any time is the balance of its synthesis and breakdown, but in most cases both processes will alter to make the enzymic adjustment. Such arguments apply to microorganisms, but isotope studies have suggested that in growing cells the turnover of cell protein is virtually zero ($0 \cdot 2\%$ per hour in yeast cells grown aerobically on 3% glucose with a mean generation time of about 90 minutes). In a culture kept stationary by starvation, the turnover of cell protein may rise to about $0 \cdot 7\%$ per hour and this is similar to the turnover rate found in mammalian cells. The rate of turnover of protein is roughly the same irrespective of the mean generation time of the cells. In the slowly dividing mammalian cell (which is never faced with the traumatic change of environment experienced by yeast in changing from aerobic to anaerobic conditions) there is time to adjust to the new situation through the mechanism of protein turnover before the necessity for cell division arises. With the microorganism the short generation times do not allow this leisurely approach and the unwanted enzymes may be removed actively. This phenomenon may be investigated by following the enzyme changes in yeast transferred from a medium requiring oxidative removal of carbon (e.g., one containing ethanol or acetate) to a medium with 10% glucose where oxidative mechanisms (i.e. mitochondrial mechanisms) becomes superfluous.

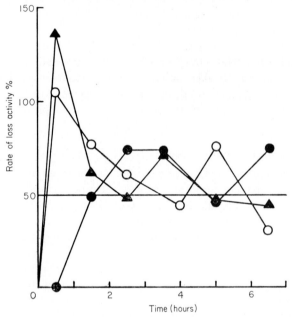

Figure 8. Changes in the activities of succinate-cytochrome c oxidoreductase (▲), NADH-cytochrome c oxidoreductase (○) and NADH oxidase (●) during adaptation of yeast to anaerobic growth on 10% glucose. On this type of plot any point above the 50% mark indicates a loss of activity that is faster than dilution by new protein

At the beginning of the experimental period the aerobic medium contains mainly ethanol (derived from the original glucose supply) and the cells have fully developed mitochondria. Activities of various mitochondrial enzymes decline following glucose addition. If it is assumed that the synthesis of a particular enzyme stops but no active degradation occurs then the specific activity of these enzymes will decline by 50% at each cell division. The enzyme will thus be diluted out. If the specific activity of the enzymes declines faster than 50% per cell division then there must be some specific process removing the enzyme. On the other hand, if the specific activity of the enzyme declines less than 50% per cell division there must be continuing synthesis in spite of a decline in activity. Whether this is a resultant of the same rate of synthesis with an increased rate of breakdown, or a lowered rate of synthesis or a change of both the rates, is impossible to say. Figure 8 shows some changes in mitochondrial enzymes. The specific activity of both NADH-cytochrome c reductase and succinate-cytochrome c reductase decreased rapidly during the lag phase and the early stages of growth; NADH oxidase behaved in the same manner but about one generation behind in time. This suggests that the electron transport chain is actively destroyed at a number of points. Whereas the enzymes feeding electrons to cytochrome oxidase were actively removed, the terminal enzyme disappeared at a rate which was less than the dilution rate and was therefore still being synthesized although it was not required.

Table 6. Percentage of original specific activity of various enzymes in *Saccharomyces cerevisae* after 3·0 hours of glycolytic adaptation

Enzyme	Percentage of original specific activity	
	Aerobic adaptation	Anaerobic adaptation
α-Oxoglutarate dehydrogenase	45	21
Succinate-cytochrome c oxidoreductase	31	17
NADH oxidase	48	18
Cytochrome c oxidase	67	41

A batch of aerobically grown cells was divided into three samples. One sample was grown aerobically on 10% glucose and another was grown anaerobically in an identical medium. (The third sample was analysed for its enzyme content.) The growth rate of both cultures was the same and after 3 hours the cells were harvested and specific activities of the enzymes were compared with those in a sample of the original culture; these control activities were taken as 100

The loss of cytochrome oxidase was influenced by the presence of oxygen in the high glucose medium. The presence of oxygen decreased the enzyme loss as it did that of the other structurally bound mitochondrial enzymes (Table 6). Of the other mitochondrial enzymes fumarase and aconitase disappear at the dilution rate but malate dehydrogenase was lost very rapidly and even before growth began some 50% of the activity had disappeared. From the loss in malate dehydrogenase activity and the known specific activity of the enzyme it can be calculated that about 1·5% of the cell protein is lost by the removal of this enzyme alone. Thus, without considering the decline in other enzymes during the lag phase, the protein loss is already more than 0·75%—the value that would be expected from the measurements of protein turnover in the non-growing cells under the conditions of starvation. Constant enzyme proportions, then, do not seem to apply to the loss of yeast mitochondrial enzymes any more than the induction of the organelles. It is possible that the retention of cytochrome oxidase is due to the persistence of relatively high synthetic activity—perhaps the messenger RNA of this protein is relatively long-lived, whereas for fumarase and aconitase, the messenger must be absent when growth is resumed. The activities which disappear most rapidly—reductase and oxidase—are complex functions, requiring the cooperation of a number of components oriented in the membranous framework; these are more likely to suffer rapid functional disarrangement than individual enzymes. These results show that the removal of unwanted enzymes is selective and is influenced by metabolic conditions. It was therefore of interest to examine the influence of metabolic inhibitors on the process particularly since Bartley and Tustanoff (1966) have shown that the development of respiration in anaerobically grown yeast (and the associated synthesis of mitochondrial enzymes) was very little affected by inhibitors of glycolysis, protein synthesis or nucleic acid synthesis. Table 7 shows the effect of a series of inhibitors on the rate of disappearance of two enzymes; one (succinic cytochrome c reductase) is a part of the mitochondrial membrane and the other, malate dehydrogenase is a soluble component of the mitochondria. The yeast was grown aerobically on low glucose concentration and then transferred to 10% glucose. The activities of the aerobic yeast cells are given as 100% and the measurement of activity subsequently was after 40 minutes exposure to the 10% glucose (i.e. just at the end of the lag phase). This minimized any complications of change in enzyme activity due to yeast growth. Arsenate, which would be expected to uncouple substrate level phosphorylation, had no effect on the destruction of the two enzymes suggesting that no energy was required for the breakdown. However, in agreement with the results of Witt, Kronan and Holzer (1966) cycloheximide abolished the breakdown of malate dehydrogenase, suggesting the necessity for protein synthesis (possibly of a proteinase) for the destruction of the enzymes. Unpublished work of Chapman and Bartley has shown that cycloheximide at the concentration used is a potent inhibitor of glycolysis and as Table 7 shows, there is a general finding that inhibitors of glycolysis stabilize the

Table 7. Effect of inhibitors on the loss of enzymes on transfer of yeast grown aerobically on a low glucose concentration to 10% glucose

Expt No	% of activity 40 minutes after transfer to 10% glucose	% of activity 40 minutes after transfer to 10% glucose in the presence of the concentration of inhibitor given in brackets						
		Arsenate	Cycloheximide	Azide	Iodoacetate	Borohydride	Bisulphite	Fluoride
		A. Succinate cytochrome c reductase						
1	84	81 (10 mM)	99 (0·1 mM)	101 (0·75 mM)	100 (1 mM)	98 (37 mM)	88 (0·4 mM)	85 (10 mM)
2	78	—	—	103 (3 mM)	71 (2 mM)	99 (9·3 mM)	70 (0·4 mM)	77 (20 mM)
		B. Malate dehydrogenase						
1	46	41 (10 mM)	99 (0·1 mM)	79 (0·75 mM)	78 (1 mM)	55 (37 mM)	99 (0·4 mM)	94 (10 mM)
2	43	—	—	100 (3 mM)	112 (2 mM)	63 (9·3 mM)	114 (0·4 mM)	96 (20 mM)

two mitochondrial enzymes. It is tempting to speculate that the rate of glycolysis is the determining factor in defining the level of mitochondrial enzymes.

From blowfly mitochondria

In the developing fly, also, there appears to be a selective removal of particular enzyme systems at a time when other enzymes are increasing in activity. The appearance early in development of a thoracic mito-chondrial system for the oxidation of fatty acids has already been described and it was pointed out that soon after emergence this capacity begins to decline rapidly. The change is not the result of a dilution of the activity by increasing amounts of other mitochondrial proteins—there is an absolute loss of activity (see Figure 5).

It was not feasible to exclude completely the possibility that the thoracic preparations contained a separate group of mitochondria (distinct from the sarcosomes whose development has already been discussed) which were responsible for these changes. However, the total mitochondrial population could not be fractionated on the basis of differences in specific gravity in such a way as to separate α-glycerophosphate and fatty acid dehydrogenase activities, although the latter was concentrated mainly in the lighter (and smaller) mitochondria—as would be expected from the activity pattern (Figure 1). The decline after emergence did not appear to be a consequence of an increasing impermeability to the substrate, as sonicated preparations were no more active than the original material. Thus there is no precise information about the reasons for the loss of activity, which may involve the whole set of enzymes or possibly, just one key enzyme.

It is interesting to speculate on the possible relation of these findings to the extremely rapid onset of senescence in adult flies. Senescence has a dramatic effect in inactivating a number of mitochondrial enzymes about eight days after adult emergence *in the male*. These changes are greatly delayed in the female, and it seems possible that they may be initiated by the inability of male flies to remove fatty acids by oxidation after the first few days of adult life. The female has an alternative pathway for the disposal of fatty acids, by channelling them into the fat reserves required for egg production. Thus in the male, but not in the female, fatty acids may accumulate in the haemolymph or in the muscle itself, until they are sufficiently concentrated to begin a generalized disruption of the mito-chondria. In turn, this will accelerate the release and activation of mitochondrial proteinases (see later), so that an autocatalytic destruction of mitochondria will occur. The consequent lowering of the capacity for

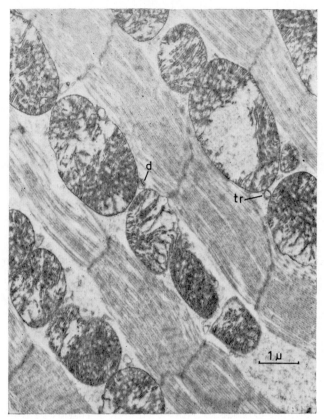

Plate 3.   A longitudinal section of *Lucilia* flight muscle at 8 days post-emergence after osmium fixation. There is considerable disorganization of the fibrils and the mitochondria. The only features still recognizable in the remaining cytoplasm are tracheoles (tr) and 'dyads' (d) of T-system and sarcoplasmic reticulum

ATP synthesis in the thorax will diminish locomotory activity and prevent the maintenance of the structure of the muscle mitochondria. These proposals are compatible with the histological appearance of the tissue in senescing insects (Gregory and coworkers, 1968; Plate 3).

Mitochondrial degradation

The loss of mitochondrial function can arise from structural damage or by loss of an essential component such as a phospholipid or protein. It is not always easy to allocate the precise reason for the loss of activity. For example, the loss of succinate-cytochrome c reductase activity on

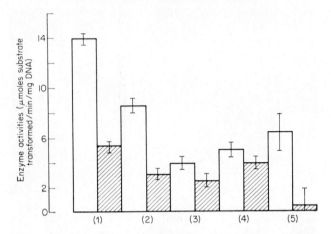

Figure 9. Comparison of some mitochondrial enzymes and glucose-6-phosphatase in normal mice liver (unshaded columns) and in the liver of mice kept under hypoxic conditions for 48 hours (shaded columns). Enzyme activities in pairs from left to right are: (1) Cytochrome oxidase $\times 10^{-3}$; (2) NADH-Cytochrome c reductase $\times 10^{-1}$; (3) Succinate dehydrogenase; (4) Malate dehydrogenase $\times 10^{-2}$; (5) Glucose-6-phosphatase

transfer of respiring yeast to a medium of high glucose content could be due to the loss of phospholipid or disorganization of the complex arrangement of the components of the enzyme. Similarly, the loss in activity of NADH-cytochrome c reductase and cytochrome oxidase that occurs in the liver of mice exposed to hypoxic conditions (Figure 9) could be due not only to the loss of the enzyme but also to a lack of essential phospholipids; this latter possibility is supported by the finding that there is a decline in the activity of glucose-6-phosphatase and a disappearance of intracellular membranes, pointing to a defect in the synthesis of phospholipids for membranes. Since the turnover of mitochondrial phospholipid is much faster than that of the mitochondrial protein, a simple defect in formation of phospholipids could have a disproportionately large effect on the activity of mitochondrial enzymes.

Mitochondrial proteinases

Besides these possibilities for mitochondrial inactivation there may be an involvement of specific proteinases that can selectively hydrolyse enzymes. Thus, if a suspension of mitochondria, isolated in the usual manner, is incubated either in sucrose or in saline media at neutral pH, there is a gradual liberation of amino acids into the medium at a rate of about 0·15 μmoles/mg dry wt/hour at 40°. This implies a complete breakdown of all the mitochondrial protein under these conditions in about 54 hours. From the studies of the turnover of mitochondrial protein (Fletcher and Sanadi, 1961; Bailey, Taylor and Bartley, 1967; Taylor, Bailey and Bartley, 1967) it is clear that *in vivo* these mitochondrial neutral proteinases must be held in check since the measured half-lives are about 9 days. However, this estimate of the rate of proteolysis does give an idea of the potentialities for hydrolysing mitochondrial protein should the need arise. It is especially interesting that there appears to be no substrate acting as a source of amino acids in these experiments other than the mitochondria themselves. However, the neutral proteinase activity is not confined to the mitochondria but is found in all cell fractions; therefore these proteinases may have a specific role in degrading

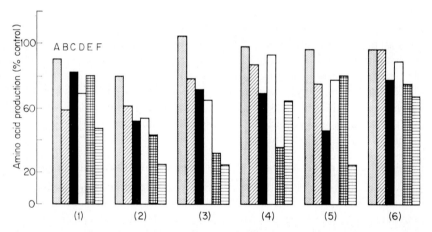

Figure 10.   Effect of inhibitors on the production of amino acids by rat liver homogenate and cell fractions. All fractions were incubated for 1 hour at 40° C aerobically. The incubation medium contained 2·5 ml of fraction in 0·25 M sucrose, 1 ml of 0·1 M tris-HCl buffer, pH 7·4 and 0·5 ml of inhibitor in water (final volume 4 ml). Amino acid production is given as a percentage of the control value without inhibitor. The inhibitors were all 1 mM (final concn), except for soya-bean trypsin inhibitor, which was present at a concentration of 0·5 mg/ml of incubation medium. Fractions: (1) whole homogenate; (2) nuclei; (3) mitochondria; (4) fluffy layer; (5) microsomes; (6) final supernatant. Inhibitors in each case: A potassium borohydride; B di-isopropyl phosphorofluoridate; C soya-bean trypsin inhibitor; D EDTA; E iodosobenzoate; F *p*-chloromercuribenzenesulphonate

proteins in all parts of the cell. In aerobic incubations in phosphate buffer at pH 7·4, about 8% of the total activity in fractions isolated from rat liver is found in the mitochondria. There does not appear to be the same range of types of proteinases in all cell fractions, as shown by the response to the series of inhibitors (Figure 10; Alberti and Bartley, 1965); the mitochondrial fraction has a distinctive pattern of response to these compounds. The measurement of proteinase activity by estimating the amounts of amino acids liberated into the medium is complicated by the fact that under aerobic conditions amino acids can be oxidized. Therefore, the proteinase activity may be underestimated; in aerobic conditions the mitochondrial proteinases are always apparently less active than under anaerobic conditions. However, the total activity of the unfractionated homogenate is almost the same under anaerobic and aerobic conditions and is always considerably less than the summed activity of the isolated fractions. Therefore, it seems probable that there are some natural inhibitors present which prevent the full activity of the proteinases from being manifest in the homogenate and which are diluted out in the fractionation procedure. In general, mitochondria from liver show a much higher proteinase activity than mitochondria from muscle. This is to be expected if the proteinases are concerned with the adjustment of the enzymic composition of a tissue, since in liver a constant change in enzymes must be made to meet changing metabolic circumstances. The presence in mitochondria of key enzymes of gluconeogenesis such as pyruvate carboxylase (whose activity is constantly adjusted by hormonal and other influences) may well require the presence of the mitochondrial proteinases to make the necessary adjustment.

Comparison of mitochondrial neutral proteinases and lysosomal cathepsins

Almost all tissues show some proteinase cathepsin activity at acid pH values. These proteinases have been implicated in tissue autolysis; in particular the lysosome has been shown to contain cathepsins. It was important, therefore, to establish that the neutral proteinase activity of the mitochondrial fraction was not simply the residual activity of contaminating lysosomes. The matter is complicated by the fact that at acid pH values the rate of amino acid liberation from the mitochondrial preparations increases greatly, being 3·5 times as much at pH 6·2 as at pH 7·4, and 6·2 times as much at pH 5·2. Beaufay and deDuve (1959) state that the lysosomal cathepsin is 'almost' inactive at pH 6·0 and from Figure 5 of Dingle (1961) it can be calculated that no more than 3% of lysosomal cathepsin activity remains at pH 7·4. Further, the stimulation of lysosomal cathepsin in passing from pH 6·5 to pH 4·5 is about 4·5-fold, whereas the stimulation of the mitochondrial proteinase is about $6 \cdot 5$-fold over the same pH range. Some estimation may be made of the maximum contribution that lysosomal cathepsin can make to the liberation of amino acids, using the data of Sawant, Desai and Tappel (1964). They incubated purified lysosome fractions with mitochondria and measured the tyrosine liberated at pH $7 \cdot 0$. Assuming that they have corrected for any amino acids produced by the mitochondria themselves it may be calculated that 8% of the protein of the mitochondrial pellets would have to be contributed by lysosomes to give the observed rate of amino acid production.

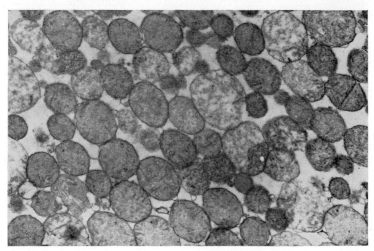

Plate 4. Electron micrograph of mitochondria isolated by the procedure described in the text ($\times$ 12,500). Most mitochondria have a well preserved matrix, outer membrane and cristae

This seems unlikely as it would imply a concentration of lysosomes in this 'heavy mitochondrial fraction'. More direct evidence can be gathered from electron microscope pictures of the mitochondrial preparations used in the experiments of Alberti and Bartley (1969). Plate 4 illustrates a typical field of a section through the mitochondrial pellet. No well defined lysosomes can be seen and even when doubtful particles are counted as lysosomes in this and many other fields inspected, the percentage is less than 1%. Wattiaux and de Duve (1956) have used the detergent Triton X-100 to disrupt lysosomes and release the lysosomal enzymes in the fully soluble form. However, as might be expected, the detergent also has a disruptive effect on mitochondria as shown in Plate 5. Measurement of the neutral proteinase activity in a mitochondrial preparation in which

Triton X-100 has been included in the washing fluid showed that the rate of amino acid production was only some 55% of the normal rate of production. At worst, then, more than half the proteinase activity must be due to mitochondria and not to lysosomes. However, since much of the mitochondrial proteinase is soluble (as will be shown later) it might be expected that it would be lost from those mitochondria that were disrupted by Triton X. Inspection of Plate 5 shows that only about half of the

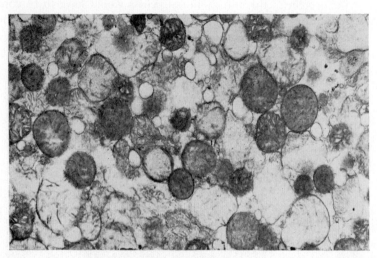

Plate 5. Electron micrograph of mitochondria isolated by the procedure described in the text and then exposed to 0·1 % Triton X-100 at 0° for 50 minutes (× 12,500). Many of the mitochondria still retain matrix, outer membrane and cristae

mitochondria retain their membrane after the detergent treatment and the loss of proteinase is what might be expected from this amount of disruption. The results also emphasize the points made previously about the heterogeneity of mitochondria (in relation to their enzymic composition); here this is shown in relation to their resistance to detergent disruption. The resistance to detergent may be a function of the mitochondrial water and solute content. Heterogeneity of isolated mitochondria in this sense has been demonstrated by Amoore and Bartley (1958) and this may be reflected by a similar heterogeneity within the cell.

Another approach to determining the contribution by lysosomes to amino acid release in mitochondrial preparations at neutral pH is to adopt methods for increasing the proportion of lysosomes in the preparations and to stabilize the lysosomes during the incubation procedure. Appelmans and de Duve (1955) have used β-glycerophosphate to stabilize lysosomes and thus it might be expected that the inclusion of this substance in the *isolation* medium might result in a greater proportion of lysosomes in the final preparation and hence a more rapid release of amino acids—if lysosomes are responsible for the proteolysis. However, no such stimulation occurred. On the other hand, if β-glycerophosphate were included in the *incubation* medium but not in the preparation medium it might be expected that the lysosomes present would be stabilized and that the amino acid production would decrease. In fact the amino acid production was increased progressively as more β-glycerophosphate was substituted for sucrose in the incubation medium.

Since lysosomes are smaller than mitochondria there is a tendency for them to sediment with the small mitochondrial particles; therefore it might be expected that the proteinase activity would be concentrated in 'light' mitochondrial fractions rather than in the 'heavy' fractions. Preparation of these different fractions according to Appelmans and coworkers (1955), followed by freezing and thawing to ensure that there were no complications due to permeability barriers, showed that acid phosphatase activity was concentrated in the 'light' mitochondrial fraction as found by de Duve and coworkers (1955). The ratio of specific activities of acid phosphatase in the two fractions was light : heavy, 3 : 1. The same ratio could be anticipated for the proteinase activity if lysosomes were responsible for the amino acid release. In fact, the ratio obtained was 1 : 3; therefore the lysosomal cathepsins cannot be making a large contribution to the mitochondrial proteinase activity.

Localization of the proteinase within the mitochondria

Earlier it was suggested that the mitochondrial proteinase functioned in the destruction of individual mitochondria or to remove unwanted enzymes to allow for the synthesis of other enzymes. It is interesting in this connection to discover whether the proteinase is attached to the insoluble framework of the mitochondria or is a soluble mitochondrial protein. It is also of interest to see whether the amino acids are produced within the mitochondria where they could contribute to the pool of endogenous mitochondrial amino acids described by Bellamy (1962). Table 8 (Alberti, 1964) shows the changes with time in the concentrations of amino acids in mitochondria incubated at three different temperatures. Each value is obtained from samples of the mitochondrial suspension which were centrifuged to separate the mitochondria from the suspending medium. The decanted supernatant fluid and the pellet were treated with 2N perchloric acid to stop enzyme action and the protein and amino acid contents of both were estimated. From these values and the measured

Table 8. Effect of incubation for 1 hour at 0°, 22° and 40°, on amino acid content, water content and protein leakage of rat-liver mitochondria

Tempera- ture	Incubation time minutes	Protein leakage % total	I/M	Total amino acid content μmole/mg dry wt	Amino acid concentration		P/S	Concentration gradient	
					Internal P μmole/ml internal water	External S μmole/ml external water		Actual μmole/ml	Calculated μmole/ml
0°	0	2·5	2·47	0·037	8·4	1·2	7·0	7·2	7·2
	15	4·6	2·45	0·041	7·5	1·3	5·8	6·2	6·1
	30	—	—	0·047	10·0	1·2	8·3	8·8	9·5
	60	9·4	2·48	0·057	10·0	1·8	5·6	8·2	8·2
22°	15	5·3	3·83	0·050	8·0	1·3	6·2	6·7	11·1
	30	16·5	3·33	0·061	9·9	2·1	4·7	7·8	11·2
	60	28·3	—	0·078	10·6	3·3	3·2	7·3	—
40°	15	34·4	5·67	0·108	25·5	1·7	15·0	23·8	56·8
	30	42·4	6·43	0·236	76·3	3·3	23·1	73·0	195·3

The 40° samples were incubated in a water bath and the 22° samples at laboratory temperature in air. Actual protein leakage at 0° was measured. Calculated concentration gradient = internal amino acid concentration minus external amino acid concentration, assuming that no swelling had occurred. I/M is the amount of mitochondrial water per unit dry wt of mitochondria amount of intramitochondrial water, the intramitochondrial concentration of amino acid and the extent of swelling of the mitochondria were calculated. Even at $0°$ there was an increase in the concentration of mitochondrial amino acid with time and after one hour $9·4\%$ of the mitochondrial protein had been solubilized. This is presumably a reflection of the spontaneous breakdown of the mitochondria. At higher temperatures the rate of protein loss was much faster and the mitochondria became much more swollen. In 15 minutes at $40°$ the mitochondria were twice their original size and had lost one-third of their protein. At this stage the entire increase in amino acids had occurred within the mitochondria; the concentration in the medium had not risen. By 30 minutes the concentration of amino acids in the mitochondria was almost ten times the initial value and sufficient had leaked into the medium to more than double the initial concentration. The concentration gradient maintained by the mitochondrial membrane at this stage was 73 mM; if the amino acids had been produced without any water uptake by the mitochondria the concentration gradient would have been almost 200 mM. Thus it appears that the amino acids are produced within the particles and that the mitochondrial membrane remains relatively impermeable to them. In view of the current ideas (Lardy and coworkers, 1965; Chappel and Haarhoff, 1967) of the involvement of amino acids in the transport of oxoacids across the mitochondrial membrane it seemed possible that the high concentration of amino acids found reflected either an active process or a specific adsorption process. This was tested by adding glutamate to a suspension containing both intact and disrupted mitochondria; little or no concentration or adsorption was found. Therefore, there seems no doubt that the amino acids produced by proteinase activity are released within the mitochondria and only appear in the medium when the mitochondrial membrane become 'leaky'. It was shown earlier that mitochondrial proteinase cannot be fully active in mitochondria *in vivo* and it appears that one of the factors inhibiting the full expression of activity is structural, since the disruption of the mitochondria by freezing and thawing doubled the rate of amino acid production during subsequent incubation.

Although most of the preceding discussion has been concerned with 'neutral proteinase' activity it is clear from the experiments with different proteinase inhibitors that there is more than one enzyme involved. Also the rate of amino acid production increases as the pH of the medium is lowered. This increase implies either a contamination by lysosomal cathepsins or the presence of mitochondrial proteinases with acid pH optima. Some light has been thrown on this problem by studies with

Table 9. Amino acid production by subfractions of rat-liver mitochondria, prepared by centrifugation

Fraction	Dry weight % broken mitochondria	% total amino acid production		Specific activity % production / % dry weight	
		pH 7·4	pH 5·8	pH 7·4	pH 5·8
Broken mitochondria	100·0	100·0	100·0	1·0	1·0
66,250 g-min precipitate	6·2	1·4	2·7	0·2	0·4
390,000 g-min precipitate .	9·7	3·1	3·6	0·3	0·4
1,800,000 g-min precipitate	18·2	7·8	9·2	0·4	0·5
3,600,000 g-min precipitate .	13·3	4·1	5·9	0·3	0·4
Final supernatant (soluble fraction) .	51·1	68·6	50·3	1·3	1·0
Total	98·5	85·0	71·7		

Precipitates from the centrifugings were made up to the required volume with 0·25 M sucrose. 1·5 ml of each fraction was incubated with 0·5 ml of 0·1 M potassium phosphate buffer, pH 7·4 or pH 5·8. Incubations were in air for 1 hour at 40°. Reactions were stopped with 1 ml 2N $HClO_4$:

mitochondria that had been disrupted in the French Pressure Cell. Table 9 shows that most of the proteinase activity both at pH 7·4 and pH 5·8 was soluble but the ratios of activity were not the same in each fraction. The experiments are complicated because the total proteinase activity was not recovered in the sum of the mitochondrial fractions. This may be due to separation of enzyme and substrate as Baird (1964) showed that such separation was possible during the isolation of submitochondrial fractions. The change in the ratio of the activities at pH 7·4 and 5·8 confirms the presence of more than one proteinase in the mitochondria. Gel infiltration of the soluble mitochondrial fraction and precipitation of some of the soluble protein by adjustment to pH 5·0 concentrated the proteinase activity and produced preparations where the ratio of activity at neutral and acid pH values showed wide variation. Fractionation of the soluble protein of the mitochondria with ammonium sulphate (40–60% saturation) produced a preparation which had a neutral proteinase activity greater than the activity at acid pH and which had roughly double the specific activity of the original soluble mitochondrial extract. From these experiments it seems probable that mitochondria contain a range of soluble proteinases, at least some of which had pH optima in the region of pH 7·0.

Metabolic function of mitochondrial proteinases

The result of the action of mitochondrial proteinase is to increase the pool of mitochondrial amino acids that are available either for resynthesis of proteins or for oxidation. The range of enzymes synthesized within the mitochondria is unknown, though there is some evidence that soluble enzymes are synthesized on the extramitochondrial cell membranes and

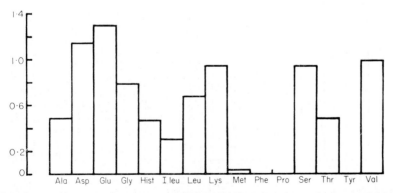

Figure 11.   Pattern of amino acids found in mitochondria immediately after isolation. Valine is set at 1

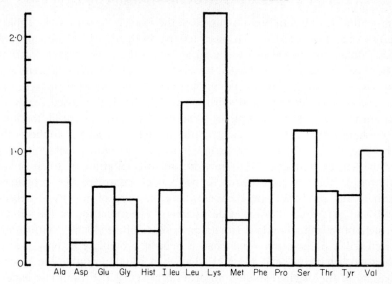

Figure 12. Pattern of amino acids liberated from mitochondria incubated at pH 7·4 and 40° in 25 mM phosphate buffer for 60 minutes. Valine is set at 1

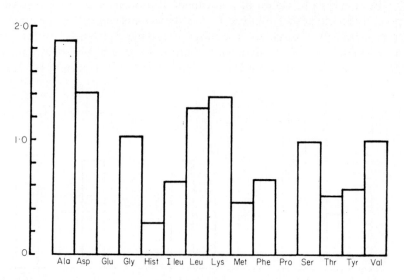

Figure 13. Pattern of amino acids liberated under the same conditions as in Figure 11 but with the addition of 10 mM succinate. Valine is set at 1

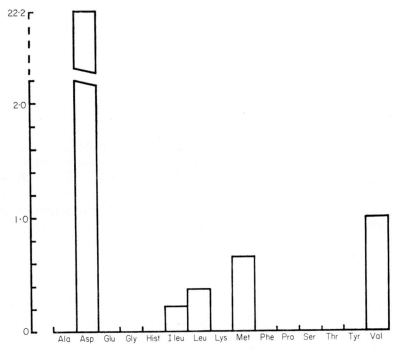

Figure 14.   Pattern of amino acids liberated when mitochondria were incubated in a medium suitable for measuring oxidative phosphorylation; viz. $MgCl_2$ 5 mM, AMP 10 mM, K phosphate buffer 12·5 mM, succinate 12·5 mM, tris buffer 12·5 mM. Valine is set at 1

transported into the mitochondria. One of the key enzymes of gluconeogenesis (pyruvate carboxylase) is located in the mitochondria; the enzyme increases in activity under the influence of corticosteroids and decreases under that of insulin. It is therefore of some interest to find that amino acid production in rat liver mitochondria is stimulated by corticosteroids or adrenocorticotrophic hormone and decreased by insulin. Addition of a number of oxidizable substrates also inhibited the release of amino acids from mitochondria. These decreases in amino acid production in the presence of substrate are in accord with observations that the enzyme–substrate complex is less liable to degradation than the free enzyme (Knox and Greengard, 1965). Under conditions where oxidative phosphorylation occurred there was a large increase in amino acid release which was abolished by added 2-4-dinitrophenol. All these observations are complicated by the observations that the degree of swelling of the mitochondria and the pH influenced the rate of amino acid production and some of the effects described may be a consequence of a primary action on mitochondrial water or pH. Nevertheless, the interactions considered here could form the basis of an elaborate control mechanism if selected enzymes are attacked bv the proteinases.

If mitochondrial proteinases are to act as metabolic control agents then they must show some selectivity that will vary according to the metabolic conditions. Figure 11 describes the pattern of amino acids found in freshly-isolated mitochondria and Figures 12, 13 and 14 can be used to compare this with the patterns of amino acid liberation when mitochondria are incubated in phosphate buffer alone, with added substrate and under conditions used for measuring oxidative phosphorylation. (It has already been pointed out that the total quantities of amino acids vary under these conditions.) It is clear that there is selectivity in the pattern of amino acids produced and this implies a selectivity of the proteins being attacked.

SUMMARY

The investigations reviewed in this paper make it clear that the biogenesis and degradation of the mitochondria of a number of types of cells are processes in which individual components can be inserted into or removed from the mitochondrial structure in response to changing physiological conditions. This behaviour is most marked in cells which can adapt to growth in a wide range of environments (yeast); it is less marked in cells which experience more stable conditions (the liver); and is not found to anything like the same extent in tissue of highly specialized function which develop in an environment which is subject to more rigid control (the flight muscle). Even in this last type, however, it seems that various kinds of protein and phospholipid are incorporated into the mitochondria at different stages during development. The time course of this process suggests that a structural matrix (of protein and phospholipids) is laid down, which can accumulate the enzymes of the mitochondria when these are made available. This matrix must be capable of imposing some degree of spatial organization on various combinations of mitochondrial enzymes. Moreover, even in this class of mitochondria, particular enzymes can be removed from the matrix without a loss of function of the entire mitochondrial system. A similar situation must apply to the incorporation of new enzymes into yeast mitochondria adapting to changes in the chemical composition of their growth medium, as the removal of particular enzymes to make room for new components does not destroy other functions of the mitochondria.

It follows from this selective removal that the degradative enzymes must themselves exhibit a considerable degree of specificity in action, and moreover, that their action must normally be held in check by some kind of inhibitory structure or component. Reasons have been advanced for believing that the most likely method of achieving specificity and control is an increased susceptibility to attack of enzymes in the absence of their substrates. Thus, the mitochondrial protease may be operative almost continually, degrading mitochondrial enzymes at a relatively steady rate; the soluble enzymes would probably be attacked most rapidly, while those that are membrane-bound may be hydrolysed only after the action of lytic agents (such as fatty acids or phospholipases) on the membranes. Under these conditions, the presence of a particular substrate is capable of converting the enzyme to a more resistant form, and there will be a close correlation between the environmental composition and the enzyme complement of the mitochondria. Moreover, as different enzymes will differ in their susceptibility to proteolysis, a range of half-lives for proteins would be anticipated during the normal life cycle of the mitochondria—as was found with rat liver mitochondria. The destruction of any part of the mitochondrial structure (by swelling or similar treatments) will expose to the direct action of proteases many enzymes which are not saturated with their substrates so that such treatments will apparently activate the proteases. The constant turnover of the mitochondrial enzymic proteins appears to be the inevitable price which the organism has to pay in order to give itself the greatest possible flexibility in its use of materials from the environment for the vital generation of ATP by oxidative processes.

References

Alberti, K. G. M. M. (1964). *D. Phil. Thesis*, Oxford.

Alberti, K. G. M. M. and Bartley, W. (1965). *Biochem. J.*, **95**, 641.

Alberti, K. G. M. M., and Bartley, W. (1969). *Biochem. J.*, **111**, 763.

Amoore, J. E., and Bartley, W. (1958). *Biochem. J.*, **69**, 223.

Appelmans, F., and de Duve, C. (1955). *Biochem. J.*, **59**, 426.

Appelmans, F., Wattiaux, R., and de Duve, C. (1955). *Biochem. J.*, **59**, 438.

Baird, G. D. (1964). *Biochem. Biophys. Acta*, **93**, 293.

Bailey, E., Taylor, C. B., and Bartley, W. (1967). *Biochem. J.*, **104**, 1026.

Bartley, W., and Tustanoff, E. R. (1966). *Biochem. J.*, **99**, 599.

Beaufay, H., and de Duve, C. (1959). *Biochem. J.*, **73**, 604.

Beattie, D. S., Basford, R. E., and Koritz, S. B. (1966). *Biochemistry*, **5**, 926.

Bellamy, D., and Leonard, R. A. (1965). *General and Comparative Endocrinology*, **5**, 402.

Bellamy, D. (1962). *Biochem. J.*, **82**, 218.

Brosemer, R. W., Vogell, W., and Bucher, Th. (1963). *Biochem. Z.*, **338**, 854.

Brunner, G., and Neupert, W. (1968). *Febs. Letters*, **1**, 153.

Bucher, Th. (1965). *Symp. Biochem. Soc.*, **25**, 15.

Bygrave, F. L. (1969). *J. Biol. Chem.*, **244**, 4768.

Chappell, J. B., and Haarhoff, K. N. (1967). In *Biochemistry of Mitochondria* (Eds. Slater, E. C., Kaniuga, Z., and Wojtczak, L.). Academic, London and New York, p. 75.

Criddle, R. S., Bock, R. M., Green, D. E., and Tisdale, H. (1962). *Biochemistry*, **1**, 827.

Crompton, M., and Birt, L. M. (1967). *J. Insect Physiol.*, **13**, 1575.

D'Costa, M. A., and Birt, L. M. (1967). *J. Insect Physiol.*, **12**, 1377.

Dingle, J. T. (1961). *Biochem. J.*, **79**, 509.

Ferguson, J. J., Boll., M., and Holzer, H. (1967). *Europ. J. Biochem.*, **1**, 21.

Fletcher, M. J., and Sanadi, D. R. (1961). *Biochem. Biophys. Acta*, **51**, 356.

Gear, A. R. L. (1965). *Biochem. J.*, **95**, 118.

Getz, G. S., Bartley, W., Lurie, D., and Notton, B. M. (1968). *Biochim. Biophys. Acta*, **152**, 325.

Gregory, D. W., Lennie, R. W., and Birt, L. M. (1968). *J. of Royal Microscopical Soc.*, **88**, 151.

Halder, D., Freeman, K., and Work, T. S. (1966). *Nature, Lond.*, **211**, 9.

Hansford, R. G., and Chappell, J. B. (1967). *Biochem. Biophys. Res. Commun.*, **27**, 686.

Kagawa, Y., and Racker, E. (1966). *J. Biol. Chem.*, **241**, 2475.

Knox, W. E., and Greengard, O. (1965). *Advances in enzyme regulation*, Pergamon, Oxford, p. 247.

Lardy, H. A., Paetkau, V., and Walter, P. (1965). *Proc. Nat. Acad. Sci., Wash.*, **53**, 1410.

Lennie, R. W., Gregory, D. W., and Birt, L. M. (1967). *J. of Insect Physiol.*, **13**, 1745.

Lennie, R. W., and Birt, L. M. (1967). *Biochem. J.*, **102**, 338.

McGivan, J. D., and Chappell, J. B. (1967). *Biochem. J.*, **105**, 15P.

Parsons, D. F., Williams, G. R., Thompson, W., Wilson, D., and Chance, B. (1966). *Febs. Letters*, **1**, 155.

Sawant, P. L., Desai, I. D., and Tappel, A. L. (1964). *Biochim. Biophys. Acta*, **85**, 93.

Swick, R. W., Stange, J. L., Nance, S. L., and Thompson, J. F. (1967). *Biochemistry*, **6**, 737.

Taylor, C. B., Bailey, E., and Bartley, W. (1967). *Biochem. J.*, **105**, 605.

Walker, A. C., Gregory, D. W., and Birt, L. M. (1969). *J. Insect Physiol.*, **15**, 519.

Walker, A. C., and Birt, L. M. (1969). *J. Insect. Physiol.*, **15**, 305.

Wattiaux, R., and de Duve, C. (1956). *Biochem. J.*, **63**, 606.

Witt, I., Kronan, R., and Holzer, H. (1966). *Biochem. Biophys. Acta*, **118**, 522.

LIFE OUTSIDE THE CELL
(OR, WHAT THE BIOLOGIST SAW)

J. S. D. Bacon

*Department of Biochemistry, Macaulay Institute for Soil Research,
Craigiebuckler, Aberdeen*

The cell theory is now generally accepted. This means that a chemist or X–ray crystallographer feels constrained to draw a circle on the blackboard, with another circle within it to represent the nucleus, before explaining the structure of nucleic acids and their importance for the processes that go on within the boundaries of each cell. No-one will deny (perceptibly) that these indispensable molecules need to be investigated in the utmost detail, but it is a good idea now and then to remember that the original description of a cell referred not to its contents, but to its bounding wall. In many animal cells this may be only two or three molecules thick, but in most plant cells it constitutes a large proportion of the dry matter, and it would be dangerous to assume that a satisfactory description of cell metabolism can be given without including the activities in this region.

It seems that biochemists have often only the vaguest ideas about the composition of the cell wall of the yeast, *Saccharomyces cerevisiae*, although this organism has played a leading role in the development of biochemistry since the time of the Buchners. Many, when pressed, hazard the doubly-wrong guess that it is composed of cellulose fibrils, and would be surprised to learn that it is 100–400 nm thick (Hagedorn, 1964) and may constitute a quarter of the cell's dry weight.

Although I should have known better, I was one of those who underestimated the toughness of this wall, in circumstances explained below, and so think that it may be useful to others to set out here in a personal and selective way some of the problems facing a cell that possesses a thick outer layer, not the least of which must be the manipulation of large quantities of constituents outside what some would consider the proper limits of the cell. All molecules with a legitimate reason for visiting the cell must be allowed to pass through this layer on their way to the cytoplasmic membrane, which presumably decides finally whether to accept or reject them. If the cell wishes to stretch for any reason it will probably have to loosen the wall structure first. If it wishes to reproduce by budding it must permit the addition of a whole new section of wall and later must seal the gap when the daughter cell leaves home. If it wishes to exercise enzymic influence on its surroundings, or secrete a protective slime coating, large molecules have somehow to be exported through the wall. Like most householders, it will doubtless find that repairs are needed frequently if the wall is to continue to fulfil its protective function. Once these needs are admitted it is clear that the cell must retain the power to modify the wall, and that the structure will have its own characteristic metabolism.

Preliminary observations

My own interest in this problem is intimately connected with the Sheffield Department of Biochemistry, although the experimental work was done several years later. My room at Sheffield was at the far end of the corridor into which the visitor stepped from the rather insalubrious lower slopes of the University site, then being very properly colonized by *Senecio squalidus*. He would pick his way along this corridor, which was lined with cupboards on one side and apparatus of the most varied kind on the other, and near the end would pass a door which led down some steps into the boiler house; here he might find over his head a muslin tray on which brewer's yeast had been spread to dry in the warm draught. A glance into the boiler house through the open door gave the feeling that one was looking into the engine room of the University. This was reinforced by the occasional ringing of a telephone, which I suppose created a subconscious idea that the Vice-Chancellor was ringing for Full Steam Ahead.

This was certainly the signal that Professor Krebs had given, and the rooms along the corridor were overfilled with biochemists attracted by his genius, all determined to make the most of their time there. At the precise moment I am describing, the three rooms at the corridor end belonged to the late Peter Nossal, from Australia, David Hughes, of the London Welsh (now repatriated), and myself, from Dorset, working my passage North.

In the course of a study of fructosyl transfer by enzymes in the Jerusalem artichoke, begun in 1948 (Bacon and Edelman, 1951) and continued with much success by Jack Edelman and his colleagues to the present time (see Edelman and Jefford, 1968), we had discovered that a commercial yeast invertase preparation catalysed the transfer of fructosyl residues from sucrose to various acceptors. It was now necessary to characterize the products more fully and to make sure that this action was not due to some enzymic impurity in the preparation. I therefore turned to fresh baker's yeast and was surprised to find how difficult it was to prepare an extract with a reasonable level of invertase activity, although cell suspensions were very active. This fact was of course well known to earlier generations of biochemists, but despite my reading I had not realised that yeast had to be allowed to autolyse for a week or more before it would release a substantial part of its invertase. I must have assumed that the autolysis was needed to make the wall sufficiently porous because I asked David Hughes for some yeast broken in the press he was then developing (Hughes, 1951), and was given a preparation that Peter Nossal was using as a source of fumarase (Nossal, 1952). I found the supernatant of this preparation to be a very active source of invertase. The thought occurred to me that it might have been prepared from a batch of yeast particularly rich in invertase, but being chiefly concerned with qualitative effects (Bacon, 1954), I did not check the point, and thought little about the matter for the next six years.

Later Professor P. J. Allen from Wisconsin, propelled to Sheffield by the famous cycle, came to work in the next room and we collaborated in a study of higher plant invertases. Some experiments were done with sugar beet plants, and from these two facts emerged, incidental to the main purpose of the work (Allen and Bacon, 1956). The first was that no invertase at all could be detected in the root tissue; the second was that treatment of the leaves with ether, which makes it possible to squeeze out most of the sap (a method due to Schryver; see Chibnall, 1966) did not release any invertase, although some was undoubtedly present and could be extracted by grinding with sand. These observations also took about six years to acquire significance for me, illustrating the capacity of biological research to throw up a multitude of subsidiary problems which for one reason or another (e.g. lethargy) one does not attempt to solve.

Soluble periplasmic enzymes in yeast

In the spring of 1958 my wife and I went to the Institute of Biology in Prague to work with Dr. Mikulas Burger, who was keen to study yeast maltase in more detail. In the previous year Myrbäck (1957), in a volume dedicated to that Grand Master of yeast biochemistry, Carl Neuberg, had described a series of experiments with yeast killed by ethyl acetate. When treated in this way the cells lost about a third of their dry matter, but none of the invertase, and he had suggested that this was because the enzyme was attached to some insoluble structure. It seemed possible that peptide linkages were involved because papain released the enzyme, though rather slowly. Thinking that treatment with ethyl acetate might help in the preliminary stages of purification of the maltase we repeated Myrbäck's procedure and confirmed that the invertase was retained.

Remembering the high activity of the crushed yeast produced in Sheffield I wondered whether Myrbäck's explanation was really correct, and we decide to smash the ethyl acetate treated cells in a Hughes press, which fortunately was available. When this was done all the invertase appeared in solution. We later found that living yeast also yielded practically all its invertase in solution when crushed in the press, or by shaking with glass beads. A brief note, made briefer by editorial insistence, appeared in 1958 (Burger, Bacon and Bacon, 1958); in this we also reported that the invertase was liberated from living cells by the action of snail digestive juice. The latter observation was extended by Dr. Burger to conditions in which the yeast protoplasts (or sphaeroplasts) survive (Burger, Bacon and Bacon, 1961), confirming the results obtained independently by Friis and Otto-lenghi (1959).

Our observations on mechanical breakage were at first treated with some reserve by Myrbäck (1960), but later he was able to confirm them in all respects (Myrbäck, 1961). However, because yeast biochemists were preoccupied with the release of protoplasts by snail digestive juice (Eddy and Williamson, 1957, 1959; Millbank, 1963; Sutton and Lampen, 1962; etc.) the main conclusion we drew was ignored and they continued to think of invertase as being bound to an insoluble cell structure, now specified as the wall; this view is still expressed by Lampen (1968). The fact is, that unless one considers that the binding of invertase is peculiarly sensitive to mechanical damage, unlike the bulk of the very similar mannan-protein complexes which remain in the broken walls, it is evident that most of the enzyme exists in a soluble form trapped between the plasmalemma and some relatively impermeable layer of the wall. The use of snail juice, which liberates the invertase while the wall is being digested, confuses the issue.

One effect of this confusion is seen in a paper by Weimberg and Orton (1964) who, assuming that acid phosphatase in *Saccharomyces mellis* is a 'wall enzyme', reject the use of mechanical breakage *because it sets the enzyme free*, and use instead a treatment with cold acetone reminiscent of the ethyl acetate treatment of Myrbäck. They are thus led to consider the effect of certain reagents on this wall preparation to be 'elution' of the acid phosphatase, whereas our interpretation would be that the permeability of the wall is being increased. A reagent that has had a pronounced effect in many experiments of this kind is 2-mercaptoethanol. Thus, it released alkaline pyrophosphatase from acetone-treated *S. mellis* cells, and facilitated the action of snail digestive juice on them (Weimberg and Orton, 1964). We found (Bacon, Milne, Taylor and Webley, 1965) that all the invertase of ethyl acetate killed baker's yeast was lost in 24 hours at pH $7·5$ in the presence of 2-mercaptoethanol, but more significantly Davies and Elvin (1964; Davies, 1967) had already shown that invertase is lost from living cells of *S. fragilis* under these conditions.

If an enzyme is released in a soluble form by mechanical breakage of living cells, and also under conditions in which protoplasts are formed by digestion of the wall, there is a *prima facie* case for assuming it to be held in a soluble form between the wall and the plasmalemma. The results of Weimberg and Orton (1964) put acid phosphatase in this category, and one could perhaps provisionally add melibiase (Friis and Ottolenghi, 1959). However, small amounts of the enzymes may be found in wall preparations (Eddy and Williamson, 1959) and, more important, in the protoplast. Gascon and Ottolenghi (1967) and Lampen (1968) have shown that although these extra and intra-cellular forms of invertase have identical kinetic properties, they differ in molecular weight, and Lampen has evidence that the greater weight of the 'extracellular' form is accounted for by its possession of a mannan moiety. It has long been known that yeast invertase is closely associated with a mannan (Fischer, Kohtès and Fellig, 1951) probably identical with the polysaccharide that makes up half the carbohydrate content of the cell wall. Lampen speculates that attachment of the mannan is necessary for the export of the enzyme. The same might be true of the acid phosphatase (Boer and Steyn-Parvé, 1966). Some other wall enzymes are discussed below.

Porosity of the yeast cell wall

It is pertinent to ask whether any measurements of the porosity of the yeast wall have been made, and if so, whether they support the hypothesis that substances would be prevented from escaping if their molecular weights were around 300,000. Gerhardt and Judge (1964) have attempted this by measuring the penetration of substances of known molecular size into densely packed wall preparations. Their measurements, assuming the homogeneity of their test substances, show the wall to be impervious to molecules of molecular weight 4,500 and upwards.

This would certainly support our hypothesis, and it would be particularly interesting to know whether treatment with thiols would make the wall more porous.

These measurements, however, apply to the bulk of the wall material, and would take little account of the presence of larger holes here and there. There seems little doubt that quite large protein molecules can penetrate rapidly to the surface of the plasmalemma (see, for example, experiments with bovine serum albumin by Ottolenghi, 1967), so it must be argued either that the cell can create temporary points of entry for such molecules or that the invertase and acid phosphatase are somehow prevented from having general access to the inside surface of the wall.

Differences exist in the degree to which yeasts release invertase into the growth medium (Dworshack and Wickerham, 1961). It would be very interesting to see whether this was correlated in any way with the porosity of the wall. Our knowledge of the chemical structure is still too elementary to distinguish between (say) the walls of *S. fragilis* and *S. cerevisiae*.

Occurrence in other organisms

Is this phenomenon peculiar to yeasts? There are reasons why it is relatively easy to demonstrate it in yeast. Yeasts usually have a very high invertase activity, far greater than that of the agents used to prepare protoplasts. Snail digestive juice fails to reveal a similar situation in higher plants because it is itself richer in invertase than the tissue treated. It seems likely that if removal of cell walls from a variety of organisms could be achieved by the use of mixtures of a few highly purified enzymes (see below) the phenomenon would be found to be more widespread.

An alternative approach, through histochemistry, has been used with *E. coli*, where alkaline phosphatase can be seen to be located between the cytoplasmic membrane and the wall (Done, Shorey, Loke and Pollak, 1965).

Failure to admit the possibility of a phenomenon often hinders its discovery. It is too readily assumed that a soluble enzyme released from a broken cell must have originated from within the cytoplasmic membrane.

Invertase in higher plant cells

The amount of invertase produced by a particular strain of yeast is subject to variation, but the factors involved are not fully understood. In higher plants invertase is often present in the cell wall region and rather more is known of the factors influencing its production there.

My own involvement in this problem also goes back to Sheffield, where our work on invertases brought us into contact with scientists working on cane (Tate and Lyle Ltd.) and beet sugar (British Sugar Corporation). The presence of the free hexoses, glucose and fructose, in beet juice leads in the refining process to the production of acids which cause losses of sucrose; any treatment that increases the free hexose has thus to be minimized. A mixture of glucose and fructose is commonly called 'invert sugar', as though it were the product of inversion (hydrolysis causing reversal of the sign of the optical rotation) of sucrose, though of course there is no particular reason why these sugars need arise in this way in the plant cell. Nevertheless, some suspicion is naturally directed at sources of invertases, and, if anything, those of microorganisms contaminating the beet roots are given the blackest looks by sugar refiners.

Discussion of this problem with G. K. G. Campbell and A. R. Trim at the Plant Breeding Institute in 1960 brought to mind two pieces of information. One was the demonstration by MacDonald and DeKock (1958) at the Macaulay Institute that sucrose was broken down quite rapidly when disks cut from sugar beet root were washed in aerated running tap water; the products formed included not only glucose and fructose, but also trisaccharides like those produced by the transfer action of plant invertases. The second was the absence of invertase from the root tissue (mentioned above). The obvious conclusion was that although there is no invertase in freshly-cut tissue it must develop when the tissue is washed.

Interference with the invertase assay by the high concentrations of reducing sugars in the disks was overcome in our earliest experiments by taking advantage of the other observation made by Paul Allen, namely that invertase was not lost from leaves treated with ether. This on reflection sounded just like the treatment of yeast with ethyl acetate, and we found that when we did this to disks of root tissue the sugars escaped but the invertase remained. These preliminary experiments showed that invertase activity appeared during the washing of the beet disks and reached levels far greater than those needed to bring about the observed hydrolysis of sucrose. This observation was reported to the Biochemical Society in 1961 (Bacon, 1961) and had been taken up by Edelman and Hall (1965) even before that date, using tuber tissue from Jerusalem artichokes. They made the very interesting observation that all the invertase formed was firmly bound to the cell wall fraction. In beet only about half is so bound, the rest remaining in the 1000 g. supernatant (Vaughan and MacDonald, 1967). Whether this soluble fraction also lies outside the plasmalemma is not known. Sacher, Hatch and Glasziou (1963) in their studies of the acid invertase of sugar cane storage tissue calculated that a substantial proportion of the enzyme was extracellular, although little was bound to the wall.

Since 1961 invertase has been found to develop in storage tissue from a number of species, and the possibility that microbial contamination might be responsible has been eliminated by preparing the tissue under aseptic conditions (Bacon, MacDonald and Knight, 1965). Changes in the invertase activity of plant cells had already been closely correlated with cell extension in roots by Wanner and Leupold (1947) and by Robinson and Brown (1952). Hatch and Glasziou (1963) also showed very clearly that there is a positive correlation between invertase activity and the rate of growth of sugar cane stems. The connection between invertase and cell walls would thus not seem to be fortuitous.

Some features of the process by which invertase activity appears in aged storage tissue have been studied by my colleagues at the Macaulay Institute (see Vaughan and MacDonald, 1968 *a*, *b*) leading to the tentative conclusion that a *de novo* synthesis of the enzyme is taking place. There seems little evidence that removal of a specific invertase inhibitor is responsible (*cf.* Pressey, 1968), although presumably some repressor substance is lost or destroyed before nucleic acid and protein synthesis can take a new course. In sliced tissue the process is sensitive to oxygen tension in the surrounding fluid, but it is likely that in intact roots oxygen supply is not limiting (MacDonald, 1968) and some other physiological control must operate. Plant growth substances (indolylacetic acid, kinetin, gibberellic acid) influence the final amounts of invertase synthesized (*cf.* Edelman and Hall, 1964).

Another situation in which invertase is associated with growth is in the dark-grown pea seedling. Confining her attention chiefly to the third internode Datko (1968) showed that the enzyme activity was highest in the distal third of the internode, which was still growing fast, and relatively low in the proximal third, which had stopped growing, while the activity in the other two internodes was still lower. Decapitation of the seedling and treatment of the cut apex with indoleacetic acid produces profound changes in the morphology of the distal segment. Increase in invertase activity ceases after 1 day and in that period seldom does more than keep pace with increases in total protein and cell wall material, but there is a 10 to 40-fold increase in cellulase activity over 3–4 days, at which stage root primordia begin to grow through the cortex (Datko and Machlachlan, 1968).

However, if a segment of the internode is detached its invertase activity at once begins to fall, despite the fact that it continues to elongate (Bacon, 1965; Datko, 1968). Vaughan (1968, unpublished) has also found that hydroxyproline will inhibit invertase synthesis in pea root segments while stimulating their rate of elongation.

One may therefore guess that there is no unbreakable connection between invertase level and cell wall extension, whether the invertase is partly bound to the wall (in beet root), or mainly soluble (in pea epicotyl). This is not to say though, that there is no functional relationship, and we may briefly turn to speculations about this.

Possible functions of higher plant invertases

Sucrose and invertase are so ubiquitous in plant tissues (*cf.* Arnold, 1968) that it is natural to suppose that one must be the substrate of the other, and that the purpose of this connection is to convert sucrose to monosaccharide. Other possible substrates, such as oligosaccharides of the raffinose or fructosan series, exist in appreciable concentrations in some plants, and it always remains a possibility that a more significant alternative substrate exists. The fructose-transferring action of the enzyme has no obvious function (Bacon, 1960) and a role in sucrose synthesis by the reversal of its action may be ruled out (Allen and Bacon, 1956).

Sacher, Hatch and Glasziou (1963) have developed the thesis that invertase is concerned in the storage of sucrose by sugar cane, and certainly it is difficult to see how sucrose could fail to suffer hydrolysis if it diffused freely through cells wall containing the enzyme. In yeasts the enzyme must usually hydrolyse all the sucrose in the vicinity of the cell, and so facilitate the uptake of the sugar by active mechanisms of absorption. In this way it would resemble other microbial enzymes whose function is to depolymerize materials of high molecular weight so that they can diffuse through the wall and be absorbed.

It would be dangerous, though, to assume too readily that enzymes found in the periplasmic region are primarily concerned with the utilization of foreign substances; their main function may be to service the wall structure, and any action they show upon other substances could be incidental.

The invertase activity of the etiolated pea epicotyl is very much higher than that of the corresponding tissue grown in full light, so that one might ask whether the enzyme is needed chiefly when the cells are dependent upon an external supply of carbohydrate. A peculiar feature of the sucrose breakdown that occurs in storage tissue disks is that hardly any fructose accumulates; after many days of ageing the tissue contains mainly glucose, which is present in an amount not very different from that combined in the original sucrose. The system would need to be analysed further before one could take this as evidence for preferential utilization of fructose, and, in fact, all other evidence seems to show that plant cells use glucose in preference to fructose.

This point might easily be dismissed from our attention if it were not that sugar analyses of maize root (Hellebust and Forward, 1962) and pea epicotyl (Datko, 1968) show similar large excesses of glucose over fructose in the regions where the invertase activity is highest. A little research might simply show a high rate of conversion of free fructose to free glucose in those situations, but could just possibly shed a little more light on why the invertase is there.

In the pea epicotyl, as I have mentioned, the invertase disappears very rapidly when the segment is chopped out, while *in situ* it may be retained for several days without much change. A segment left attached to the

C

lower part of the seedling (internodes, cotyledons and roots) loses invertase more slowly; if left attached to the growing shoot tip it behaves much as if completely excised (Bacon, unpublished).

Such a rapid destruction implies that the enzyme is within easy reach of control mechanisms, and it is perhaps not surprising to find that practically all the invertase in this tissue is released in solution when the cells are disrupted. Whether the destruction takes place inside or outside the plasmalemma remains to be investigated.

Periplasmic enzymes bound to the cell wall

Attachment within a wall structure would not be expected to hinder the action of invertase on sucrose (m.w. = 342). In the yeast wall there is evidently an abundance of structural elements (mannan–protein complexes) closely related chemically to yeast invertase, so that even though we may not yet know exactly how the wall mannan–protein complexes are cross-linked we can see in principle no difficulty in anchoring some of the invertase to the wall.

A situation more difficult to visualize is that of the β-glucanase(s) of the yeast wall. Brock (1965a) and more recently Abd-el-Al and Phaff (1968) have described and partly purified soluble β-glucanases from several species of yeast. These act upon the non-reducing chain-ends of $\beta(1\rightarrow3)$ and $\beta(1\rightarrow6)$ glucans, liberating glucose (i.e. they are exoglucanases). These enzymes are lost into the growth medium from *S. fragilis* and *Hansenula anomala* but not from *S. cerevisiae* or *S. carlsbergensis*, behaviour recalling the differing extent to which invertase is lost from various yeasts. The effects of their action on the glucans of the yeast wall would be expected to be limited, and not likely to lead to any 'softening' of the structure, such as might be needed as a preliminary to bud growth by insertion of new material.

We have recently obtained evidence that another type of β-glucanase is bound to the yeast wall. When broken wall preparations are incubated with laminarin, a mainly $\beta(1\rightarrow3)$ glucan, a series of oligosaccharides is produced, indicating that an endoglucanase is present. This could have a much more profound effect on the wall, because it is now well established that endo $\beta(1\rightarrow3)$ glucanases from other organisms attack the wall glucans very extensively (Phaff, 1963). It still remains something of a puzzle, though, how an enzyme fixed in the wall could reach out and bite any but the glucan molecules nearest to it. This may of course, be what is intended, so that no wholesale demolition can occur. The increase in the permeability of yeast walls caused by slow drying, or by autolysis with cell poisons, may be due to the action of this wall enzyme. The wall has no action on lutean, a mainly $\beta(1\rightarrow6)$glucan, but we must be careful not to ascribe this to the specificity of an active centre before we are sure that the lutean molecules can enter the wall structure.

Wall-modifying periplasmic enzymes

Glucanases have also been found in the walls of filamentous fungi (Mitchell and Sabar, 1966). The production of a glucanase capable of hydrolysing one of the cell wall components of *Schizophyllum commune* has been related to the sexual morphogenesis of this species (Wessels and Niederpruem, 1967). Brock (1965*b*) had already speculated on a connection between the yeast exoglucanase and cell fusion processes. In fact, from what we know of the wall composition of many fungi and higher plants we would expect that glucanases would be needed to modify or destroy them, and this could occur as much under physiological as under pathological conditions. The dissolution of the β-glucan in the cell walls of the endosperm is a well-known feature of the germination of barley (Preece, 1957). The presence of several different structural systems in a single wall would permit a multiplicity of controls over its strength and porosity. Thus in yeast one could list upwards of ten different linkages open to modification by enzyme action (glycosides, peptides, glycopeptide bonds, phosphodiesters, etc.).

As I argued earlier, it does not follow that all these enzymes will be found to be attached to the wall structure; they may be present in a soluble form in the periplasmic region. To establish this is a peculiarly difficult problem, because the most elegant way of establishing their location is to prepare protoplasts, a process requiring the use of similar wall-attacking enzymes. Some means must therefore be found of distinguishing, for example, the foreign glucanases from the (hypothetical) soluble periplasmic glucanases. This will call for the use of highly purified and well-characterized lytic enzymes.

These will find important uses for other purposes. An indication of the benefits that would follow is given by the work of Shapiro, Grossman and Marmur (1968) who wished to prepare mitochondrial DNA in undegraded form from yeast cells. Snail digestive juice has been used to prepare protoplasts which can then be lysed very easily, avoiding the brute force needed to break the cell wall (Duell, Inoue and Utter, 1964). Unfortunately this digestive juice contains enzymes irrelevant to the job of protoplast formation and damaging to DNA. There being at present no known method of separating the minimal mixture of wall-destroying enzymes from snail juice (cf. Anderson and Millbank, 1966) Marmur and his colleagues were obliged to use instead a mixture of microbial enzymes, probably no less complex, but less damaging to DNA. We might hope eventually to use only two or three highly purified lytic enzymes, and so open the way to much gentler procedures for examining the contents of the yeast cell.

I need hardly add that these lytic enzymes would also have potential applications in the treatment of diseases caused by fungi, but we shall need to know a great deal more about the structural components of fungal cell walls before we can decide which enzymes are the most promising for these purposes.

Mechanisms of wall synthesis

I come last to the question that really stands first among the problems raised by the possession of a massive cell wall. How is a structure of such dimensions and rigidity assembled outside the cytoplasmic membrane?

It is worth looking briefly at the cell walls of higher plants, because there the problem is seen at its greatest. Roelofsen (1959; also 1965) has given a very detailed description of much of the earlier research, and later accounts have been written, for example, by Setterfield and Bayley (1961), Preston (1965); and Mühletahler (1967).

An important difference between the walls of yeasts and those of most other plant cells is that the latter contain fibrils. These are usually composed of cellulose but in fungi chitin often takes its place.

The first stage in the building of higher plant cell walls chiefly consists of the production of a meshwork of these fibrils; later more fibrils are incorporated, usually in a very regular manner, and a great deal of matrix material is added, the final structure having some of the characteristics of reinforced concrete. We have therefore to consider two types of product: fibrils and amorphous matrix.

The structure of the fibrils is not known with certainty. Until recently each was generally believed to be composed of about 40 cellulose molecules packed side by side; X-ray evidence indicated that alternate chains were arranged in opposite directions. Both features made it difficult to understand why such a structure should be the basic unit of cellulose synthesis. Recently Manley (1964) has proposed that the fibril structure is formed by the coiling of a single folded cellulose molecule. The biochemical unit would then be required to operate on one molecule at a time. Preston (1965) thinks that he can see these units, with fibrils still attached, on the inner surface of some algal cell walls, and has suggested how they could be packed together to give the characteristic changes of direction of the fibrils in adjacent layers. Our knowledge of the biochemistry of cellulose synthesis in higher plants is still in a very primitive state (see Hassid, 1967; Ordin and Hall, 1968) and it is doubtful whether we yet have techniques refined enough to study synthetic processes in which the spatial arrangement of the products probably depends upon associations with molecules of diverse chemical structure.

In cellulose synthesis by the bacterium *Acetobacter xylinum* evidence has been obtained that the fibrils are assembled outside the cell, from precursors that have a lipid component (Colvin and Beer, 1960). This idea, which seemed to be in conflict with what little is known about cellulose synthesis in plants now receives support from some observations on synthesis of complex bacterial polysaccharides (see e.g. Higashi, Strominger and Sweeley, 1967) and it has been suggested that a building unit requires to be linked to lipid so that it can be passed through the bacterial cytoplasmic membrane. (It may be recalled that Lampen proposed that a polysaccharide moiety had to be attached to an enzyme before it could be exported from the yeast cell.)

Fibrils may thus be extruded by sub-units attached to the outside of the plasmalemma, or conceivably assembled from soluble precursors synthesized within the cytoplasm. The matrix materials could be secreted by either type of process. For example, Matile, Moor and Mühletahler (1967) have described small particles attached to the plasmalemma of yeast, which they believe to be concerned in wall synthesis.

The alternative idea, that precursors are elaborated in the cytoplasm and then secreted has also depended much on circumstantial microscopic evidence, rather than on the precise location of biochemical events within the cell. The Golgi apparatus, in particular, has been seen to be associated with wall synthesis in plant cells (see the summary by Northcote, 1968). Electron microscopy of ultrathin sections shows Golgi vesicles close to the plasmalemma, and occasionally emptying through it into the wall region.

The most direct implication of these events with wall synthesis has been given by some ingenious experiments of Northcote and Pickett-Heaps (1966). After feeding a pulse of tritiated glucose to wheat root tips they fixed the tissue and cut thin sections which were stained and subsequently coated with photographic emulsion and examined in the electron microscope. Grains of silver marking the presence of labelled substances moved from the interior of the cell to the wall as the incubation proceeded. Parallel measurements of the incorporation of label into polysaccharide showed that galactose was the most abundant labelled sugar present, so that what was being 'watched' in the radioautographs was essentially matrix material. The silver grains were seen to be concentrated over the Golgi apparatus, supporting the view that this structure is concerned with wall synthesis.

It would be possible to follow this theme further, in the manner of some reviewers, stumbling forward into more and more barren territory, where the soil is too fact-deficient even for speculations to take root. Instead I shall leave the reader to consider whether he or she has not something to contribute to a solution of these problems. We are still very dependent upon plant growth for our survival as a species, and it is time that biochemists began to make their contributions to this side of the balance sheet. Up to now they have helped more to increase the number of hungry mouths than to find the means of filling them.

A confession and some ruminations

The more observant among my readers will by now have realized that despite its title this essay is mainly about invertase, which is what my Sheffield colleagues were expecting anyway. Here is another example of nature's compensatory processes; twenty years ago I should have resented the suggestion that I was destined to spend years of my life on a subject that then seemed as dead for me as the dodo. Its revival has been due to the pursuit of a number of essentially biological problems.

During this period the purely chemical approach to yeast invertase (purification, physical properties, kinetics, action of inhibitors, etc.) has been taken up from time to time by workers in many laboratories, but without any advance in knowledge commensurate with the efforts expended. Some hoped that through a study of this easily obtained enzyme they might learn something of the mechanism of enzyme action in general, and of glycosidases in particular. Because of its rather unusual nature (more like a polysaccharide than a protein; cf. Fischer and Kohtès, 1951) it has proved difficult to purify by the techniques of protein chemistry, and this hope has not been realized.

Let us suppose, though, that the efforts had been successful, so that we knew the full structure of the enzyme and understood its catalytic mechanism. What would this have told us of its place in the economy of the yeast cell? What could we have deduced about the properties of invertase in other fungi, or in higher plants? Not much, it would seem, and so without looking further than a single hydrolytic reaction we find ourselves faced with a problem central to modern biology: how to assimilate the achievements of biochemistry. Put more simply: what can the biochemist do, and what can he not do, for his fellow biologists? The successful organization of biological research and teaching depends very much on finding the correct answers to these questions. Can anything be learnt from earlier discussions of the place of biochemistry in biological thought?

Cambridge and Sheffield

I happen to be one of the few who were fortunate enough to spend longish periods in two Departments of Biochemistry that had a very considerable influence on the development of the subject in Britain, and I have naturally wondered if, apart from being led by scientists of outstanding ability, they had any other features in common which contributed to this influence. Both had a complete conviction that biochemistry was a discipline in its own right, and that it had great contributions to make to biology, and through this to human welfare. This conviction in itself was enough to explain the enthusiasm that pervaded both laboratories. The differences between them arose partly from their different positions in the historical development of the subject, and partly of course from the different personalities of the Professors.

Hopkins' laboratory was filled with pioneers, whose research covered almost the whole of biology, and he himself continually emphasized the practicability of investigating all living processes at the chemical level. In his lectures outside the Department he devoted much of his efforts to overcoming the resistance of organic chemists, particularly those in England, to the idea that the activities of protoplasm were a respectable, and perhaps more important, a profitable subject for research. The reluctance of the chemists to participate was evidenced by the staff of his Department, many of whom were biologists by training or inclination, but, as subsequent events showed, a healthy chemical tradition was always maintained.

Hopkins in 1937 tried to show in his autobiography 'that it is not altogether my own fault if I have remained . . . intellectually an amateur. In research I have at no time worked under, or with an expert senior to myself.' Refusing to accept this claim to amateur status, Marjory Stephenson suggested that his unique contribution was that 'he alone among his contemporaries succeedeed in *formulating* the subject'. The consequence of this was that his Department attracted everyone who felt the power of this formulation, whether it was expressed in his own writings or in the teaching of his staff.

To those who now see in this formulation only a set of familiar biochemical concepts it is difficult to convey the suspicion with which they were regarded as little as thirty years ago, and, lest it might be thought that only the chemists are referred to, the story of A. C. Chibnall (1966) is worth reading, with its flashback to Hopkins' early days in Cambridge.

Krebs' Department in Sheffield was representative of the next stage in the development of biochemistry. Hopkins had pictured 'cell life as an ordered sequence of events governed by specific catalysts' and lived to see important features of fermentation and respiration explained in these terms, but his Department by the very diversity of its research had only a limited stake in the development of studies of intermediary metabolism. As we know, Krebs might have discovered the citric acid cycle in Cambridge, but Sheffield instead gained the honour, and became a new centre of attraction.

By this time biochemistry was gaining acceptance (Krebs' inaugural lecture in 1946 was entitled 'The Advent of Biochemistry') and the attraction of Sheffield was more specific; it was based on a desire to learn more about the methods that had led to the establishment of the citric acid cycle. Most of those attracted were biologists, hoping to apply these techniques to their own particular problems, but there were also chemists of a new, less sceptical generation, and (a sign of the times) graduates in biochemistry.

It seems unlikely that Krebs has ever thought of himself as an amateur, even intellectually, and he has always acknowledged a great debt to his teacher, Otto Warburg (Krebs, 1964, 1967). One might therefore have expected to find marked differences in the style of his Department.

In fact, these differences were not obvious, and the reason was not simply Krebs' feeling of admiration for the Cambridge Department, to which he had come as an exile from Germany (cf. Krebs, 1964), but the identity of his philosophical standpoint with that of Hopkins. Inevitably the smaller size of the Department and the accelerating growth of the subject tended to restrict the scope of the research, but the professionalism Krebs brought to it, in particular the extensive use of technicians, helped to offset this. The Department was in no way a 'school', if by that term is meant 'a whole laboratory . . . working on aspects of the professorial problem by the professorial methods'. The relative independence of the research workers was the basis for a democratic form of organization reminiscent of that in Cambridge.

What differences there were probably reflected the difference between the 'amateur', i.e. the pioneer prepared to turn his hand to anything, and the professional, whose job was to make the dreams of the pioneers come true. Anyone who had worked in Sheffield would have recognized Krebs in this quotation: 'to all members of the research department he was ever available for consultation and advice', but not in this one: 'Newcomers quickly lost their awe of him and learnt to drift into his room and, in the opinion of all the rest, to waste his time; it was, in fact, the opinion of each member of his department that everyone else traded on the Professor's good nature and woefully wasted his time.'

In this period biochemistry above all was beginning to demonstrate its power and there was always plenty to be done in the laboratory; philosophical discussions, though not entirely absent, were less important than they had been a generation before. It does not follow from this though that all the philosophical problems have been solved, so let us return to the questions that prompted this digression.

Biochemical unity and biological diversity

In their efforts to establish biochemistry as a distinct scientific discipline biochemists used often to emphasize the biochemical unity underlying the diversity of living forms. The discoveries of the last few decades have done much to substantiate their views. Sometimes this idea of unity was implicit in their actions, as in the well-known liver and horseradish biochemistry, at other times spelled out for popular consumption:

'The biochemist finds that considerable resemblances exist between the chemical substances in different cells and tissues, not only when these are derived from the same animal, but also when the tissues compared are from organisms as distinct as cats and cabbages, or mushrooms and millipedes. This knowledge is most encouraging because it suggests that the life of each is based on the same fundamental processes . . . and leads one to hope that information gained . . . in one organism will be of use . . . in all living organisms' (Bacon, 1944).

'Very true', said the Duchess: 'flamingoes and mustard both bite. And the moral of that is—"Birds of a feather flock together". '

'Only mustard isn't a bird', Alice remarked.

'Right, as usual', said the Duchess: 'what a clear way you have of putting things!'

It is doubtful whether in view of her next remark we should be prepared to rely upon Alice, but can we, in fact, say anything useful and permanent about the differences between flamingoes and mustard without invoking biochemistry? It is my contention that we can. Hopkins discussed this general question in the second Purser Memorial lecture in 1932 and again in his famous address to the British Association in 1933. He asked his audience not to suspect him of 'claiming that all the attributes of living systems or even the more obvious among them are necessarily based upon chemical organization alone', but expressed the belief that 'this organization will account for one striking characteristic of every living cell—its ability, namely, to maintain a dynamic individuality in diverse environments.'

With the advantage of a further thirty-five years' study of cellular structure we must be careful in interpreting his statements. In particular it is difficult to understand exactly what he meant by 'chemical organization', and how he would have reacted to what has now been discovered about the fine structure of cell organelles. Undoubtedly he visualized intracellular catalysts as being 'organized' to the extent that some were fixed to membranes, but it would seem that by chemical organization he meant the linking of individual enzymes through the extreme specificity of their catalytic reactions, His assertion was in part a response to those who denied that an *in vitro* study of intracellular enzymes could explain how they acted in the highly-structured cell system.

Similarly, from its context, 'all the attributes of living systems' seems to refer to the general properties of living matter, and it is not intended to include all biological phenomena. Growth, reproduction and heredity were among the attributes that 'it is not illogical to believe . . . are based upon organization which is in some sense higher than the chemical level'.

Now that biochemistry has begun to reach into these fields some may feel that 'chemical organization' is here also a sufficient explanation (hence the peculiar hybrid term, 'molecular biology') but others of us will seize upon the phrase 'in some sense higher' as a better representation of our point of view. As the technique of electron microscopy advances we shall eventually be able to study the morphology of quite small molecules, so that there will be no real gap in our observations anywhere between chemical structure and the gross anatomy of living organisms. Although at first this might appear to add to the confusion it should in the end simplify matters, because it will then be clear to each biologist that he must choose the level of structure at which his research will be centred. At present, largely as a result of the fascinating developments in nucleic acid biochemistry there is a tendency for biologists to become demoralized, and to believe that because each molecule of DNA carries messages the only real advances in biology can be made by reading them chemically, forgetting that the living cell contains the only means by which the messages can be translated into structure and activity. We still know very little about a multitude of biological phenomena. All *can* be examined at the molecular level, but this does not mean that nothing of significance can be said about them at higher levels of organization.

When we are immensely better informed about the structures and interactions of macromolecules we shall be able to explain the possible ways in which they can combine to produce cell organelles and larger anatomical structures, but this will still leave us with the necessity of discovering which particular structures have been selected, and which rejected, by the evolutionary process. The biochemistry that puts us in this position will be a very much more sophisticated science than the one we know today, and it would be optimistic to the point of madness to believe that we can afford to abandon other fields of biology while we wait for it to arrive.

Recommendations

Nevertheless, the non-biochemists will have to do some hard thinking about the teaching of biology, drop their well-intentioned but half-baked ideas about the training of integrated biologists or cell biologists (? semi-integrated biologists) and move over a bit to make room for the biochemists. Generally speaking, the rise of biochemistry as a teaching subject took place outside the departments of 'pure' biology, and often created a very uneasy situation. Believing, rightly, that biochemistry was a part of biology, some biologists tried to teach it in their own degree courses instead of welcoming it as an independent subject, drawing students from the physical sciences as well as biology. Cambridge was particularly fortunate in having a course structure that permitted the elementary teaching of biochemistry to have its independence as early as 1935. In many universities rigidity of thinking and of organization were such that contrived solutions emerged, not very satisfactory to anyone concerned; at the back of them lay the reluctance of chemists and biologists alike to relinquish some of their academic territory (and students). Thus although everyone was ready to join in exclamations of praise and gratitude for the successes of biochemistry its rise to power has left biology in a badly disturbed state. I am convinced that this is in part due to a neglect in recent years of the philosophical arguments used by Hopkins in formulating the discipline of biochemistry.*

To the biochemists, dizzy with success, it should be sufficient to offer one last quotation from his 1933 address to the British Association: 'If the biochemist should at any time be inclined to overrate the value of his contributions to biology, or to underrate the magnitude of problems outside his province, he will do well sometimes to leave the laboratory for the field, or to seek even in the museum a reminder of that infinity of adaptation of which life is capable. He will then not fail to work with a humble mind, however great his faith in the importance of the methods which are his own.'

A moral

In this essay I have tried to draw attention away from the nucleus to the boundary of the cell, and to show that each cell wall will have its own characteristic metabolism, although 'outside' the cell. We have noticed that the enzyme invertase has a close association with plant cell walls, but

* The uncited quotations in this essay may easily be found by reading the whole of 'Hopkins and Biochemistry' (1949). Ed. by Needham, J., and Baldwin, E., Cambridge; W. Heffer and Sons Ltd.

knowledge of its catalytic properties does not explain the association, nor does it seem likely that a fuller knowledge of the chemical structure of the enzyme would help at present. What is presumably needed is a better understanding of the organization of structures and events in the wall region, and so we have been led to consider levels of organization in living systems, and have come near to accepting the dangerous task of defining the point at which chemical structure passes into fine structure. At this point the biochemist should be willing to hand over some of the responsibility to his fellow biologists, and they should be willing to accept it. Analogous points exist at which chemical energy passes into other forms of energy. All that is required for a harmonious development of biochemistry alongside the other biological sciences is for everyone to recognize these boundaries.

But here is the Duchess digging her chin into my shoulder again.

'And the moral of that is—"The grass always looks greener on the other side of the fence".'

'And sometimes it is, too!' thought Alice.

References

Abd-el-Al, A. T. H., and Phaff, H. J. (1968). *Biochem. J.*, **109**, 347.
Allen, P. J., and Bacon, J. S. D. (1956). *Biochem. J.*, **63**, 200.
Anderson, F. B., and Millbank, J. W. (1966). *Biochem. J.*, **99**, 268.
Arnold, W. N. (1968). *J. Theoret. Biol.*, **21**, 13.
Bacon, J. S. D. (1944). *The Chemistry of Life*, p. 5. London: Watts and Co.
Bacon, J. S. D. (1954). *Biochem. J.*, **57**, 320.
Bacon, J. S. D. (1960). *Bull. Soc. Chim. Biol.*, **42**, 1441.
Bacon, J. S. D. (1961). *Biochem. J.*, **79**, 20P.
Bacon, J. S. D. (1965). *Biochem J.*, **96**, 38P.
Bacon, J. S. D., and Edelman, J. (1951). *Biochem. J.*, **48**, 114.
Bacon, J. S. D., MacDonald, I. R., and Knight, A. H. (1965). *Biochem. J.*, **94**, 175.
Bacon, J. S. D., Milne, B. D., Taylor, I. F., and Webley, D. M. (1965). *Biochem. J.*, **95**, 28C.
Boer, P., and Steyn-Parvé, E. P. (1966). *Biochim. Biophys. Acta*, **128**, 400.
Burger, M., Bacon, E. E., and Bacon, J. S. D. (1958). *Nature, Lond.*, **182**, 1508
Burger, M., Bacon, E. E., and Bacon, J. S. D. (1961). *Biochem. J.*, **78**, 504.
Brock, T. D. (1965a). *Biochem. Biophys. Res. Commun.*, **19**, 623.
Brock, T. D. (1965b). *J. Bact.*, **90**, 1019.
Chibnall, A. C. (1966). *Annu. Rev. Biochem.*, **35**, 11.
Colvin, J. R., and Beer, M. (1960). *Canad. J. Microbiol.*, **6**, 631.
Davies, R. (1967). *Abh. dt. Akad. Wiss. Berl., Klässe für Medizin, Jahrgang 1966*, No. **6**, p. 195.
Davies, R., and Elvin, P. A. (1964). *Biochem. J.*, **93**, 8P.
Datko, A. H., and Machlachlan, G. A. (1968). *Plant Physiol.*, **43**, 735.
Datko, A. H. (1968). *Ph.D. Thesis, McGill University, Montreal, Canada.*

LIFE OUTSIDE THE CELL   65

Done, J., Shorey, C. D., Loke, J. P., and Pollak, J. K. (1965). *Biochem. J.*, **96**, 27C.

Duell, E. A., Inoue, S., and Utter, M. F. (1964). *J. Bact.*, **88**, 1762.

Dworshack, R. G., and Wickerham, J. L. (1961). *Applied Microbiol.*, **9**, 291.

Eddy, A. A., and Williamson, D. H. (1957). *Nature, Lond.*, **179**, 1252

Eddy, A. A., and Williamson, D. H. (1959). *Nature, Lond.*, **183**, 1101.

Edelman, J., and Hall, M. A. (1964). *Nature, Lond.*, **201**, 296.

Edelman, J., and Hall, M. A. (1965). *Biochem. J.*, **95**, 403.

Edelman, J., and Jefford, T. G. (1968). *New Phytol.*, **67**, 517.

Fischer, E. H., and Kohtès, L. (1951). *Helv. Chim. Acta*, **34**, 1123.

Fischer, E. H., Kohtès, L., and Fellig, J. (1951). *Helv. Chim. Acta*, **34**, 1132.

Friis, J., and Ottolenghi, P. (1959). *C. R. Lab. Carlsberg*, **31**, 259.

Gascon, S., and Ottolenghi, P. (1967). *C. R. Lab. Carlsberg*, **36**, 85.

Gerhardt, P., and Judge, J. A. (1964). *J. Bact.*, **87**, 943.

Hagedorn, H. (1964). *Protoplasma*, **58**, 250.

Hassid, W. Z. (1967). *Ann. Rev. Pl. Physiol.*, **18**, 267.

Hatch, M. D., and Glasziou, K. T. (1963). *Plant Physiol.*, **38**, 344.

Hellebust, J. A. ,and Forward, D. F. (1962). *Canad. J. Bot.*, **40**, 113.

Higashi, Y., Strominger, J. L., and Sweeley, C. C. (1967). *Proc. Nat. Acad. Sci., Wash.*, **57**, 1878.

Hughes, D. E. (1951). *Brit. J. Exp. Path.*, **32**, 97.

Krebs, H. A. (1964). *Biochem. J.*, **80**, 231.

Krebs, H. A. (1967). *Nature, Lond.*, **215**, 1244.

Lampen, J. O. (1968). *Leeuwenhoek Ned. Tijdschr.*, **34**, 1.

MacDonald, I. R. (1968). *Plant Physiol.*, **43**, 274.

MacDonald, I. R., and DeKock, P. C. (1958). *Ann. Bot., Lond.*, **22**, 429.

Manley, R. St J. (1964). *Nature, Lond.*, **204**, 1155.

Matile, P., Moor, H., and Mühletahler, K. (1967). *Arch. Mikrobiol.* **58**, 201.

Millbank, J. W. (1963). *Exp. Cell Res.*, **29**, 422.

Mitchell, R., and Sabar, N. (1966). *J. Gen. Microbiol.*, **42**, 39.

Mühletahler, K. (1967). *Ann. Rev. Pl. Physiol.*, **18**, 1.

Myrbäck, K. (1957). *Arch. Biochem.*, **69**, 138.

Myrbäck, K. (1960). In *The Enzymes*, Vol. **4**, p. 382. Ed. by Boyer, P. D., Lardy, H., and Myrbäck, K., London: Academic Press.

Myrbäck, K. (1961). *Brauwissenschaft*, **14**, 82.

Nossal, P. M. (1952). *Biochem. J.*, **50**, 349.

Northcote, D. H. (1968). *Brit. Med. Bull.*, **24**, 107.

Northcote, D. H., and Pickett-Heaps, J. D. (1966). *Biochem. J.*, **98**, 159.

Ordin, L., and Hall, M. A. (1968). *Plant Physiol.*, **43**, 473.

Ottolenghi, P. (1967). *C. R. Lab. Carlsberg*, **36**, 95.

Phaff, H. J. (1963). *Annu. Rev. Microbiol.*, **17**, 15.

Preece, I. A. (1957). *Cereal Carbohydrates*. London: Royal Institute of Chemistry.

Pressey, R. (1968). *Plant Physiol.*, **43**, 1430.

Preston, R. D. (1965). *In Biosynthetic Pathways in Higher Plants*. Ed. by Pridham, J., and Swain, T., London: Academic Press.

Robinson, E., and Brown, R. (1952). *J. Exp. Bot.*, **3**, 356.

Roelofsen, P. A. (1959). *The Plant Cell Wall. Encyclopaedia of Plant Anatomy*. Ed. by Zimmerman, W., and Ozenda, P. G., Berlin: Borntrager.

Roelofsen, P. A. (1965). *Advances in Botanical Research*, **2**, 69.

Sacher, J. A., Hatch, M. D., and Glasziou, K. T. (1963). *Plant Physiol.*, **38**, 348.
Setterfield, G., and Bayley, S. T. (1961). *Annu. Rev. Pl. Physiol.*, **12**, 35.
Shapiro, L., Grossman, L. I., and Marmur, J. (1968). *J. Mol. Biol.*, **33**, 907.
Sutton, D. D., and Lampen, J. O. (1962). *Biochim. Biophys. Acta*, **56**, 303.
Vaughan, D., and MacDonald, I. R. (1967). *Plant Physiol.*, **42**, 456.
Vaughan, D., and MacDonald, I. R. (1968a). *J. Exp. Bot.*, **18**, 578.
Vaughan, D., and MacDonald, I. R. (1968b). *J. Exp. Bot.*, **18**, 587.
Wanner, H., and Leupold, U. (1947). *Ber. schweiz. botan. Ges.*, **57**, 156.
Weimberg, R., and Orton, W. L. (1964). *J. Bact.*, **88**, 1743.
Wessels, J. G. H., and Niederpruem, D. J. (1967). *J. Bact.*, **94**, 1594.

THE REGULATION OF PURINE NUCLEOTIDE METABOLISM IN BACTERIA

Kenneth Burton

Department of Biochemistry, University of Newcastle upon Tyne

A remarkable basic feature of cell metabolism is the versatility of the purine nucleotides which act as energy carriers, as precursors of nucleic acids and as components of many enzyme systems. In general, and especially in growing bacteria, net synthesis of RNA is the major process that consumes purine nucleotides as distinct from just changing the state of phosphorylation. Although bacteria may appear to be poorly developed organisms, their low ecological niche does not imply biochemical naivety. Indeed, they have been exposed to more generations of evolutionary selection than higher organisms and have quite obviously acquired sophisticated mechanisms of biochemical regulation appropriate to their natural habitats. Many of them, such as *Escherichia coli*, are particularly notable for their ability to adapt quickly to a variety of changes when oxygen or the various sources of carbon or nitrogen become exhausted. Since these changes might directly affect the biosynthesis of ATP and GTP, we can expect nucleic acid synthesis to be regulated by the availability of purine nucleotides. Thus, it is appropriate to ask how far the cellular processes may compete with each other for the available purine nucleotides.

REGULATORY MECHANISMS

Metabolism can be controlled either by regulating enzyme biosynthesis or by directly controlling enzyme activity. The latter method is a fine control that acts quickly and is likely to be more immediately involved in regulating the levels of purine nucleotides. Regulation of enzyme biosynthesis can reduce a metabolic flux only slowly but it can, of course, act more quickly when an enzyme is being induced or de-repressed in response to a new demand.

Abbreviations: r-RNA, ribosomal RNA; m-RNA, messenger RNA; t-RNA, amino acid transfer RNA; P-ribose-PP, 5-phosphoribosyl-1-pyrophosphate; PEP, 3-phosphoenolpyruvate; 3-PGA, 3-phosphoglycerate.

Krebs and Kornberg (1957) emphasized the idea that metabolic path-ways are regulated by relatively few pacemaker steps. This view is still held but there may perhaps be rather more regulatory substances or modulators than were initially thought to be involved. There are various degrees of complexity in the interactions with the pacemaker enzymes but the controls typically involve oligomeric enzymes with distinct modulator and catalytic sites and often a sigmoid relationship between the enzyme activity and the concentration of the modulator or critical substrate. The sigmoid relationship can increase the precision and sensitivity of the con-trol by amplifying the effects of small changes in the concentration of a regulating metabolite.

We can imagine several possible general control mechanisms for nucleic acid synthesis, one of them being a direct regulation of the activity of the polymerases by the concentrations of the four nucleotide substrates. The detailed kinetics of these enzymes are poorly understood and most atten-tion has naturally been paid to the influences of the templates rather than to the concentrations of the substrates. Before examining the possibility of substrate-level control, it seems important to examine other information about the way in which the nucleotide pools and the synthesis of nucleic acids are regulated in *E. coli* and similar bacteria.

Regulation of purine nucleotide biosynthesis

Roberts and coworkers (1955) first gave clear evidence for effective con-trols in the biosynthesis of nucleotides. Their elegant isotope competition experiments showed that pre-formed nucleosides or bases were taken up by bacteria and inhibited endogenous synthesis from simpler precursors. Later work (McCarthy and Britten, 1962; Buchwald and Britten, 1963) showed clearly that uptake of the nucleic acid bases was limited—presum-ably by the level of endogenous nucleotides. Even now, little is known about the regulation of the uptake but direct controls of enzyme activity are known to occur at certain critical steps in the biosynthesis (Figure 1).

The amidation of glutamic acid and the pyrophosphorylation of ribose-5-phosphate are preliminary steps which are both more important in the synthesis of bacterial nucleic acid than in the synthesis of bacterial protein (Table 1). Glutamine synthetase is inhibited by CTP and AMP (Stadtman and coworkers, 1968) while phosphoribosyl pyrophosphoryl transferase is inhibited by ADP or possibly AMP (Switzer, 1967; Atkinson and Fall, 1967; Klungsøyr, Hagemen, Fall and Atkinson, 1968). It is interesting to note that there is evidence for the level of P-ribose-PP affecting the rate of purine biosynthesis in mammalian tissues (Rajalakshmi and Handschumaker, 1968; Rosenbloom and coworkers, 1968).

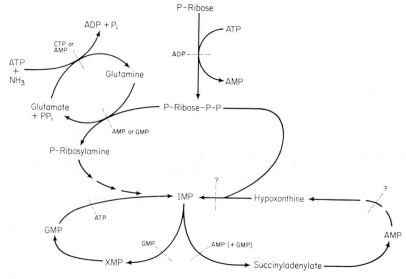

Figure 1. Feedback control of the synthesis and interconversion of purine nucleotides in bacteria. Based on literature information for *E. coli*, *A. aerogenes* and *S. typhimurium* (see text)

Table 1. Metabolic intermediates needed for protein and nucleic acid synthesis in bacterial growth

Precursor	End product	
	Nucleic Acid	Protein
Group A. Sources of C or C and N		
Aspartate	0·33	1·2
Glutamate	—	0·80
P-ribose-PP	0·67	0·08
PEP or 3PGA	—	1·17
Erythrose 4-P	—	0·26
Group B. Used as sources of N only		
Glutamate	0·33	2·61
Aspartate	0·50	0·25
Glutamine (amide-N)	1·0	0·46
NH_3	0·33	0·18

Calculated from compositional data (Roberts and coworkers 1955) and known pathways for *E. coli* growing aerobically on a glucose ammonium salts medium. The values are the mMoles needed to synthesize the components in 1 gram of dry cells

The amination of P-ribose-PP is essentially the first specific step in the biosynthesis of purine nucleotides although this and the next four steps are also used in bacteria for the biosynthesis of thiamine. Since thiamine is made only in very small amounts, it is not surprising that the amination step is controlled by GMP and AMP (Nierlich and Magasanik, 1965). Later steps do not appear to be controlled by feedback inhibition until beyond IMP, the branch point of the pathway (Magasanik and Karibian, 1961). There might also be a degree of cross-activation since ATP is needed for the last step in the formation of GMP while GTP is required for the first step of the conversion of IMP to AMP:

$$IMP + GTP + aspartate \rightarrow adenylosuccinate + GDP + P_i$$

Several nucleotides including AMP and GMP have been found to inhibit the enzyme from *E. coli* (Wyngaarden and Greenland, 1963).

Of the two steps to GMP, the first is controlled by GMP itself (Mager and Magasanik, 1960; Buzzee and Levin, 1968):

$$IMP + NAD^+ \rightarrow XMP + NADH + H^+$$

There is no direct evidence for regulation of the second step:

$$XMP + NH_4^+ + ATP \rightarrow GMP + AMP + PP_i$$

However, it is inhibited by an adenosine analogue, psicofuranine, and some features of this inhibition suggest that the enzyme might be an allosteric protein with psicofuranine being an analogue of an unknown natural modulator (Kuramitsu and Moyed, 1966; Fukuyama, 1966).

Interconversion of purine ribonucleotides

Interconversion proceeds via IMP involving at least two additional controlled reactions that act in the reverse direction to each branch of the synthetic pathway. GMP is converted to AMP with the aid of GMP reductase which is inhibited by ATP (Mager and Magasanik, 1960). AMP is not converted directly to IMP in *S. typhimurium* (Zimmerman and Magasanik, 1964), a possible route being via adenosine, inosine and hypoxanthine (Mans and Koch, 1960). There is little information about the regulation of these latter steps in bacteria but they are probably regulated by the nucleotide levels, if only to prevent useless cycling.

Regulation of DNA synthesis

The formation of deoxyribonucleotides appears to be an important control step in DNA synthesis and the pools of deoxynucleotides are generally much lower than those of the ribonucleotides. Reduction occurs at the diphosphate level in *E. coli* or at the triphosphates in *Lactobacillus leich-manii* (see reviews by Larsson and Reichard, 1967; Blakley and Vitols, 1968). In each case a single, oligomeric enzyme can reduce ribonucleotides of adenine, guanine, uracil and cytosine and there is a complex control involving inhibition and activation by ATP and by different deoxyribonucleotides.

Maaløe and Hanawalt (1961) made an important contribution by showing that RNA and/or protein synthesis was needed for the initiation of each cycle in the replication of DNA. Once initiated, a cycle can be completed without RNA and protein synthesis. The distinction between initiation and growth was amplified by the replicon hypothesis (Jacob, Brenner and Cuzin, 1963) and by Pritchard and Lark's discovery (1964), that thymine deficiency does not at first affect the frequency of initiation. Since DNA synthesis is regulated primarily by its initiation (Cooper and Helmstetter, 1968) and since the levels of the deoxynucleotide triphosphates alter during thymine deficiency (Neuhard, 1966), it seems unlikely that these nucleotides are important in regulating the initiation of DNA synthesis.

Amino acids and RNA synthesis

In the early 1950's several workers showed that RNA synthesis was suppressed when the essential amino acid was withdrawn from amino acid auxotrophs. There was no reason to think that nucleotide biosynthesis was affected and so it was assumed that the effects represented a physiological control of RNA synthesis. Stent and Brenner (1961) discovered that different strains of *E. coli* showed different responses depending upon the presence of the relaxed control mutation (designated *rel* or *RC*). *Rel* strains can accumulate large amounts of RNA when protein synthesis is inhibited by amino acid deficiency whereas strains with the 'wild-type' gene (*rel*$^+$) show little net synthesis of RNA under these conditions and are termed 'stringent'.

Despite much detailed study, the mechanism of the amino acid control in stringent strains is not clear (see review by Edlin and Broda, 1968). Although the accumulation of RNA is suppressed, m-RNA is made at a very high rate from operons which are either fully reduced or fully derepressed (Morris and Kjeldgaard, 1968; Edlin, Stent, Baker and Yankofsky, 1968; Lavallé and De Hauwer, 1968). This fact excludes mechanisms based on the general inhibition of either RNA polymerase or the synthesis of nucleoside triphosphates. Recent studies of RNA polymerase (Burgess, Travers, Dunn and Bautz, 1969) open the exciting possibility that an associated protein might regulate its initiation at different sites on the

DNA. The enzyme is evidently more complex than it was previously thought to be and it is therefore not out of the question for the amino acid control to operate by selective inhibition of RNA polymerase.

The occurrence of the amino acid control does not mean that RNA synthesis is necessarily linked to simultaneous protein synthesis since many potent inhibitors of protein synthesis, such as chloramphenicol or terramycin, do not inhibit RNA synthesis and can even stimulate it, perhaps by causing the accumulation of amino acids when protein synthesis is inhibited. It seems quite clear that RNA synthesis in stringent bacteria requires a full complement of the various aminoacyl t-RNA's (Eidlic and Neidhardt, 1965) but the available evidence does not favour a simple control of RNA synthesis by acylated or unacylated t-RNA (Ezekiel and Valulis, 1966). Quite apart from the experimental evidence presented by Ezekiel and Valulis, it is difficult to imagine how a deficiency of any single amino acid might directly inhibit the controlling step when the t-RNA's for the other 19 amino acids are all in the acylated form. Direct studies of RNA polymerase activity *in vitro* do not support the view that the activity of this enzyme is controlled by the charging of t-RNA (Bremer, Yegian and Konrad, 1966).

One inhibitor of protein synthesis, trimethoprim, has a different effect from the others so far investigated. Trimethoprim inhibits RNA synthesis in *rel*$^+$ (stringent) strains but not in *rel* (relaxed) ones and the effect is not relieved by supplying amino acids (Shih, Eisenstadt and Lengyel, 1966). Its action is to inhibit dihydrofolic acid reductase and thus to prevent the initiation of protein synthesis by N-formylmethionyl t-RNA although it might well also affect the maturation of nascent r-RNA by methylation. Together with the other evidence involving t-RNA in the amino acid control, the action of trimethoprim suggests that net synthesis of RNA in a *rel*$^+$ strain may depend upon the presence of ribosome–m-RNA–peptidyl t-RNA complexes. This idea has not yet been clearly confirmed because there is no general agreement about the effects of amino acid deficiency on the size and number of polysomes in *rel*$^+$ and *rel* bacteria (Morris and De Moss, 1966; Ron, Kohler and Davis, 1966; Friesen, 1968).

Further analysis of the control is confused by the present lack of agreement about the nature of the effect on the synthesis of r-RNA. It is generally agreed that when the net synthesis of RNA is inhibited, m-RNA accumulates in preference to r-RNA and t-RNA. Indeed, after allowing for the reduced entry of radioactive labels into the precursor pools, the total rate of m-RNA synthesis does not appear to be reduced by a very large factor (Nierlich, 1968). It is often suggested that the control might prevent the synthesis or r-RNA but DNA–RNA hybridization experiments after a pulse label (Friesen, 1966, 1968; Stubbs and Hall, 1968) indicate that this is not so and therefore suggest that the stringent control might operate by degrading the newly synthesized r-RNA.

Whether or not this is so most evidence is against the amino acid control operating by limiting the supply of the triphosphate precursors of RNA. It is not supported by several direct analyses for the ribonucleoside triphosphates (Goldstein, Brown and Goldstein, 1960; Neidhardt and Fraenkel, 1961; Edlin and Neuhard, 1967; Bagnara and Finch, 1968), and moreover, if triphosphates did limit RNA synthesis, they would reduce the transcription of m-RNA from fully de-repressed operons. Nevertheless, limitation of the triphosphate precursors has been strongly advocated as a mechanism for the control (Gallant and Cashel, 1967; Cashel and Gallant, 1968), a strong line of evidence being a large fall of UTP and CTP on amino acid exhaustion. In view of other analyses (Goldstein and coworkers, 1960; Edlin and Neuhard, 1967; Bagnara and Finch, 1968; Edlin and Broda, 1968), the change found by Cashel and Gallant (1968) cannot be generally important.

Although Edlin and Broda (1968) have not given any nucleotide analyses for relaxed strains, their analyses of stringent strains show a considerable fall in GTP and comparison with other analyses mentioned above confirms that GTP is the only one of the four triphosphate precursors of RNA that could conceivably be involved in the amino acid control. Even so, the argument for this possibility is very weak.

Balanced synthesis of different types of RNA

Since the amino acid control reduces the proportion of r-RNA to m-RNA, it is one way in which the content of ribosomes might be adjusted when bacteria exhaust preferred nutrients. Although the rel^+ gene is an advantage to wild-type bacteria when amino acids become exhausted from the growth medium (Alföldi, Stent, Hoogs and Hill, 1963), it is not the only mechanism involved in regulating the levels of ribosomes. Neidhardt (1963) has shown that rel mutants can adjust their rates of RNA synthesis quite normally when they are transferred to richer media, to a poorer carbon source, or from ammonium salts to tryptophan as a source of nitrogen. Several attractive explanations have been suggested involving control by either free ribosomes or ribosomal subunits but there is as yet little direct positive evidence for any particular mechanism.

Nucleoside triphosphates and RNA synthesis

Although net synthesis of nucleic acids is halted by removing the source of purines from adenine or guanine-requiring mutants, the cells cannot be entirely depleted of their adenine nucleotides because glucose is oxidized normally (Pardee, 1954) and because precursors of purine nucleotides can accumulate in these mutants despite the need for ATP in their synthesis.

In this laboratory, Mrs. G. Thomas has investigated the nucleotide pools in a strain of *E. coli* (NE-1) which requires both adenine and guanine. This organism has the genotype F^-: *proA$^-$ lac y$^-$ purB$^-$ guaA$^-$ mal$^-$ xyl$^-$ str^r* and was obtained as a *his$^+$str^r* recombinant between a HfrH: *guaA$^-$* strain and the F^-: *purB$^-$ his$^-$ str^r* strain AB1325. Strain NE-1 lacks both adenylosuccinase and XMP aminase and so it cannot synthesize IMP or convert IMP into either AMP or GMP. On transfer to a medium deficient in both adenine and guanosine, ATP and ADP fell after the first 10 minutes. A greater and much more rapid fall occurred when guanosine was supplied without adenine (Figure 2), apparently

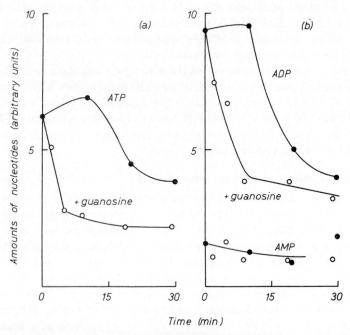

Figure 2. Adenine nucleotides in a double purine-requiring strain NE-1, grown on aerated glucose ammonium salts medium at 25° C supplemented with thiamine, [^{14}C]adenine, guanosine, proline and histidine. At 0 minutes it was transferred by centrifuging into medium lacking purines, guanosine then being added to one portion. Adenine nucleotides were determined by their radioactivity after extraction by trichloroacetic acid, de-salting with charcoal and two-dimensional separation on paper, (a) ATP; (b) ADP or AMP as indicated.
○, with added guanosine; ●, no purine added

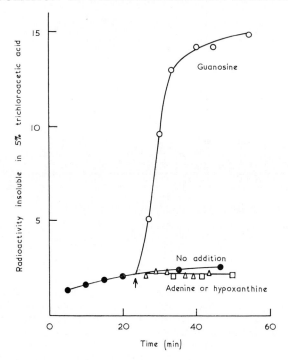

Figure 3. Effects of individual purines or nucleosides on the incorporation of uracil into the acid-insoluble fraction of the double mutant NE-1. The culture was grown as for Figure 2 but with unlabelled adenine and with uracil. At 0 minutes it was transferred by filtration into medium lacking adenine and guanine but containing [^{14}C]uracil (●). Adenine (△), hypoxanthine (□) or guanosine (○) was added to portions at 24 minutes

because of a dramatic stimulation of nucleic acid synthesis (Figure 3) affecting both RNA and DNA. Addition of adenine without guanosine does not induce incorporation of precursors into nucleic acids. Hence, in this mutant at least, GTP appears to be much more important than ATP in limiting nucleic acid synthesis.

In other experiments with the parent adenylosuccinase mutant, there was an analogous behaviour, allowing for the presence of XMP aminase. Hypoxanthine would similarly stimulate nucleic acid synthesis and there was a large accumulation of guanine mononucleotides, the greatest effect being in GTP (Figure 4). Nucleic acid synthesis was most rapid at about 5 minutes after the addition of hypoxanthine and yet by this time there was only a small increase in GTP and none in GDP or GMP. The guanine nucleotides increased as the nucleic acid synthesis stopped, suggesting

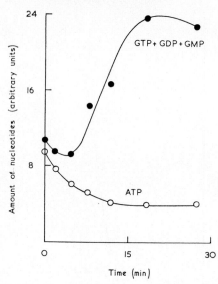

Figure 4. Amounts of purine nucleotides in cultures of an adenylosuccinase mutant. Strain AB-1325 was grown on aerated glucose-salts medium at 25° with thiamine, 2, 8-[³H]adenine, proline and histidine. It was transferred by filtration at 0 minutes to medium in which the adenine was replaced by [³H]hypoxanthine of the same specific activity. Nucleotides were extracted by trichloroacetic acid and estimated by the radioactivity after separation with correction for the absence of ³H at position 2 in guanine

that the synthesis of nucleic acids is sensitive to small changes in the GTP pool and that the enzymes which make GTP overshoot when nucleic acid synthesis stops for lack of ATP. Hypoxanthine or xanthine nucleotides cannot be involved directly in stimulating RNA synthesis since these bases have no effect in the NE-1 strain. When no source of purine was supplied, the fall of GTP was comparable with that of ATP but represented a larger fraction of the initial amount (Table 2).

Table 2. Changes of ATP and GTP in purine-starvation of an adenylosuccinase mutant

Time of starvation (minutes)	ATP	GTP
0	32	15
10	27	9·0
20	25	8·7
30	19	4·3

Amounts are given as percentage of the total initial adenosine and guanosine phosphates

Compartments in the nucleotide pools

A striking feature of the nucleotide analyses is the low level of GMP in exponentially growing bacteria (e.g. Table 3). The only probable way to make GDP from GMP is by guanylate kinase (Oeschger and Bessman, 1966):

$$ATP + GMP \rightleftharpoons GDP + ADP$$

Since the equilibrium should be similar to that of adenylate kinase ($K = 2 \cdot 2$), it is difficult to see how GMP can be converted to GDP so effectively unless ATP and ADP can be distributed very unevenly throughout the cell.

Table 3. Distribution of purine nucleotides in log-phase cells

	Amount (% of total purine mononucleotides)
ATP	27
ADP	25
AMP	17
GTP	13
GDP	15
GMP	3

Strain AB-1325 grown on glucose-salts medium aerated at 25° and supplemented with adenine, histidine, proline and thiamine

Private pools of nucleotides have previously been suggested by McCarthy and Britten (1962) and by Buchwald and Britten (1963) on the basis of evidence that exogenous precursors are incorporated into nucleic acids before complete admixture with internal nucleotide pools. Although their arguments have been questioned (Nierlich and Vielmetter, 1968; Nierlich, 1968; Salser, Janin and Levinthal, 1968) it is still necessary either to invoke private pools or to assume considerably higher levels of m-RNA than are indicated by DNA–RNA hybridization experiments (Friesen, 1966; Pigott and Midgley, 1968; Midgley, 1969). The existence of private pools has recently been confirmed by kinetic studies of the incorporation of pyrimidines into the RNA of E. coli (Mueller and Bremer, 1968).

Effects of purine deficiency on protein synthesis

In the adenine and guanine requiring strain, guanosine alone permits an appreciable synthesis of protein (Figure 5) which falls off after the period

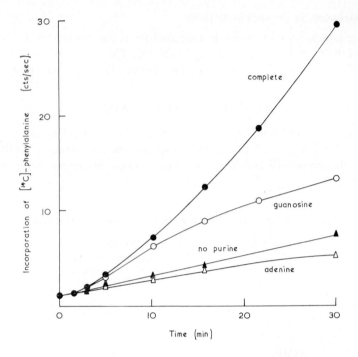

Figure 5. Protein synthesis by the double purine-requiring strain NE-1, grown on sodium lactate medium at 37° with supplements as for Figure 2. At 0 minutes it was transferred to media containing U-[^{14}C]-L-phenylalanine and in which adenine and/or guanosine may have been omitted. Acid-insoluble radioactivity was measured at intervals

of rapid nucleic acid synthesis. In contrast, adenine alone does not allow protein synthesis and even suppresses it below that observed with no purine. In a similar manner, β–galactosidase was not induced in the absence of guanosine but guanosine would allow an appreciable synthesis of enzyme even in the absence of adenine (Figure 6). Hence protein synthesis *in vivo* resembles nucleic acid synthesis in being limited more by the availability of GTP than by the availability of ATP. There is not enough evidence to show whether this occurs solely because of its dependence on m-RNA or because not enough GTP is available for the polymerization of amino acids.

An important deduction from Figures 5 and 6 is that m-RNA is readily made with guanosine in the absence of adenine.

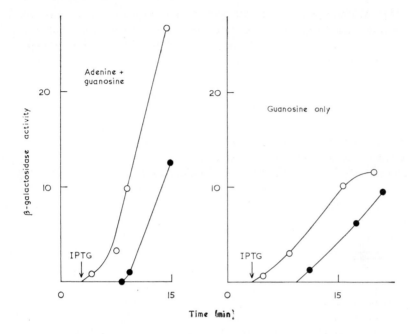

Figure 6. Synthesis of β-galactosidase. After growth as for Figure 5, strain NE-1 was transferred to fresh media at 0 minutes and isopropylthiogalactoside (IPTG) was added at 3 minutes. Following Kepes (1963) samples were removed at the times indicated and β-galactosidase was measured directly ($\bullet$) or after diluting out the inducer in complete medium ($\bigcirc$). The difference between the two curves is a measure of m-RNA that had been initiated at the time of dilution as well as any incomplete β-galactosidase. No β-galactosidase was formed with adenine alone

Nucleotide pools and energy metabolism

In this laboratory, most types of purine-requiring strains of E. *coli* have been found to oxidize glucose normally in the absence of purines, the only effect on the oxygen consumption being to prevent the increase in rate that would have accompanied normal growth. However, conditions which severely deplete the ATP pool also inhibit the oxidation of glucose by 30–60%. This can occur in several ways, for example by giving only hypoxanthine to an adenylosuccinase mutant or by starving an IMP trans-formylase mutant of purine in the absence of histidine. In the latter case, the de-repression of histidine biosynthesis converts ATP into amino-imidazole carboxamide ribotide which cannot be re-utilized to make

AMP. Mutants which lack adenylosuccinate synthetase are in a special position because removing adenine is expected to lead immediately to a guanine/adenine imbalance. In one such mutant the oxygen consumption was reduced by about 80% on removing adenine with an even greater effect when histidine was also removed.

The effect appears to be in the glycolytic pathway since it will inhibit the oxidation of glucose but not that of lactate by lactate-grown *E. coli*. Anaerobic utilization of glucose and the aerobic utilization of mannitol are also affected. Glucose oxidation is hardly affected at 25°, possibly because bacteria grown at this temperature have a higher content of adenine nucleotides (Franzen and Binkley, 1961). Any secondary effects due to defective energy metabolism in adenine-starved bacteria may therefore be obviated by using lactate medium or by using a glucose medium at 25°.

The mechanism of the effect on glycolysis is not yet known. When it was discovered, it seemed reasonable to expect an inhibition either of glucose uptake or of one of the kinases in the Embden–Meyerhof pathway, especially since the activity of *E. coli* phosphofructokinase might fall when the concentrations of both ATP and ADP are reduced (Blangy, Buc and Monod, 1958). Nevertheless, a primary effect on the uptake and phosphorylation of glucose appears to be eliminated by the finding of a marked rise of fructose-1,6-diphosphate with falls in the levels of hexosemonophosphates (N. F. Varney, unpublished). So far, no effect has been found on the viability of the depleted bacteria.

At first sight, any purpose of this effect seems to be even more obscure than the mechanism. It could reflect a normal control of glycolysis by adenine nucleotides or it could be a complete artefact, since the extreme conditions of adenine deprivation might have no counterpart in the natural environment of wild-type bacteria. Nevertheless, it is an indication that uncontrolled synthesis of RNA can deplete adenine nucleotides to a degree where glycolysis is inhibited.

GTP as a regulator of RNA synthesis?

It is suggested that severe depletion of adenine nucleotides is normally avoided because the synthesis of RNA is more sensitive to changes in the level of GTP than to changes of ATP. There is also the possibility that the ATP and GTP which act as nucleic acid precursors are in a separate compartment from the bulk of the adenine nucleotides.

Although adenylosuccinase mutants can convert adenine nucleotides to guanine nucleotides, this conversion does not appear to be activated during purine starvation. Presumably it only occurs when there is an excess of adenine nucleotides as well as a deficiency of guanine nucleotides. RNA synthesis in 'wild-type' bacteria will therefore be expected to stop by deficiency of guanine nucleotides before there is serious depletion of adenine nucleotides.

Even so, net synthesis of RNA seems to be very sensitive to small changes in the level of GTP. A large part of the GTP could well be segregated from the sites of RNA synthesis or it could be that the RNA polymerase shows a sigmoid concentration dependence upon GTP. There is not yet enough evidence to evaluate this latter possibility. Several authors (e.g. Steck, Caicuts and Wilson, 1968) have found sigmoid substrate concentration curves particularly in the presence of Mn^{2+} ions but these effects are possibly due to metal-binding artefacts or to slow initiation of RNA chains under the conditions used.

The idea that GTP is important in controlling the rate of RNA synthesis helps to suggest a function for the partial inhibition of aspartate carbamoyl transferase by GTP (Gerhardt and Pardee, 1962). GTP might have been expected to act like ATP and to activate the enzyme, thus increasing the synthesis of pyrimidine nucleotides when there is an excess of purine nucleotides. However, temporary imbalances of the nucleotide precursors of RNA are probably a common feature of bacterial growth as individual substrates in complex media become exhausted. If it developed that ATP was low and GTP high, RNA would still be synthesized, thus consuming ATP and creating an unstable situation. Also, aspartate would be used for pyrimidine synthesis despite the possibility that it might be better deployed for converting GTP to ATP. These possible difficulties could be avoided by the inhibition of aspartate carbamoyl transferase by GTP. Low ATP coupled with high GTP might then release more aspartate for adenylosuccinate synthetase and might also reduce the utilization of adenine nucleotides by limiting the supply of UTP and CTP for RNA synthesis. In the converse situation when ATP is high and GTP low, no similar problem will arise because aspartate is not needed to convert ATP to GTP and because the low GTP would limit RNA synthesis.

At present, it seems important to establish whether the control of RNA synthesis by GTP levels affects the synthesis of different types of RNA to the same extent. It also seems necessary to investigate whether there could be a direct control on the RNA polymerase and whether this is at the initiation of transcription or on the process of chain elongation. Although many questions obviously remain, regulation of RNA synthesis by GTP levels would appear to be a potentially valuable mechanism for avoiding severe depletion of adenine nucleotides in 'wild-type' bacteria.

References

Alföldi, L., Stent, G. S., Hoogs, M., and Hill, R. (1963). *Z Vererbungslehre*, **94**, 285.

Atkinson, D. E., and Fall, L. (1967). *J. Biol. Chem.*, **242**, 3941.

Bagnara, A. S., and Finch, L. R. (1968). *Biochem. Biophys. Res. Comm.*, **33**, 15.

Blakley, R. L., and Vitols, E. (1968). *Ann. Rev. Biochem.*, **37**, 201.

Blangy, D., Buc, H., and Monod, J. (1968). *J. Mol. Biol.*, **31**, 13.

Bremer, H., Yegian, C., and Konrad, M. (1966). *J. Mol. Biol.*, **16**, 94.

Buchwald, M., and Britten, R. J. (1963). *Biophysic. J.*, **3**, 155.

Burgess, R. R., Travers, A. A., Dunn, J. J., and Bautz. E. K. F. (1969). *Nature*, **221**, 43.

Buzzee, D. H., and Levin, A. P. (1968). *Biochem. Biophys. Res. Comm.*, **30**, 673.

Cashel, M., and Gallant, J. (1968). *J. Mol. Biol.*, **34**, 317.

Cooper, S., and Helmstetter, C. (1968). *J. Mol. Biol.*, **31**, 519.

Edlin, G., and Broda, P. (1968). *Bact Rev.*, **32**, 206.

Edlin, G., and Neuhard, J. (1967). *J. Mol. Biol.*, **24**, 225.

Edlin, G., Stent, G. S., Baker, R. F., and Yanofsky, C. (1968). *J. Mol. Biol.*, **37**, 257.

Eidlic, L., and Neidhardt, F. C. (1965). *J. Bacteriol.*, **89**, 706.

Ezekiel, D. H., and Valulis, B. (1966). *Biochim. Biophys. Acta*, **129**, 123.

Franzen, J. S., and Binkley, S. B. (1961). *J. Biol. Chem.*, **236**, 515.

Friesen, J. D. (1966). *J. Mol. Biol.*, **20**, 559.

Friesen, J. D. (1968). *J. Mol. Biol.*, **32**, 183.

Fukuyama, T. T. (1966). *J. Biol. Chem.*, **241**, 4745.

Gallant, J., and Cashel, M. (1967). *J. Mol. Biol.*, **25**, 515.

Gerhardt, J. C., and Pardee, A. B. (1962). *J. Biol. Chem.*, **237**, 891.

Goldstein, D. B., Brown, B. J. , and Goldstein, A. (1960). *Biochim. Biophys. Acta*, **43**, 55.

Jacob, F., Brenner, S., and Cuzin, F. (1963). *Cold Spr. Harb. Symp. Quant. Biol.*, **28**, 329.

Kepes, A. (1963). *Biochim. Biophys. Acta*, **76**, 293.

Klungsøyr, L., Hagemen, J. H., Fall, L., and Atkinson, D. E. (1968). *Biochemistry*, **7**, 4035.

Krebs, H. A., and Kornberg, H. L. (1957). *Ergebn. Physiol.*, **49**, 212.

Kuramitsu, H., and Moyed, H. S. (1966). *J. Biol. Chem.*, **241**, 1596.

Larsson, A., and Reichard, P. (1967). In *Progress in Nucleic Acid Research and Molecular Biology*, Vol. 7. Ed. by J. N. Davidson and W. E. Cohn. Academic Press, London.

Lavallé, R., and De Hauwer, G. (1968). *J. Mol. Biol.*, **37**, 269.

Maaløe, O., and Hanawalt, P. (1961). *J. Mol. Biol.*, **3**, 144.

Magasanik, B., and Karibian, D. (1960). *J. Biol. Chem.*, **235**, 2672.

Mager, J., and Magasanik, B. (1960). *J. Biol. Chem.*, **235**, 1474.

Mans, R. J., and Koch, A. L. (1960). *J. Biol. Chem.*, **235**, 450.

McCarthy, B. J., and Britten, R. J. (1962). *Biophysic. J.*, **2**, 35.

Midgley, J. E. M. (1969). *Biochem. J.*, **115**, 171.

Morris, D. W., and De Moss, J. A. (1966). *Proc. Nat. Acad. Sci.*, *Wash.*, **56**, 262.

Morris, D. W., and Kjeldgaard, N. O. (1968). *J. Molec. Biol.*, **31**, 145.

Mueller, K., and Bremer, H. (1968) *J. Molec. Biol.*, **38**, 329.
Neidhardt, F. C. (1963). *Biochim. Biophys. Acta*, **68**, 365.
Neidhardt, F. C., and Fraenkel, D. G. (1961). *Cold Spr. Harb. Symp. Quant. Biol.*, **26**, 63.
Neuhard, J. (1966). *Biochim. Biophys. Acta*, **129**, 104.
Nierlich, D. P. (1968). *Proc. Nat. Acad. Sci., Wash.*, **60**, 1345.
Nierlich, D. P., and Magasanik, B. (1965). *J. Biol. Chem.*, **240**, 352.
Nierlich, D. P., and Vielmetter, W. (1968). *J. Molec. Biol.*, **32**, 135.
Oeschger, M. P., and Bessman, M. J. (1966). *J. Biol. Chem.*, **241**, 5452
Pardee, A. B., (1954). *Proc. Nat. Acad. Sci., Wash.*, **40**, 263.
Pigott, G. H., and Midgley, J. E. M. (1968). *Biochem. J.*, **110**, 251.
Pritchard, R. H., and Lark, K. G. (1964). *J. Molec. Biol.*, **9**, 288.
Rajalakshmi, S., and Handschumaker, R. E. (1968). *Biochim. Biophys. Acta*, **155**, 317.
Roberts, R. B., Cowie, D. B., Abelson, P. H., Bolton, E. T., and Britten, R. J. (1955). In *Studies of Biosynthesis in E. coli.* Carnegie Institution of Washington Publication, Washington D.C.
Ron, E. Z., Kohler, R. E., and Davis, B. D. (1968). *Proc. Nat. Acad. Sci., Wash.*, **56**, 471.
Rosenbloom, F. M., Henderson, J. F., Caldwell, I. C., Kelley, W. N., and Seegmiller, J. E. (1968). *J. Biol. Chem.*, **243**, 1166.
Salser, W., Janin, J., and Levinthal, C. (1968). *J. Molec. Biol.*, **31**, 237.
Shih, A.-Y., Eisenstadt, J., and Lengyel, P. (1966). *Proc. Nat. Acad. Sci., Wash.*, **56**, 1599.
Stadtman, E. R., Shapiro, B. M., Kingdon, H. S., Woolfolk, C. A., and Hubbard, J. S. (1968). In *Advances in Enzyme Regulation* Vol. 6. p. 257. Ed. by G. Weber. Oxford: Pergamon Press.
Steck, T. L., Caicuts, M. J., and Wilson, R. G. (1968). *J. Biol. Chem.*, **243**, 2769.
Stent, G. S., and Brenner, S. (1961). *Proc. Nat. Acad. Sci., Wash.*, **47**, 2005.
Stubbs, J., and Hall, B. D. (1968). *J. Molec. Biol.*, **37**, 289.
Switzer, R. L. (1967). *Fed. Proc.*, **25**, 560.
Wyngaarden, J. B., and Greenland, R.A. (1963). *J. Biol. Chem.*, **238**, 1054.
Zimmerman, E. F., and Magasanik, B. (1964). *J. Biol. Chem.*, **239**, 293.

SHEFFIELD AND SECRETIONS, KREBS
AND CONTRACTIONS

R. E. Davies

Department of Animal Biology, University of Pennsylvania

On All Fools' Day, April 1 1945, I made a potentially traumatic transfer from Chemistry to Biochemistry in spite of the advice of an eminent chemist that a position with Dr. H. A. Krebs would prejudice my later career in an English Department of chemistry. Such was the antagonism between Chemistry and Biochemistry that an old and common insult was 'Tierchemie ist Schmierchemie'.

However, after helpful advice from Dr. Brynmor Jones, I made my decision and became a founder member of the newly formed Medical Research Council Unit for Research in Cell Metabolism which occupied just one office and one laboratory. I had worked for three and a half years on wartime problems involving synthetic organic chemistry but despite membership in the Home Guard and the National Fire Service, still had a little free time. This was because of the one night a week we all had to spend at the University 'fire-watching' in case of an air raid with incendiary bombs. I used to spend these nights in the library learning what was happening in the world of science. This allowed informal contacts with Dr. H. A. Krebs who was then senior lecturer in biochemistry and with Dr. and Mrs. Bielschowsky, two refugees who were working on cancer and shock and living on duck eggs and a pittance.

MEDICAL   RESEARCH   COUNCIL

UNFIT FOR RESEARCH IN CELL METABOLISM

TELEPHONE NO. 27451

FROM

H. A. KREBS, M.A CAMB., M.D. HAMBURG

PROFESSOR OF BIOCHEMISTRY

I was pleased that Krebs offered me a position on the staff of the Medical Research Council despite my lack of formal preparation in biochemistry, but some people had doubts even about Krebs who was made a professor with the formation of the M.R.C. Unit. The Figure shows

D   85

how a typesetter felt about it. This letterhead was used for many days before it was read carefully. It also led to another problem. An industrial firm thought that the Unit was headed by a troika and sent advertising material to all three of H. A. Krebs, M. A. Camb. and M. D. Hamburg.

A first problem on joining the Unit was to decide what to do. I had read in Perspectives in Biochemistry about Laidlaw's sewage organisms which looked like saphrophytic viruses, required haemin as a cofactor and might be a simple form of life to study (Holmes and Pirie, 1937). Prof., as we all called him, thought it was too difficult and suggested either the synthesis of citromalic acid, a possible missing component of the citric acid cycle, or the mechanism of hydrochloric acid production in the stomach.

Citromalic acid seemed less attractive, which was lucky for me since, unknown to us, it had already been synthesized and shown to be inactive in the cycle. Thus, the problem of the secretion of hydrogen ions was chosen. The general outlines of the intermediary metabolism were clear by then. What was unknown was how ATP is used to synthesize compounds, drive half-reactions backwards and generally do the work required for living things to live. The plan was quite obvious. Incubate gastric mucosa in (Krebs–Henseleit) bicarbonate saline in a Warburg manometer and look for a liberation of carbon dioxide as the hydrochloric acid was secreted. A rapid trip to the abattoir showed that the fourth stomach of a sheep had long thin flaps of gastric mucosa that could easily be prepared in sheets suitable for a Warburg cup. However, they steadfastly refused to give off the expected amount of carbon dioxide, despite histamine or other possible stimulants or extracts. This went on for five months together with the advice not to bother with the literature because there was nothing of interest in it.

Eventually, I took some time off to delve into history and soon found papers by Gray (1943) and Delrue (1930) which showed how the 'obvious' plan was flawed. They had set up the gastric mucosa of a frog so that it separated two chambers and had found that the pH on one side was lowered and on the other side was raised. Clearly, if the stomach secreted as much alkali as acid, then there would be no net liberation of carbon dioxide. The basis of this idea was already in the finding of Bence-Jones in 1845 that there is an alkaline tide in the urine following a meal, but this had all escaped us. The products of secretion had thus to be separated from the rest of the solution.

I developed a method to dissect away the muscle layer from the frog's stomach to leave a very thin tube or bag of gastric mucosa that could be washed out and tied at both ends with silk thread. When this was put into a Warburg apparatus and stimulated with histamine, there was a dramatic uptake of carbon dioxide and the bag of mucosa filled up with a clear, highly-acid fluid. We had obtained the very opposite of the effect for which we had been searching and I had learned a valuable lesson. One of the hardest things to find in a biological research programme is a clear effect to study, but if you do not get that effect, or even get a misleading one, this may be because your own 'obvious' plan is at fault.

I had completed the first successful experiment on August 8, 1945 and then gone for a short vacation. On returning, I worked out methods for studying mucosa turned inside out that should transfer bicarbonate ions like a kidney. I also convinced Dr. E. Eva Crane, a physicist, interested in bees and biological potentials, that the electric potential across the gastric mucosa was worth investigating. We cleaned up a dirty, brick-walled cellar in the Physics Department, built a suitable apparatus, did some controls and started off. We soon found that the observed electric potential varied with the current passed through a partially-submerged light bulb, which acted as a heater, and that no hydrochloric acid was secreted. A gas heater solved the first problem, but the second was insoluble. We kept on and on in the belief that the first good experiment could not have been wrong. But it was not until spring 1946 that the mucosa began to secrete lots of acid again. It was only then and later that we discovered the remarkable seasonal variations in the secretory activity of frogs at high latitude. In general, the gastric mucosa responded to histamine in spring and autumn, secreted spontaneously in summer and was achlorhydric during the winter hibernation (Bradford, Crane and Davies, 1950).

Nowadays in America, lots of large, fresh, live frogs can be obtained from dealers, but just after World War II in England we had to catch our own. The best sources were the numerous water tanks or dams that the National Fire Service had built all over the city as emergency water supplies in case air raids damaged the main water pipes. The frogs jumped in to breed, but could not get out. They just sat around on floating debris and could be caught easily with a net. Everyone, including Prof., his children, faculty and technicians went out on frog forays. Once Charlie Terner and I dropped the frog box and had to go chasing frogs all over the road in the centre of Sheffield. Eventually, we were helped by lots of boy scouts and then built a froggery with night lights at ground level. The lights attracted insects which kept the frogs well fed and healthy.

Work progressed for some years on the relation between the oxygen uptake, electron transport and acid secretion and the exact site of acid secretion, the role of carbonic anhydrase, gastric urease and the chemical and electrical energy relations (see Davies, 1951). Many sorts of gastric mucosa were looked at. The best mammalian one for work with isolated tissue was the polecat which we got from a local poacher. Prof. even lent us his car and some rationed petrol so David E. Hughes, Trevor D. Ford and I could go off to an underground maze in a Derbyshire cave called Jug Holes. There we caught 50 bats and their gastric mucosa respired, secreted acid moderately well and had a typical electric potential. However, they were not much better than mice, which need high-pressure oxygen for the best results.

Prof. once suggested that mitochondria might be more directly involved in ion transport than was then believed, so Walter Bartley and I did some experiments and found that they really were (Bartley and Davies, 1952). This first finding of the secretory activities of mitochondria and the relation to metabolically determined swelling and contraction (Price, Fonnesu and Davies, 1956) led, after a lag period of several years, to an explosive interest in this topic which continues even now. Other fields were entered. The role of gastric urease (see Kornberg and Davies, 1955) ion movement in kidney slices (Whittam and Davies, 1954) and several others. I seemed well established in the study of secretion until 1952. By that time the biochemistry labs at Sheffield had become a 'must' for touristical scientists and we had moved to some new laboratories partially converted from a large lavatory and a men's cloak room. We all took turns in showing visitors around and talking to them. It was important to speak first and ask them about their researches, otherwise, you didn't learn anything because they wanted to know what you were doing. It was my turn when Professor Albrecht Fleckenstein, a pharmacologist from Heidelberg who was visiting Oxford, decided to come to the 'Krebs Institute'. He told me of his calculations that the movements of sodium and potassium might be the energy source for muscle contraction, but a great difficulty was that he needed 70 potassium ions to be moved for the oxidation of one glucose molecule. He became very excited when I told him that Sandy Ogston and I had worked out a theory of secretion that could lead to 72 ions being moved during this oxidation. This theory (Davies and Ogston, 1950) was elaborated at a symposium on nervous tissue (Davies and Krebs, 1952) and, eventually became a precursor of what is now often called the Mitchell chemiosmotic theory (Mitchell, 1967). With a P/O ratio of 3 and 2 ions moved per ATP split, this gave 12 ions per O_2 and hence 72 for the 6 O_2 required to oxidize glucose.

However, I also told him that, since all biochemists 'knew' that adenosine triphosphate was the energy source for muscle contraction, no one would believe him unless he could show that muscles could contract without splitting ATP. It so happened that, just then, in Prof.'s lab. many people were studying oxidative phosphorylation and had worked out methods for analysing adenine nucleotides in tissue. I discussed the problem with Prof. and he decided to invite Albrecht to Sheffield, before returning to Heidelberg, to see what really happened to ATP.

I borrowed some muscle levers from David Smyth in Physiology and thus became involved in a direct interest in work on muscle which has continued ever since.

We soon found that the ATP didn't change at all in single contractions of frog rectus abdominis muscles. Albrecht then left for Heidelberg determined to see if phosphorylcreatine also stayed constant. Apparantly it did at 0°C and in the Spring of 1954, I went to be a guest professor in the Pharmacology Institute in Heidelberg to help investigate the turnover of radioactive phosphate in muscle.

We could find no evidence for an increased turnover of the terminal two phosphorus atoms of ATP during a single contraction of muscle at 0°C but this was not conclusive nor was any evidence forthcoming that phosphorylcreatine broke down under these conditions, though it was possible that some extra inorganic phosphate appeared, but the increase was not statistically significant.

Prof. was in America just then and found that Wilf Mommaerts, at Western Reserve, Cleveland, Ohio, U.S.A., had also found conditions where muscles could contract without any measurable change in ATP or phosphorylcreatine. We decided to publish simultaneously in *Nature* (Fleckenstein, Janke, Davies and Krebs, 1954; Mommaerts, 1954).

Prof. was then invited to Oxford. The Medical Research Council Unit went with him but I left for Philadelphia after 18 months. Prof. had lectured at the University of Pennsylvania some years before and had invited Sam Gurin over for a sabbatical summer at Sheffield in 1949 where he taught us about ^{14}C and learned about the techniques for the study of intermediary metabolism. Sam had asked if I was interested in going to Penn. and, as I was going to a meeting at Madison, Wisconsin on active transport in 1955, I called on him at Penn. to discuss the situation. Sam met me at the 30th Street railway station with the news that I had already been appointed as Professor of Biochemistry and all I had to do was come. I took a year's leave of absence in 1956. This was extended for another year and, somehow, I'm still there.

During the next several years much effort was put into trying to find a certain chemical change in muscle during a single contraction, but it all failed. At one point, all possible phosphorus-containing compounds were excluded, these included phosphorylcreatine, all the adenosine, inosine, guanosine and cytosine phosphates, phosphoenolpyruvate, all the phosphoglyceric acids, the phosphorus in the total acid-insoluble residue of muscle including phosphatido-peptide phosphorus, phospholipid phosphorus, ribonucleic and deoxyribonucleic acids (see Davies and Cain, 1961). Something seemed to be wrong. It was! There had seemed good reason to study a slow muscle at $0°C$ where we might freeze the muscle quickly before recovery metabolism had restored everything. The rectus abdominis was temporarily abandoned in favour of a muscle for which there were good psychological reasons for it being very slow. This was the paired retractor penis of the male turtle. It is not easy to separate the two muscles without damage and it's best to check for the long claws of the male, since the ovipositor muscles are very similar, as Dennis Cain and I once discovered to our surprise. This muscle of the male turtle was the one which showed the very first certain chemical change to be found during a single working contraction—the appearance of inorganic phosphate (Cain and Davies, 1960). However, it was soon confirmed in the slow rectus abdominis and even in the quick sartorius. Further work showed that, after all, it came from phosphorylcreatine. There were by then, much better ways of measuring inorganic phosphate, creatine and phosphorylcreatine than we had used in Heidelberg. Even so, a repeat of the experiments using exactly the original techniques showed a clear breakdown of phosphorylcreatine. Albrecht who was by then in Freiburg also was able to observe such a breakdown, but why the original experiments failed is still a mystery to me. Wilf also, and virtually simultaneously, found that the work done could be accounted for by the breakdown of phosphorylcreatine on reasonable estimates of the free energy released from its cleavage.

This put us all back to 1934 when Lundsgaard had shown that for a series of contractions, the external work could be correlated with the change in phosphorylcreatine.

There had been all sorts of red herrings and blind alleys. The Dritte Fraktion (Fleckenstein and coworkers, 1954), a highly stable phosphorus compound, the possibility of a highly labile precursor of the inorganic phosphate which appeared on the runs after electrophoresis of the radioactive muscle extracts (Davies, Cain and Delluva, 1959) for some months only to disappear again as techniques improved or the season changed—a will-o'-the-wisp (or Wilfried o' the wisp) (Davies, 1961). Carnosine phosphates came and went (Cain, Delluva and Davies, 1958). It was all very confusing and it must be admitted that our experiments started with about eight years (really thirty man years) of irreproducible results, bad experiments, blind alleys, despair, desperation, false hopes and sheer frustration.

Research had thrown a flood of darkness on the whole field, but at least by now we were able to find out what phosphorylcreatine was used for in single contractions. No detectable amount was needed for activation or shortening *per se*. It was needed for work, and in the right amounts (Cain, Infante and Davies, 1962). However, we were no nearer solving Professor A. V. Hill's 1950 'Challenge to Biochemists' which was to show that ATP really is directly involved as an energy source in muscle contraction.

The solution came as follows: When looking through the abstracts of the 1959 meeting of the Federation of American Societies of Experimental Biology, I noted in abstract number 1057 of Kuby and Mahowald that dinitrofluorobenzene could irreversibly inhibit both creatine phospho-kinase and myokinase. However, this material, often known as the Sanger Reagent, is very aggressive, reacts with free amino and some other groups, and seemed to have little chance of having any specificity. I noted by the abstract 'try it sometime', and thought it would be only a last resort. It was. No one else in the world bothered with it, and two years later when we had nowhere else to go, Dennis Cain suggested that it had become time to try it.

It worked. It really worked. After 40 minutes at 0°C in a saline containing an 0·38 mM solution, frog muscles used only ATP. The 'Challenge' had been met (Cain and Davies, 1962).

Much work followed which led to a 'molecular theory of muscle contrac-tion: calcium-dependent contractions with hydrogen bond formation plus ATP-dependent extensions of part of the myosin–actin cross-bridges'. This paper (Davies, 1963) was conceived and written in outline during the days Helen and I were travelling to the Tetons in Wyoming in the summer of 1962. We drove alternate hours and I dictated the basis of it all during several days while driving the long straight roads to the West.

Sometime after this the University of Pennsylvania celebrated the 200th anniversary of the founding of its School of Medicine. I was honoured to be a speaker on the same programme with Prof. who had been invited over for the occasion. The session was devoted to the 'Control of Energy Metabolism' and my contribution concerned the 'Bioenergetics of Muscular Contraction'. This is part of what I said (Davies, 1965):

'Our experiments have been done in collaboration with Drs. Delluva, Cain, Infante, Kushmerick and Minihan and have been mainly on frog muscles at 0°C. Experiments have usually lasted about one second with a home-made apparatus. This apparatus has the peculiar property that virtually everything in it was borrowed. Professor Krebs may recognize the stimulator and stopwatch borrowed from Oxford. Professor Brobeck may recognize the kymograph we scavenged from his stockroom and Professor Chance lent us the ergometer for the experiments. The total apparatus cost me only $2.50. Its purpose was to make it possible to freeze the muscle rapidly *in situ*. This was done by this little device which is an old automobile pump operated by a derelict washing machine relay which lifts some liquid Freon and rapidly freezes the muscle. With this apparatus the muscle can be frozen *in situ* at any point in the contraction–relaxation cycle.'

During the subsequent discussion Prof. gave me all the things I had borrowed from Oxford. They are still in constant use.

The 'Challenge' had been part of the Festschrift for O. Meyerhof. In the Festschrift for H. H. Weber, A. V. Hill (1950) made 'A Further Challenge to Biochemists' concerning the heat of shortening of muscle and its relation to the concomitant breakdown of ATP. Marty Kushmerick, Roy Larson and I had already begun work on this but followed Hill's protocol exactly and showed as was predicted by the theory, that this particular heat had no counterpart in an ATP splitting. The paper answering the 'Further Challenge' (Davies, Kushmerick and Larson, 1967) was dictated in outline, just in case, as I was waiting to have some surgery done at the hospital of the University of Pennsylvania.

Since then we have examined the catch mechanism in an invertebrate muscle (Nauss and Davies, 1966), found how the thermodynamic efficiency of muscle varies with the velocity of contraction (Kushmerick and Davies, 1969), investigated the dithering, or to-and-fro movement of sarcomeres, in whole muscle during an apparently smooth isometric tetanus (Larson, Kushmerick, Haynes and Davies, 1968), and followed the strange ability of tetanized muscle during a slow stretch to develop large tensions for long periods with almost no usage of ATP above that apparently needed for pumping calcium (Curtin, Drobnis, Larson and Davies, 1969).

It has been a long trail since starting at Sheffield and in retrospect I agree with the advice given by Professor Sir Hans Krebs' teacher, Otto Warburg.

This came about as follows: we were having weekly seminars on great scientists in the general field of Biochemistry and Molecular Biology to find out why they were great and how it happened. Mr. Buckley, a Graduate Student in Molecular Biology at Penn., was assigned Otto Warburg so he wrote and obtained the following reply:

November 14, 1967

'Dear Mr. Buckley!

Thank you for your letter of November 8. If you wish to become a scientist you must ask a successful scientist to accept you in his laboratory, would it be at the beginning only to clean his test tubes. If you observe carefully, what he does you will learn how discoveries are made.

It is not necessary that you know already much, before you go to the master.

The earlier you go, the greater will be your chance to become a discoverer too.

I am yours sincerely

(signed) Otto Warburg'

> How I worked on
> ATP and contraction,
> Not forgetting
> Stomach acid action,
>
> Kidney bicarbonate,
> Research on swelling,
> Electron to ion rate
> Buffers—Krebs and Henseleit,
> Seeking answers, I hope they're right.

References

Bartley, W., and Davies, R. E. (1952). *Biochem. J.*, **52**, p. xx.

Bence-Jones, H. (1845). *Philos. Trans.*, p. 333.

Bradford, N. M., Crane, E. E., and Davies, R. E. (1950). *Proc. zool. Soc. Lond.*, **120**, 471.

Cain, D. F., and Davies, R. E. (1960). In: *Muscle as a Tissue*, p. 84. Ed. Rodahl, K., and Horvath, S. M. McGraw-Hill, N.Y. (1962). Proceedings of a Conference at the Lankenau Hospital, Nov. 3–4, 1960.

Cain, D. F., and Davies, R. E. (1962). *Biochem. Biophys. Res. Commun.*, **8**, 361.

Cain, D. F., Delluva, A. M., and Davies, R. E. (1958). *Nature, Lond.*, **182**, 720.

Cain, D. F., Infante, A. A., and Davies, R. E. (1962). *Nature, Lond.*, **196**, 214.

Curtin, N. A., Drobnis, D. D., Larson, R. E., and Davies, R. E. (1969). *Fed. Proc.*, **28**, 711.

Davies, R. E. (1951). *Biol. Rev.*, **26**, 87.

Davies, R. E. (1961). *Circulation*, **24**, 429.

Davies, R. E. (1963). *Nature, Lond.*, **199**, 1068.

Davies, R. E. (1965). In: *Control of Energy Metabolism*. Ed. Chance, B., Estabrook, R. W., and Williamson, J. R. Academic Press, N.Y.

Davies, R. E., and Cain, D. F. (1961). *Biophysics of Physiological and Pharmacological Actions*, Ed. Shanes, A. Amer. Assoc. Adv. Sci., Washington, D.C.

Davies, R. E., Cain, D. F., and Delluva, A. M. (1959). *Ann. N.Y. Acad. Sci.*, **81**, 468.

Davies, R. E., and Krebs, H. A. (1952). *Biochem. Soc. Symp.*, **8**, 77.

Davies, R. E., Kushmerick, M. J., and Larson, R. E. (1967). *Nature, Lond.*, **214**, 148.

Davies, R. E., and Ogston, A. G. (1950). *Biochem. J.*, **46**, 324.

Delrue, G. (1930). *Arch. int. Physiol.*, **33**, 196.

Fleckenstein, A., Janke, J., Davies, R. E., and Krebs, H. A. (1954). *Nature, Lond.*, **178**, 1081.

Gray, J. S. (1943). *Gastroent.*, **1**, 390.

Hill, A. V. (1950). *Biochim. Biophys. Acta*, **4**, 4.

Holmes, B., and Pirie, A. (1937). In: *Perspectives in Biochemistry*. Ed. Needham, J., and Green, D. E. Cambridge University Press.

Kornberg, H. L., and Davies, R. E. (1955). *Physiol. Rev.*, **35**, 169.

Kuby, S. A., and Mahowald, T. A. (1959). *Fed. Proc.*, **18**, 267.

Kushmerick, M. J., and Davies, R. E. (1969). *Proc. Roy. Soc. Lond. B*, **174**, 315.

Larson, R. E., Kushmerick, M. J., Haynes, D. H., and Davies, R. E. (1968). *Biophys. J.*, **8**, A8.

Lundsgaard, E. (1934). *Biochem. Z.*, **269**, 308.

Mitchell, P. (1967). In: *Comprehensive Biochemistry*, **22**, 167. Ed. Florkin, M., and Stotz, E. H. Elsevier, Amsterdam.

Mommaerts, W. F. H. M. (1954). *Nature, Lond.*, **174**, 1088.

Nauss, K. M., and Davies, R. E. (1966). *Biochem. Z.*, **345**, 173.

Price, C. A., Fonnesu, A., and Davies, R. E. (1956). *Biochem. J.*, **64**, 754.

Whittam, R., and Davies, R. E. (1954). *Biochem. J.*, **56**, 445.

SOME STUDIES ON CYTODIFFERENTIATION IN MICROBES

D. E. Hughes

Microbiology Department, University College, Cardiff

This essay is mainly devoted to a brief discussion of differentiation, the relationship between the process in the metazoa, the metaphyta and microbes. It advances some reasons for believing that studies of the type now in progress in Cardiff on cytodifferentiation in eukaryotic microbes is of significance to the process of morphogenesis in higher organisms.

Since, however, these essays are primarily intended as personal tributes to Sir Hans Krebs another reason for the form of this essay is to make clear, perhaps even to myself for the first time, the influences gained from association with a great scientist, his cosmopolitan colleagues and collaborators attracted by him to Sheffield and later Oxford. This association has directed the choice not only of my own research interests but also the manner and form which the Microbiology Department in Cardiff has taken, not only in its research interests but also its teaching. This problem of scientific development and the making of scientists has been discussed recently by Sir Hans himself (Krebs, 1967).

Having accepted a Chair of Microbiology in 1964 in Cardiff, the next few months were spent attempting to decide both the form and role that such a Department should play in a University set in a highly industrialized society. The final decision was almost entirely based on previous conversations with Krebs which were summarized quite briefly and in a form which we now use as introduction to our handbook for intending students. It was that Biochemistry, and here I would include also Microbiology, was a Biological subject, that is, the questions it poses arise in the first place from biological systems and that the sharpest tools of physics and chemistry are used to gather data and to answer the problems. The occasion, so clearly in mind, that I would hazard a guess that I am using the exact words, was a debate as to whether the Biochemistry Department in Oxford should continue in the Faculty of Physical Sciences or join that of Biological Sciences. I cannot now understand why a bridging position could not have been taken rather than the final decision to remain in Physical Sciences; but Krebs' argument was advanced against this decision. Biological questions and their significance is discussed by Krebs in several different contexts and particularly striking is a recent description of his own formulation of the TCA and urea cycles which he attributes quite firmly to this philosophical approach. This insistence of the Biological origin of our Microbiology has in fact taken us into seemingly odd places, where Biology was previously thought to play little part. For instance, we recently described the microbial ecology of steel making (Hughes and Hill, 1969) where microbial infections cause high losses of steel products. The growth and chemical effects of microbes in such industrial plant and its prevention presents fascinating fundamental and applied problems of a wide range of disciplines in addition to Microbiology, and which, I suspect, would have stimulated Sir Hans' interest and curiosity.

Krebs has always insisted on the special significance in the development of novel 'tools for the job' and instances the influence of Warburg's ingenuity in this respect. The development of apparatus can, of course, become an end in itself if their main purpose is lost sight of and gadgeting is a common activity in many University departments. Nobody, however, could claim that Krebs' own infinite care in the design of a small item like a manometer fluid or manometer flask ended in this way, each new invention, by him or his team, was exploited fully.

His insistence on the choice of the correct experimental material is another mark of his approach to a problem. His accounts of the role of pigeon breast muscle slices, liver homogenates and bacteria in the development of his formulation of both Krebs' cycles and the glyoxalate shunt are fascinating object lessons in the history of Biochemistry. Once learnt at first hand they cannot be ignored or forgotten and have consciously influenced our choice of particular microbes such as a colourless algae for the specific problems of differentiation (Lloyd, 1969).

In training for research, few could have passed through the school in Sheffield without calibrating their own Warburg manometers and cups, even their own pipettes and other volumetric apparatus. Learning the precision of manometer reading and how many one could read, in a minute, to record and calculate during readings and to consider the results for designing the next experiment were all a part of Krebs' insistence on the supreme importance of laboratory skills. New pieces of equipment would appear to be tested especially after his trips to U.S.A. and I may be correct in believing that the first DU spectrometer appeared in this country after such a trip. Not all were equally useful and I can remember vividly one particularly ingenious but fragile ice breaker.

Thus, the formulation of the problem in Biological terms, selection of the most suitable experimental material, the adaptation and development of specific tools coupled with an intimate familiarity with their advantages and limitations, seems to me the essence of Krebs' teaching.

DIFFERENTIATION

As usually employed, this term is applied to processes during which a wide diversity of cell types develop from a single fertilized egg from an animal, seed or other cells in plants. Each specialized cell type is associated with specific functions which emerge as the result of diversification and restriction. The process of morphogenesis is essentially the same in the metazoa and metaphyta even when judged mainly by the morphological criteria, which were overwhelmingly used until recently. The relative simple morphology of prokaryotic cells limits the range of morphogenetic changes and there is a general reluctance by the more classical morphologists to speak of such processes as sporulation, the formation of flagella or slime layers in the eubacteria as comparable to differentiation in higher organisms. This objection does not altogether apply to eukaryotic microbes where the intracellular organization is at least as highly developed as in metazoa. More recently however, because of the failure to account for differentiation in morphological terms or quasibiophysical terms in models based on concentration gradients etc. which were fashionable some decades ago (*cf*. Spiegleman, 1948), there has been a tendency to regard differentiation merely as a switching on of new metabolic pathways and the loss of others. The newly formed enzymic systems are concerned mainly with the formation of macromolecules on which the observed morphological changes are based, for example, the synthesis of a cell component, such as haemoglobin, keratin or some other specialized product characterizing the cell type, such as amylase or insulin, both of which are formed within a single organ but by different pancreatic cell types (Krebs, 1957; Grobstein, 1963). More recently the current theories concerning the initiation and regulation of enzyme synthesis, particularly in prokaryotes (Jacob and Monod, 1963; Harris, 1968) have integrated both genetic and phenotypic interactions, so that differentiation may be discussed almost entirely in the absence of morphogenetic change. Thus, Bullough (1967) sees the essence of differentiation as that displayed by two genotypically similar prokaryotic organisms whose phenotype differs merely by one enzyme, due to a change in gene expression brought about by their exposure to different stimuli which may be either internal or external. The unit of differentiation is thus the gene translation and transcription system which leads to the synthesis or repression of a single enzyme. Even the most complicated differentiations of higher organisms may thus be described in terms of cycles or networks of enzyme systems, activated or repressed by a single trigger mechanism. The trigger initiates a chain reaction or sequential synthesis of enzymes and the consequent suppression of others. At its simplest this is expressed during the growth of a prokaryotic during a single reproductive cycle, such as can now be studied with synchronously dividing continuous cultures. The morphogenesis of multicellular organs and of whole plants and animals can be represented by a flow diagram in which a change of cell type is triggered at each branching point and follows a pathway of restriction, growth and cytodifferentiation until a highly committed, restricted and differentiated cell arises at the end of each twig. This end product may or more often, may not be able to reproduce (Abercrombie, 1967). Classical embryology is largely concerned with tracing such morphogenetic steps and representing them as elaborate networks (*cf.* Mangold, 1961; Coulombre, 1965; Heslop-Harrison, 1967). Microbiological differentiation represents one or at the most, two or three branchings of such a network, as well as being space-dependent. It is obvious that such processes are extremely time-dependent and eminently amenable to the application of the mathematics of network and systems analysis. Advances in this approach will undoubtedly lead to the formulation of much simpler mathematical models, which besides giving meaningful expression to experimental results, will give rise also to fruitful experimentation (Dean and Hinshelwood, 1966; Goodwin, 1963; Painter and Marr, 1968).

Growth and Differentiation

Growth, meaning cell reproduction and not merely protein synthesis or increase of cell size, often, but not always, inhibits differentiation. This relationship often is shown by the loss of ability to synthesize DNA in differentiating cells, which is often used as an indication of viability. The special function associated with a differentiated cell, such as the synthesis of collagen by cultures of fibroblasts often decreases during the exponential phase of growth: in contrast hyaluronidase synthesis increases. (Green and Goldberg, 1965.) The amounts of such end products of enzyme chains would be expected to be affected not only by enzyme concentrations, but also by other factors such as substrate concentration, and a multitude of competitive states must exist during differentiation when many new enzymes are being synthesized and pool sizes become limiting. No simple relationship would thus be expected between growth and differentiation. When morphogenesis is completed some tissue components are incapable of further reproduction, while others can reproduce differentiated cells at a high rate: (so called 'mitotic tissues'). This latter is probably analogous to the growth cycle of a eukaryotic microbe in its most stable state. The regulation of tissue growth is complicated by hormonal effects and the effects of cell exudates, surface phenomena, serum components, etc. These effects may be regarded as analogous to population effects in microbial cultures (Dean and Hinshelwood, 1966). The loss of response to such regulatory processes often results in an embryonic type cell growth, often viewed as a first stage in carcinogenesis (Iverson, 1965; Roe and Ambrose, 1966).

Nucleus, cytoplasm interactions in morphogenesis

It is now well established that the limitations and range of differentiation in metazoa must depend on the amount of expressible DNA in the genome (Kennell and Kotoulas, 1968). From the results of nuclear transfer and the development of whole plants from highly differentiated plant cells, it seems probable that no major modification of genome occurs in development and morphogenesis (Harris, 1968). Thus morphogenesis in metazoa is in general non-reversible especially in cells located in organs and even in some differentiated cells maintained through thousands of cell divisions in culture (Coon, 1966). This contrasts with the situation in prokaryotes where, as already briefly discussed, differentiated states are labile and often very rapidly reversed. So-called 'de-differentiation' is also found in stable cell lines from organs grown in isolation as 'micro-organisms' (Green and Todardo, 1967). Rapid loss of differentiation is often associated with overgrowth of other cells in a heterogenous population or nutritional factors and in the latter case can often be restored by reversing the unfavourable environmental conditions by the addition of specific factors (Ichikawa, Pluznik and Sachs, 1966).

While the Jacob–Monod, or similar, models of gene expression, translation and protein synthesis are satisfactory in highly labile pro-karyotes and in many eukaryotes such as the yeasts, the model is less satisfactory when applied to morphogenesis in some eukaryotic microbes and in higher organisms.

In most eukaryotic cells differentiation once triggered or initiated by gene derepression often becomes entirely independent of further nuclear control (Harris, 1968). This is difficult to explain in terms of an unstable m-RNA as found in prokaryotes and makes it necessary to search for other regulatory processes controlling the chain of events of differentiation. There is growing evidence that these factors may be intracellular stable components (Chalones, organizers) to be found in the cytoplasm in addition to plasmagenes; in the case of metazoa the hormones also play such a regulatory role (Bullough, 1967). Extrachromosomal DNA in organelles such as chloroplasts and mitochondria also play a role in organelle morphogenesis (Lloyd, 1969). They may, perhaps, be regarded as analogous to the plasmids of prokaryotes which control differentiated states related to conjugation, phage reproduction and drug resistance (Hayes, 1968; Richmond, 1967).

Microbial Differentiations

It seems reasonable to divide microbial differentiation in two separate but interrelated systems. Firstly there are the cytological changes associated with the normal growth cycle, that is the changes that occur in individual cells between each cell division. These will include the synthesis of those minimal structures on which growth and reproduction depend. In prokaryotic cells, the most apparent are cell wall and membrane synthesis, DNA replication, ribosome and mesosome formation. The synthesis of such components in a population reach a steady state during exponential growth. In many cases other structures such as mucoid layers, flagella, spores and reserve granules, etc. often are only made under conditions of 'unbalanced' growth and thus often do not appear in exponentially growing cells. More complicated structures such as those of the stalked and sheathed bacteria, sheath and microcyst formation in the myxobacteria and spores in the actinomycetes are also associated mainly with phenotypic response to unbalanced growth conditions. These, however, may be regarded as changes of cell types and thus analogues of cytodifferentiation in higher organisms. For instance, *Sphearotolus* may be grown as single bacterial unsheathed cells, either flagellated or not; its sheathed forms may also exist as separate or colonial forms, neither of which is motile and all forms may be found together in the same culture. The synthesis of membrane components in prokaryotes offers fascinating material in which the control of phenotypic response and genome expression can be readily studied. Typical of such studies are those of my colleague, Wimpenny and his group on the regulation of membrane-bound terminal respiratory systems in facultative bacteria (Venables, Wimpenny and Cole, 1968; Venables and Guest, 1968; Wimpenny, 1969).

In eukaryotic microbes, cytodifferentiation during the normal growth cycle involves the regulation of biosynthesis of intracellular organelles, such as mitochondria, chloroplasts, lysosomes, etc. which represent more highly organized membrane systems possibly evolved from those in prokaryotes, and which contain specific extra-nuclear DNA and RNA. There is good evidence to believe that the regulation of the structural components of these organelles is under both nuclear and extranuclear control (Lloyd, 1969).

Some changes involving the formation of new cell types, again often under conditions of unbalanced growth include phagosome, food vacuole, spore, ascospore and kinetosome formation and encystment and excystment. Changes from single cell to colonial forms as in the slime moulds from amoeboid to ciliates, such as *Neiglearia* can be easily controlled in the laboratory. Factors controlling the formation of diatom, foraminifera or radiolaria tests have barely begun to be studied but offer material in which highly specific and very intricate geometrical forms are constantly reproduced (Lewin, 1967).

ZONAL CENTRIFUGATION

As already mentioned the ability to appreciate significant technical advances is one of the outstanding characteristics of Krebs' approach to science and one which is constantly referred to by former workers in the Cell Metabolism Unit. Zonal centrifugation developed mainly by Anderson and his group at Oak Ridge is in our opinion one such recent major advance in cell biology, and for this reason we have paid particular attention to its exploitation and development over the last three years.

Zonal centrifugation is an extension of centrifugal density gradient separation of cell components, but it allows the essential scale-up, and at the same time increases resolution of separation. Full accounts of the biology, engineering and physics of zonal centrifuges are given in the book edited by Anderson (1966). All the commercially available heads are based on the 'A type' rotors for larger particles and 'B rotors' for smaller particles. Both types deal with single batches but continuous heads are also in use at Oak Ridge. Most rotors can be used for rate sedimentation or alternatively for isopycnic separations. This latter method separates cell particles by reason of their differences in buoyant density. The design aims of the A and B series of rotors are (*a*) ideal sedimentation and maximum resolution, (*b*) rapid gradient loading in a rotating rotor without stirring or convection, (*c*) sharp zonal development, (*d*) high 'g' forces to reduce running time, (*e*) recovery of zones without loss of resolution. Recently developed B rotors not yet commercially available achieve most, if not all, of these aims.

Until recently, most studies in analytical cytology have concentrated on the isolation of single cell components such as mitochondria, lysosomes, etc. The main significance of the zonal centrifugation is that in a single experiment most of the sedimentable organelles (density $> 1\cdot10$ cm) can be separated and resolved from one another. In addition, and this is now becoming apparent in our own work, cytodifferentiation is accompanied by ordered changes in distribution between sedimentable and non-sedimentable (density $< 1 \cdot 100$) material. This process can be studied in detail by this technique already and will be extended as newer rotors become available.

The scale-up made possible by zonal centrifugation has made us consider again the question of cell disintegration. Most of the classical tools, homogenizers, grinders, ultrasonics, etc. were developed empirically and with the exception of ultrasonics there is as yet little understanding of the physical forces involved when cells are disintegrated, nor of the effects of these forces on cell components. In most cases the effects are produced by hydrodynamic shear which fatigues structural components. Shear gradients of the order of $10^5 \times \sec^{-1}$ are needed to break cells with weak walls, such as most metazoal cells or protozoa. In the case of bacteria the gradient may be as high as $10^8 \times \sec^{-1}$ (T. Coakley, personal communication). In unpublished experiments by Hughes and Lloyd, we have shown that gradients of approximately $10^4 \times \sec^{-1}$ can rapidly uncouple well coupled mitochondria from various sources and release enzymes normally considered as bound. Gradients of the order of $10^{4-5} \times \sec^{-1}$ are needed to break biopolymers such as DNA (Pritchard, Peacocke and Hughes, 1965). The study of the time dependence of such process gives valuable clues as to the location and binding of enzymes but is also of extreme importance in designing new and more predictable apparatus for cell disintegration. This problem is discussed fully elsewhere (Hughes, Wimpenny and Lloyd, 1969) but is raised here in order to stress the importance of this first step in studies on analytical cytology, and which is too often neglected.

Although the various techniques of zonal centrifugation are well described they do not make apparent the considerable effort needed for fractionation procedures in studies on differentiation. Each fractionation yields large numbers of samples to be assessed enzymically, chemically and by microscopy—the latter generally in the electron microscope. Thus automated analysis systems are essential for such studies as well as the active collaboration of several workers and technicians in growing and disintegrating the cells and in the actual centrifugation runs which themselves may take several hours. It is worthwhile recalling in this respect Krebs' intense interest in automated analysis as well as his belief in value of team work in the Laboratory. This was extended to the consideration of laboratory design especially in favour of open planning rather than the more generally accepted individual private cell seen even now in some of the new University departments.

STUDIES OF CYTODIFFERENTIATION IN PROGRESS IN CARDIFF

The foregoing brief outline of the problem of differentiation is the background against which the choice of a limited number of eukaryotic microbes were chosen as being likely to be suitable experimental material for studies on cytodifferentiation. Our choice has been determined in part on the ability to grow relatively large amounts of cells under controlled conditions to control cytodifferentiation by altering these conditions and to isolate from them intracellular organelles in a reasonably intact functional and structural condition. Thus, in the case of the colourless alga *Prototheca zopfii* and the flagellate *Polytomella* and ciliate *Tetrahymena* and the protozoan *Hartmanella* cell disruption was carried out by methods employing low hydrodynamic shear gradients made possible by the low tensile strength of the outer envelopes of these organisms. This is an important factor which is not always recognized (Hughes and Cunningham, 1963; Hughes, Wimpenny and Lloyd, 1969). Recently following unpublished work on the effect of hydrodynamic shear on mitochondria, Klucis, Lloyd and Roache (1968) have shown how hydro-dynamic shear during isolation may affect the heterogeneity of isolated liver mitochondria as judged on morphological grounds and by measurements of respiratory control and other biochemical parameters. Enzymic methods to isolate components from yeasts and microfungi have also been adapted for these studies. Particular attention was paid initially to the isolation and maintenance of axenic cultures, especially of the protozoa. It was felt that many of the earlier studies made elsewhere might be invalidated by the presence of bacteria on which the organisms often grow and can be seen in large numbers in the food vacuoles. It was found impossible to produce axenic cultures of *Naeglieria* in which preliminary studies had been made of the amoeboid to flagellate transformation (Wilmer, 1963), although small quantities of cells could be obtained by outgrowth from penicillin or other antibiotics, the amounts were insufficient. Recently the necessity of axenic cultures has been raised sharply by the confusion between bacterial ribosomes and those of the slime mould during studies on differentiation (Ashworth, 1966; Ceccarini and Maggio, 1968).

Encystment in Hartmanellid amoeba

No satisfactory taxonomic system is available for deciding speciation in the hartmanellid soil amoeba (Griffiths, 1967). The strain used in most of the following work was a strain described by Neff as *Hartmanella castellanii.* In most of the earlier work the axenic cultures of the organisms were grown on 4% v/v Mycological peptone (Oxoid Ltd) at 30° in a shaking incubator. Log phase cells were obtained after 2–3 days, growth was measured by absorbency at 400 mμ: (E = 0·5 = approximately 4 mg dry weight/ml). Yields of approximately 12–16 mg dry weight were usual after 40–60 hours growth. More recently a satisfactory defined medium consisting of amino acids and B group vitamins has been developed.

Induction of encystment

Cultures of *Hartmanella* encyst when growth is prolonged beyond the log phase (approximately 4 days) but the numbers encysting are variable and viability often low. More or less synchronous encystment may be achieved by placing washed log phase cells in a replacement medium. Those used previously were found to yield large numbers of non-viable cysts, that is they did not outgrow or excyst when replaced into growth medium. This loss of viability was associated with the loss of cell protein, RNA and reserve materials, and can be partly prevented in a replacement medium of 5 $\times$ 10^{-2} M MgCl$_2$. Under these conditions encystment is complete in about 72 hours and most cysts are viable. The effect of Mg^{2+} is specific, other divalent ions are ineffective. The Mg^{2+} must be present continuously for about 8–9 hours. If withdrawn prior to this, encystment is arrested and many cells revert to amoebae or lyse. Amino acids, added either singly or in mixtures to the replacement medium are inactive, with the exception of glutamic acid or histidine which inhibit encystment if added before 8–9 hours have elapsed. After this they do not inhibit and cells thus stopped encysting usually lyse. In contrast, the addition of mycological peptone in the same 8–9 hour period inhibits encystment and the cells usually revert to the amoeboid form. The addition of glucose or 2-oxoglutarate improved encystment. Inhibitors of protein synthesis such as tetracycline or chloramphenicol inhibited encystment as did arsenite and iodoacetate: NaF, malonate and 2-4, dinitrophenol were without effect.

Morphological changes during encystment

By light microscopy, the onset of encystment is seen as an initial rounding of the cells followed by a shrinking due to dehydration and the loss of cell material. Internally, the food vacuoles disappear, and this is followed by the disappearance of the contractile vacuoles and mito-chondria. Stored materials such as lipid and glycogen often disappear but sometimes may increase in amount. The secretion of a three-layered cyst wall is usually complete after 40 hours but resistance to heat or the disruption effects of ultrasound are not fully developed until about 72 hours. By electron microscopy the mitochondria first appear to associate with the endoplasmic reticulum and sometimes to elongate. Subsequently they become vacuolated and the inter-cristae granules swell and appear as vesicles of $3\text{--}5 \times 10^3$ Å diameter. Localized concentrations of RNA granules (80 Å diameter) appear to be associated with cellulose synthesis (Schuster, 1963; Vickerman, 1962; Tomlinson and Muhlethaler, 1965) and is possibly associated with a loss of nuclear RNA.

Measurement of encystment

Originally cysts and amoebae were counted microscopically or by methods which depend on the differential uptake of dyes by the two forms, their response to lytic agents or the effects of ultrasound. In the later studies, the degree of encystment was correlated with the amount of

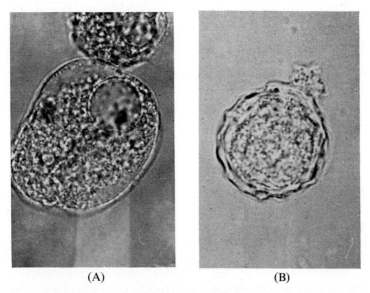

(A)   (B)

Figure 1.   Phase contrast micrographs of (A) Vegetative log-phase *Hartmanella*; (B) Cyst after 50 hours in encystment medium (A $\times$ 2·5, B $\times$ 3·75)

cellulose which is a major component of the cyst wall (Tomlinson and Jones, 1962): fully developed cysts contain about 0·14 mg cellulose/mg dry weight cyst. The cyst wall consists of a double layer of sheets or fibres 100 Å thick which buckles as the cell shrinks. Other material may be embedded between the two layers (Figure 1).

Metabolic changes during the encystment of Hartmanella

Immediately following the transference of log phase cells to the encystment medium, there is an abrupt increase in endogenous respiration which reaches a peak at about 10–12 hours and usually declines to an almost undetectable level at 50–60 hours. Hexoses and pentoses increase to a maximum value at 18–24 hours, while the onset of cellulose synthesis occurs at approximately 10–12 hours and continues to increase up to about 40–50 hours. The protein and dry weight of the cells decreases immediately and continues to fall to about 60% of the initial values at about 10–12 hours. There was also a loss of RNA but not DNA.

Experiments to determine the source of endogenous respiration were carried out by growing cells in the usual medium to which ^{14}C labelled acid-hydrolysed algal protein was added. After 40 hours growth the cells were washed and the distribution of label between the CO_2 collected during growth and encystment, the nucleic acid, the protein, the lipid and the 5%TCA soluble fractions was estimated at various times during encystment. The results strongly suggested that the bulk of the material used for endogenous respiration during encystment was derived from protein and not lipid, and also that protein was the source of hexose used for cellulose synthesis (Griffiths and Hughes, 1969).

Cell organelles and encystment in Hartmanella

Mitochondria isolated from vegetative amoebae oxidized succinate, malate, pyruvate plus malate, NADH, 2-oxoglutarate, 3-hydroxybutyrate and glutamate. Respiration with these substrates is tightly coupled to phosphorylation, as indicated by respiratory control measurements. The phosphorylating ability of mitochondrial preparations is stable for some hours and the respiration rates in the presence and absence of ADP were fairly reproducible for different mitochondrial preparations (Lloyd, Griffiths and Hughes, unpublished results) (Lloyd and Griffiths, 1968).

During the first 24 hours of encystment, isolated mitochondria show a progressive decrease in oxidative and phosphorylating ability as measured polarographically. It seems likely that these changes in their activity do not arise from damage caused to the mitochondria during their isolation. These properties and changes in mitochondrial metabolism are consistent with the changes found in electron micrographs in viable and encysting cells where it was found that there is a progressive loss of mitochondrial internal organization during encystment. Mitochondria appear to be absent in fully developed cysts.

More recently these studies have been extended to the isolation of

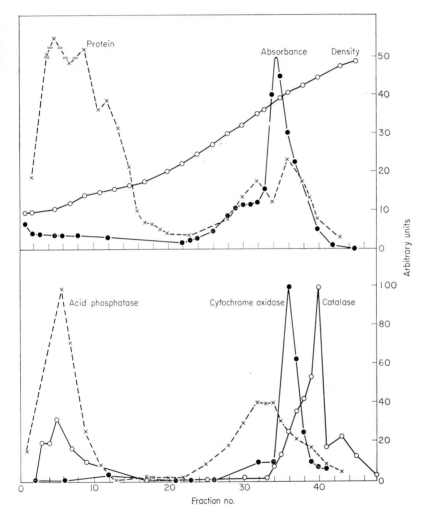

Figure 2. Profile of a zonal centrifugation separation of a homogenate from log phase *Hartmanella*. Linear sucrose gradient; B XIV rotor at 35×10^3 rpm for $2\frac{3}{4} = 6 \times 10^6$ g min

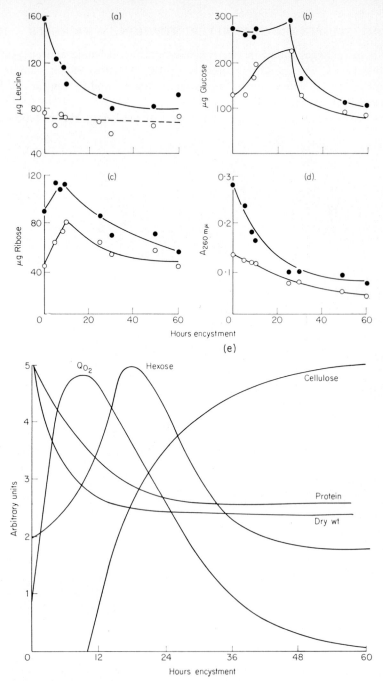

Figure 3. Progress of encystment in *Hartmanella castellani*. Log phase cells were collected, washed aseptically, and shaken gently at 25° C. (a) Free amino acids; (b) carbohydrates; (c) ribonucleotides; (d) A_{260} of hot TCA soluble material; ● μg/mg dry wt cells, ○ μg/ml supernatant medium; (e) overall progress (Ordinate adjusted to scale)

mitochondria and other membrane-bound organelles such as lysosomes and peroxisomes during early stages of encystment by zonal centrifugation on sucrose gradients. Enzymes of the glyoxalate cycle such as malate synthase and isocitrate lyase were absent in vegetative cells but appeared during encystment. They were closely associated with the peroxisome fraction which is characterized also by its high catalase content. Hydrolytic enzymes associated with lysosomes such as acid phosphatase and ribonuclease were associated with a large lysosomal fraction in vegetative cells but with small lysosomes in the encysting cells (Figure 2).

These experiments on encystment in *Hartmanella* present a process similar to that of sporulation in the eubacteria (Mandelstam, 1968), especially as the cyst appears also to be a resistant cell. Firstly the trigger mechanism sets in train a number of enzymic processes which for a period at least, do not altogether commit the cell. In the case of *Hartmanella*, this period (8–12 hours), is somewhat longer than that in bacteria. It is accompanied by changes which are connected with the need to utilize internal pools of material and even normally what are essential parts of the cell such as mitochondria, both as a source of energy and as inter-mediates for cyst wall synthesis. These include hexoses and pentoses largely derived from protein and to a lesser extent lipid. Cyst wall synthesis sets in towards the end of this preparatory stage and the cell then becomes fully committed and the process is no longer reversible (Figure 3).

The details of the trigger mechanism are as yet unclear. The evidence suggests that the exhaustion of glutamic acid and histidine play an important role. This now can be tested on a completely synthetic growth medium. The role of Mg^{2+} is also uncertain but it seems to be connected at least in part, with preventing the excessive loss of intracellular protein, carbohydrate and nucleic acids which can lead to death or at least to cysts which are not viable.

The encystment differs from sporulation in that the change in organiza-tion of cellular morphology is of the same order as occurs in changes during differentiation in higher organisms. In this sense therefore it offers a better model. The process of excystment is particularly interesting since those organelles which disappear completely during encystment and the lysosomes which become greatly modified rapidly are restored to a state normal in a vegetative cell. It appears that this depends almost entirely on exogenous material since the encysting cell leaves the cyst wall apparently intact. The organelles are also apparently reformed without a single cell division.

Genetic analysis in the hartmanellid amoebae, as for instance in the slime moulds (Sussman and Sussman, 1969), is difficult since generally no sexual fusion takes place as, say, in some strains of *Tetrahymena*. This may limit to some extent the analysis of differentiation in this organism in the future. However there is the possibility of transformation by externally added DNA as has been found possible with some cell lines from higher organisms. There is also the possibility of developing lines from defective mutants such as have proved so useful in studies on sporulation.

Lloyd (1969) has recently outlined questions that are of immediate relevance to disappearance of organelles and their biosynthesis and which now seem eminently feasible to study in such systems as described in *Hartmanella* and other organisms and in the following sections. These questions are concerned with (*a*) organelle structure, its biosynthesis and assembly (*b*) the turnover of organelles during growth and differentiation (*c*) the control mechanisms, especially the interrelationship between nucleus and cytoplasmic factors (*d*) the modification of organelles without mass increase. It will be readily appreciated that the essential underlying feature behind these questions is the fluidity and constant change both of structure and function in even the simplest cells.

Cytodifferentiation in *Polytomella* and *Prototheca*

The studies with the colourless alga *Polytomella caeca* have mainly been concerned with the morphogenesis of mitochondria. Following the discovery of a new pathway for propionate metabolism in *Prototheca zopfii* (Callely and Lloyd, 1964) it was subsequently established that the same pathway was present in *Polytomella* and that it was induced in non-proliferating cells which had been grown on acetate, by incubating them with propionate (Evans and Lloyd, 1967). As judged by oxygen uptake the induction of the pathway was completed in about 4 hours and the specific activity of at least two enzymes, β-hydroxypropionate dehydrogenase and malonic semialdehyde dehydrogenase paralleled the increases in oxygen uptake. A high proportion of the β-hydroxypropionate dehydrogenase (60%) and a lower proportion of the second enzyme (20–30%) and of propionyl CoA synthase (20%) was in the mitochondria. Similar proportions were found in cells grown in propionate. In these experiments mitochondria were prepared by breaking the cells in a Kontes type hand homogenizer with a tight fitting plunger. About 60% of the cells were broken by this method but cells could also be broken (40%) by four passages through a sintered glass filter. Mitochondria were separated from the homogenates by normal differential centrifugation methods. Their physiological state was judged by their ability to oxidize intermediates of the TCA cycle, their retention of an internal pool of pyridine nucleotides and the degree of respiratory control as measured polarographically (Lloyd and Brookman, 1967). Failure to carry out these activities was attributed either to the use of excessive hydrodynamic shear during cell disruption or to the presence of reserve carbohydrate which can be controlled during growth. Such intact mitochondria show latency, that is the rate of oxidation of added substrates is slower than in preparations which are partly damaged or become swollen. The appearance in electron micrographs of thin sections of pellets is never exactly similar to those in intact cells. However physiologically intact mitochondria have well developed cristae while in others the cristae are often grossly distorted.

In intact mitochondria from propionate grown cells, the oxidation of propionate is coupled to ATP generation. In mitochondria from induced cells, coupling is not found when the propionate oxidizing system is fully formed (4 hours) but develops during subsequent incubation, to values approaching those from cells grown on propionate. The location of inducible enzymes appeared to be within the NAD-impermeable barrier and both (β-hydroxypropionate dehydrogenase, malonic semialdehyde dehydrogenase) were membrane bound. The formation of these enzymes is inhibited by cycloheximide and by actinomycin D but not by chloramphenicol, suggesting that the enzymes are made on cytoplasmic ribosomes rather than on mitochondrial ribosomes. The passage of the enzymes from cytoplasm to the inner membranes of mitochondria forms an intriguing problem. To study this, the enzymes have been highly purified by Dr. A. Charles and it is proposed to form ferritin-labelled antibodies from them and to follow enzyme transfer by electron microscopy by this means.

Evans and Lloyd have also examined the effects of chloramphenicol on the synthesis of mitochondrial components in *Polytomella*. The synthesis of cytochromes b and a $+$ a$_3$ were inhibited but the synthesis of several enzymes of the TCA cycle, oxidation of propionate and rotenone-sensitive NADH-cytochrome c reductase were not affected. This latter system has been located on the outer membrane system (Lloyd and Chance, 1968). Similar results were found with chloramphenicol accompanied by a decrease in size and disorganization of the cristae which is restored on removing the inhibitor. The changes occurred, as far as could be seen, in the whole mitochondrial population (Lloyd and Turner, unpublished). These results and those on the induction of the propionate system are consistent with the idea that mitochondria grow by the accretion of new membrane components and reproduce by division (Luck, 1962), possibly synchronously with cell division. This latter idea is being tested here with synchronously growing cultures of *Tetrahymena*. At the same time

Doctors Brightwell and Lloyd are examining the synthesis and turnover of
other membranous organelles such as the lysosomes, autophagosomes and
peroxisomes. This work is in a very preliminary stage at the moment, but
it is quite clear that these systems, as judged by enzymic and density
measurements after zonal centrifugation, do not significantly change
during the life cycle. This is being tested further by labelling experiments
and by changing the organelles' density. On the other hand, during starvation a new lysosome component appears which differs in density from both
food vacuoles and the lysosomes initially present and may be associated
with autosomal activities (Figures 4 and 5).

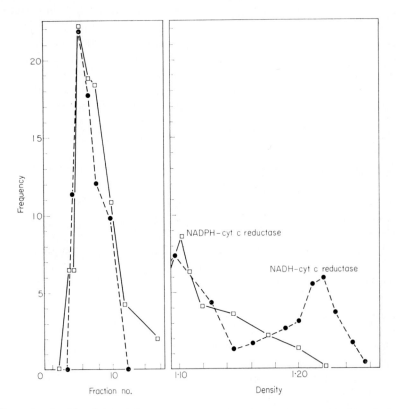

Figure 4. Profile of a separation by zonal centrifugation of a homogenate from
Tetrahymena pyriformis. Linear sucrose gradient; B XIV rotor; 35×10^3 rpm
for $2\frac{3}{4}$ h $= 6 \times 10^6$ g min. The profile is expressed as suggested by deDuve
(1967) and modified by Brightwell here so as to include material not sedimented,
i.e. Density $= < 1 \cdot 100$

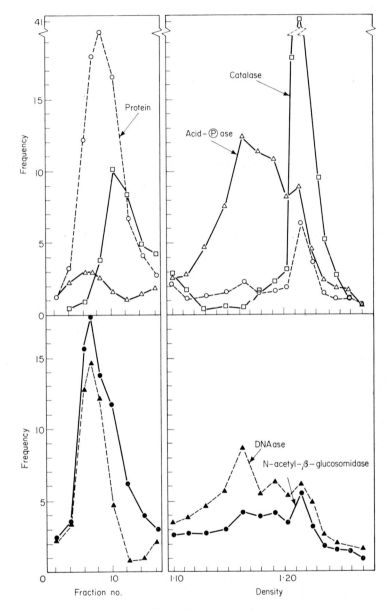

Figure 4—*continued*

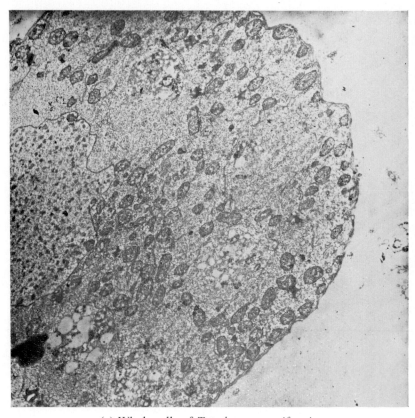

(a) Whole cells of *Tetrahymena pyriformis*

Figure 5. Electron micrographs of fractions separated by zonal centrifugation as described for Figure 4. Each fraction was fixed in glutaraldehyde, dehydrated in ethanol and embedded in methacrylate. Sections were cut in the Reichert ultratome. The choice of methacrylate as embedding agent was determined by the need to process large numbers of fractions speedily; Araldite is used when higher resolution and preservation of fine structure is needed. See also pages 115–117.

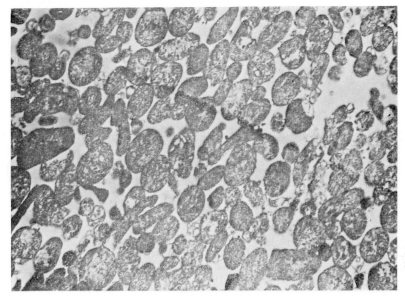

(b) Mitochondria

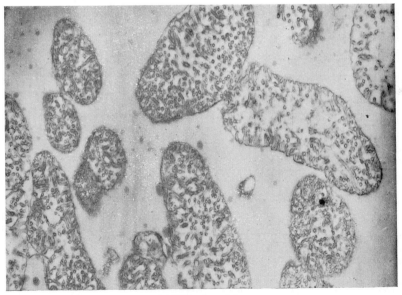

(c) Mitochondria

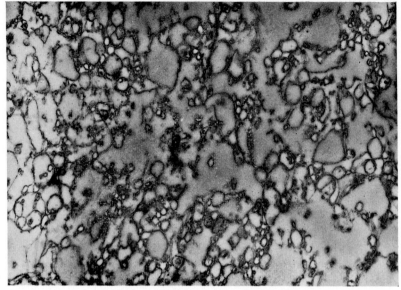

(d) Lysosomes from log phase cells

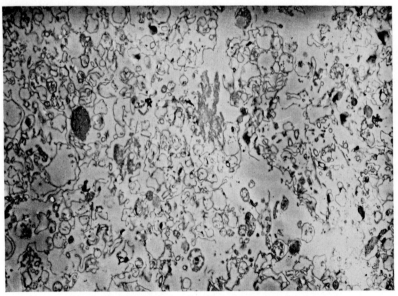

(e) Acid phosphatase fraction from starved cells

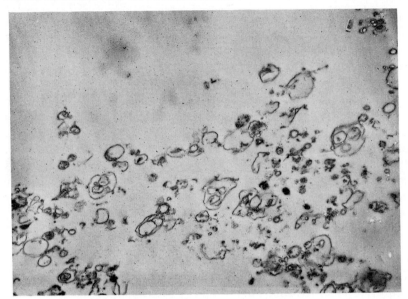

(f) DNAase fraction from starved cells

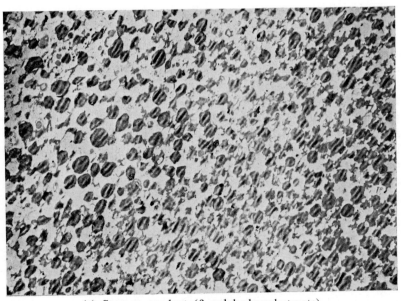

(g) Storage product (? polyhydroxybutyrate)

E

Differentiation in yeast

The application of the zonal centrifuge to study differentiation in yeast follows on the pioneer work of Polakis, Bartley and Meek (1964), Linnane (1968). The immediate aim is to extend the finding that oxygen and catabolite repression regulate the form and function of yeast mitochondria, by following the changes between the sedimentable and non-sedimentable components. The relationship between these changes and the lysosomes can also be relatively easily included. The yeasts have been grown with or without glucose or galactose and under aerobic or anaerobic conditions. Preliminary results support the idea, that both anaerobic conditions and catabolite repression by glucose, lead to a loss of enzymes and other components normally bound to the mitochondria and that these appear in the non-sedimentable fractions.

This work is also of significance to us for another reason. Krebs in discussing the 'Training of a Scientist' (1968) has again re-emphasized the complementary nature of teaching and research available only in University Departments when they reach a 'viable' size. It has, therefore, been our deliberate policy to involve all undergraduates, even from the first year, to some extent in our research. In the first year this is limited to a short period after examination, normally the students use simple microbiological methods with which they have already become familiar. By the third year, however, the students take up for two terms a project and attempt, with their supervisor, to solve a short-range but significant problem. Increasingly, it is our experience that the problems best suited for this training are those involving considerable team work, and consequent logistical planning. Separations by zonal centrifugation present problems of this type and the work on yeast summarized above was, in fact, carried out by a group of students collaborating with the supervisors and their research group. This kind of 'community of the laboratory' was another theme that Krebs often discussed, and one which I know he felt was of particular importance to the development of science in Universities. It calls for, of course, the maximum of student participation and trust between student and staff. It is not easy for the staff; but is perhaps of special significance in relation to the present unrest in the Universities.

CONCLUDING REMARKS

In this essay I have described very briefly some research in progress in Cardiff where the basic approaches seemed to me to stem directly from my long apprenticeship with Sir Hans Krebs as a member of the Cell Metabolism Unit, first in Sheffield and later in Oxford. There can, in fact, be very few active Biology Departments not influenced in some way, however indirectly, by his own research and many in this country, especially influenced as directly as our Department in Cardiff. Krebs has indicated his own indebtedness to his time with Warburg and Gowland Hopkins and thus established a kind of lineage fairly narrow and unbranched in his own case, but now much branched and expanding as Biochemistry develops. This personal contact as Krebs pointed out (Krebs 1967) is the basic process by which a scientist is made. It, of course, carries no guarantee of success or of individual progress but is at least a starting point, and one which must be guarded as the whole role of University research becomes questioned. The process seems common to all creative activities and often results in classical periods. I call especially to mind, the individually brilliant school of twelfth-century Chinese landscape painters and their long and rigorous training by their masters in brush strokes (Sumi-e), whose combination created such poetical elegance. I hope, of course, that I have learned to use at least a few of these masterly strokes wielded so effectively by Sir Hans Krebs, whose birthday we are celebrating.

References

Abercrombie, M. (1967). *Cell Differentiation*. London: Ciba Foundation.
Anderson, N. G. (1966). *The Development of Zonal Centrifuges*. U.S. Public Health Service, Monograph 21, Washington.
Ashworth, J. M. (1966). *Biochim. Biophys. Acta*, **129**, 211.
Bullough, W. S. (1967). *The Evolution of Differentiation*. New York: Academic Press.
Callely, A. G., and Lloyd, D. (1964). *Biochem. J.*, **92**, 338.
Ceccarini, C., and Maggio, R. (1968). *Biochim. Biophys. Acta*, **166**, 134.
Coon, H. G. (1966). *Proc. Natl. Acad. Sci. U.S.*, **55**, 66.
Coulombre, A. J. (1965). *Organogenesis*. New York: Holt, Rinehardt & Winston.
Dean, A. C. R., and Hinshelwood, C. (1966). *Growth, Function and Regulation in Bacterial Cells*. Clarendon, Oxford.
deDuve, C. (1967). *Enzyme Cytology*. New York: Academic Press.
Evans, D., and Lloyd, D. (1967). *Fed. Europ. Bioch. Soc. Proc.* A820.
Goodwin, B. C. (1963). *Temporal Organisation in Cells*. New York: Academic Press.
Griffiths, A. (1967). Ph.D. Thesis, University of Wales.
Griffiths, A. J., and Hughes, D. E. (1969). *J. Protozool.* (In Press.)
Green, H., and Goldberg, B. (1965). *Proc. Natl. Acad. Sci. U.S.*, **53**, 1360.
Green, H., and Todardo, G. J. (1967). *Ann. Rev. Microbiol.*, **21**, 573.
Grobstein, C. (1963). *Cytodifferentiation and Macromolecular Synthesis*. New York: Academic Press.
Hayes, W. (1968). *The Genetics of Bacteria and their Viruses*. Blackwell, Oxford.
Harris, H. (1968). *Nucleus and Cytoplasm*. Oxford: Clarendon Press.

Heslop Harrison, J. (1967). *Ann. Rev. Plant Physiol.*, **18**, 325.

Hughes, D. E., and Cunningham, V. C. (1963). *Biochem. Soc. Symposium*, **23**, 8.

Hughes, D. E., Wimpenny, J. W. T., and Lloyd, D. (1969). *Techniques in Microbiology*. (In Press.)

Hughes, D. E., and Hill, E. C. (1969). Ninth Commonwealth Mining and Metallurgical Congress. Abstracts, London.

Ichikawa, Y., Pluznik, D. H., and Sachs, D. H. (1966). *Proc. Natl. Acad. Sci. U.S.*, **56**, 488.

Iverson, O. H. (1965). *Prog. Biocybern*, **2**, 76.

Jacob, F., and Monod, J. (1963). *Ibid.* New York: Academic Press.

Kennel, D., and Koloulas, A. (1968). *J. Mol. Biol.*, **34**, 71.

Klucis, E., Lloyd, D., and Roach, G. I. (1968). *Biotech. and BioEng.*, **10**, 321.

Krebs, H. A. (1957). *Endeavour*, **16**, 125.

Krebs, H. A. (1967). *Nature, Lond.*, **215**, 1441.

Lewin, R. A. (1967). *Physiology and Biochemistry of the Algae*. New York: Academic Press.

Linnane, A. W. (1968). Round Table Conference on the Biogenesis of Mito-chondria. Bari; Adriatica Editrice. (In Press.)

Lloyd, D., and Brookman, S. J. G. (1967). *Biotech. and BioEng.*, **9**, 271.

Lloyd, D., and Chance, B. (1968). *Biochem. J.*, **107**, 829.

Lloyd, D., and Griffiths, A. J. (1968). *Exp. Cell Research*, **51**, 291.

Lloyd, D. (1969). *Soc. Gen. Microbiol. Symposium*, **19**, 299.

Luck, D. J. L. (1962). *Proc. Natl. Acad. Sci. U.S.*, **49**, 233.

Mandelstam, J. (1969). *Soc. Gen. Microbiol. Symposium*, **19**, 403.

Mangold, O. (1961). *Acta Genet. Med. Gennell*, **10**, 1.

Pritchard, N. J., Peacocke, A. R., and Hughes, D. E. (1966). *Biopolymers*, **4**, 259.

Painter, R. R., and Marr, A. J. (1968). *Ann. Rev. Microbiol.*, **22**, 519.

Polakis, E. S., Bartley, W., and Meek, G. S. (1964). *Biochem. J.*, **90**, 369.

Richmond, M. (1967). *Advances in Microbiol. Physiology*, **2**.

Roe, F. J. C., and Ambrose, E. J. (1966). *The Biology of Cancer*. London: Van Nostrand.

Schuster, F. (1963). *J. Protozool*, **10**, 313.

Spiegleman, S. (1948). *E. B. Symposia*, **2**, 286.

Sussman, M., and Sussman, R. R. (1969). *Soc. Gen. Microbiol. Symposium*, **19**, 403.

Tomlinson, G., and Jones, E. A. (1962). *Biochim. Biophys Acta*, **63**, 194.

Tomlinson, G., and Muhlethaler, K. (1965). *J. Tenn. Acad. Sci.*, **40**, 68.

Venables, W. A., Wimpenny, J. W. T., and Cole, J. A. (1967). *Biochem. J.*, **106**, 36.

Venables, W. A., and Guest, J. A. (1968). *Mol. Genetics*, **103**, 127.

Vickerman, K. (1962). *Exptl. Cell Res.*, **26**, 497.

Wilmer, E. N. (1963). *Symp. Soc. Exp. Biol.*, **17**, 215.

Wimpenny, J. W. T. (1969). *Soc. Gen. Microbiol. Symposia*, **19**, 161.

Acknowledgements

I would like to record thanks to my colleagues, especially Doctors A. Griffiths, D. Lloyd and R. Brightwell, who have allowed me to give an account of their work, some of which is as yet unpublished.

THE MICROBIAL METABOLISM OF
SIMPLE CARBON COMPOUNDS

H. L. Kornberg

Department of Microbiology, University of Sheffield

J. R. Quayle

Department of Biochemistry, University of Leicester

Of all forms of living matter, microorganisms manifest the highest degree of chemical facility. Already over 40 years ago, den Dooren de Jong (1926) listed well over a hundred compounds that could be used by bacteria as sole source of carbon for growth, and this list can be extended to include virtually all organic materials. Fortunately for our understanding, this catholicity of diet is not accompanied by a similar complexity of metabolic reactions; it is now clear that the processes of energy release from the majority of catabolic fragments, and the means whereby these fragments are assembled into the macromolecular constituents of the cell, involve relatively few steps, which are common to all organisms. The revelation of this underlying unity owes much to the work of Hans Krebs who showed in 1937 that the tricarboxylic acid cycle accounts for the combustion of food materials, with concomitant energy release, and, 15 years later, that the same cycle provides the carbon skeletons of many cell components. The establishment of the dual role of this cycle also posed, clearly and for the first time, the problems which we discuss in this survey: how can this cycle fulfil its double function in microorganisms growing on simple carbon sources? How can substances containing two carbon atoms or less, or those at an oxidation level higher than the C_2-units that enter this cycle, yield energy and the intermediates of the cycle? And how is the operation of the various metabolic routes used for these processes regulated in the cells?

Such contributions as we have been able to make to a solution of these questions owe far more to Hans Krebs than the mere posing of the problems. He was not only responsible for initiating our work but, over its first six years, he provided all the help that we could possibly have desired. In part, this help was material in form: any needs for equipment, for facilities and for supplies were met without stint and apparently without question. But equally important was the help 'Prof' gave us in

Abbreviations: Fd and FdH, oxidized and reduced ferredoxin; **PEP**, phosphoenol pyruvate; THFA, tetrahydrofolic acid.

less obvious ways: he encouraged without interfering, stimulated without driving, and inspired by example and not by precept. Despite his many commitments, as Head of a large Department, Director of a Research Unit and member of many committees, he was never too busy to talk, to offer (with touching diffidence) advice in our frequent difficulties, and to warm us with his genuine pleasure when, less frequently, things went well. It was characteristic of him that he spent many weary hours in re-writing the first drafts of our papers; it was equally characteristic that he took no credit for this or for the work reported in them.

Although it is already many years since we left Hans Krebs' laboratory, we are proud of his continued interest in our work. We therefore offer this survey to him as a token of our gratitude, affection and good wishes on his seventieth birthday.

I. ENERGY PRODUCTION

Sequences of Diminishing Complexity

1. The tricarboxylic acid cycle

(a) *Acetate*

The tricarboxylic acid cycle is a means of totally oxidizing acetate units to carbon dioxide (Figure 1). Thirty years of research, following the initial discovery by Krebs and Johnson (1937), have shown that the role of the cycle in cell metabolism is far wider than might have been predicted for the oxidation of a single intermediary metabolite. Most aerobic cells that have been examined so far are found to funnel the carbon skeletons of carbohydrate, fat and protein through the cycle as the terminal pathway of respiration (Krebs and Kornberg, 1957). The direction of such a wide variety of substrates into the same terminal oxidative sequence by way of the common intermediate acetyl-coenzyme A, clearly results in great economy of enzymic make-up. Further economies in cell metabolism are also achieved by the use of some of the intermediates of the cycle, for example, α-oxoglutarate, succinyl-coenzyme A, and oxaloacetate, as carbon skeletons for the biosynthesis of other cell constituents. It is thus to be expected that the breakdown of simple compounds which can be directly catabolized to acetate, as well as acetate itself, should proceed through the tricarboxylic acid cycle rather than through a direct linear sequence, for example acetate $\rightarrow$ glycollate $\rightarrow$ glyoxylate $\rightarrow$ formate $\rightarrow$ carbon dioxide. Such a sequence would demand four or five specific degradative enzymes. This would be wasteful in a cell which already

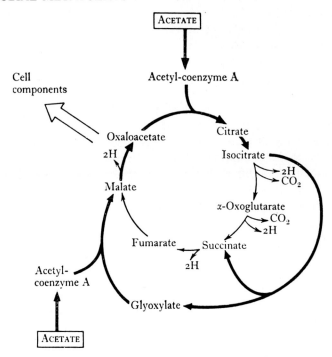

Figure 1. Routes for the provision of energy and of cell components during microbial growth on acetate. The catabolic route (tricarboxylic acid cycle) is shown as light arrows; the anaplerotic pathway (glyoxylate cycle) as heavy arrows. (Reproduced from *Symp. Soc. Gen. Microbiol.* (1965) **15**, 8, by permission of the Society of General Microbiology)

possessed a functional tricarboxylic acid cycle for biosynthetic purposes. Despite the obvious appeal of economy, unequivocal proof of the operation of the cycle in microbial cells turned out to be difficult owing to problems of cell impermeability. Indeed, the discoverer of the cycle himself argued against acceptance of the views that the cycle represented the main pathway of oxidation of acetate in yeast cells (Krebs, Gurin and Eggleston, 1952). It was some years before the problems raised by cell impermeability were satisfactorily answered, enabling the wide generality of the cycle to be established with respect to microbial oxidation of acetate (see Kornberg, 1959; Krebs and Lowenstein, 1960).

It should be noted that oxidation of acetate via the tricarboxylic acid necessitates the input of one ATP equivalent, in order to prepare the substrate for entry to the cycle as acetyl-CoA. The energy necessary for making this acyl-CoA group is not conserved, as free coenzyme A is liberated during entry of the C_2-unit into the cycle by way of the reaction catalysed by citrate synthase.

(b) Glycollate and glyoxylate

Both these substrates are at a higher oxidation level than acetyl-CoA and hence any oxidation of them through the tricarboxylic acid cycle necessitates a preliminary reduction. The reduction of a hydroxymethyl group to methyl, although it may be accomplished in organic chemistry with a single powerful reducing agent, for example phosphorus and hydriodic acid, it is not so easily accomplished biologically in one step. Indeed, Kornberg and Morris (1965) discovered that *Micrococcus denitrificans* uses a remarkably complex series of reactions to effect the reduction:

$$2CH_2OH \cdot CO_2H \rightarrow 2CHO \cdot CO_2H + 4H \quad (1)$$
$$CHO \cdot CO_2H + NH_3 + 2H \rightarrow CH_2NH_2 \cdot CO_2H + H_2O \quad (2)$$
$$HO_2C \cdot CH_2NH_2 + OHC \cdot CO_2H \rightarrow HO_2C \cdot CHNH_2 \cdot CHOH \cdot CO_2H \quad (3)$$
$$\text{erythro--}\beta\text{--hydroxyaspartic acid}$$
$$HO_2C \cdot CHNH_2 \cdot CHOH \cdot CO_2H \rightarrow HO_2C \cdot CH_2 \cdot CO \cdot CO_2H + NH_3 \quad (4)$$

Reactions (1) to (4) accomplish the condensation of two molecules of glycollate to one of oxaloacetate by way of the novel intermediary metabolite, hydroxyaspartic acid. Reduction of one pair of carbon atoms to the level of acetate is then indirectly achieved by successive loss of two molecules of carbon dioxide from the C_4-dicarboxylic acid. It is assumed that this proceeds by the familiar steps (5) to (7)

$$HO_2C \cdot CH_2 \cdot CO \cdot CO_2H + ATP \rightarrow$$
$$CH_2 \cdot C(OPO_3H_2) \cdot CO_2H + CO_2 + ADP \quad (5)$$
$$CH_2 \cdot C(OPO_3H_2) \cdot CO_2H + ADP \rightarrow CH_3 \cdot CO \cdot CO_2H + ATP \quad (6)$$
$$CH_3 \cdot CO \cdot CO_2H + NAD + CoASH \rightarrow CH_3 \cdot COSCoA + CO_2 +$$
$$NADH_2 \quad (7)$$

If appropriate interconversions of adenosine nucleotides are made, as well as interconversion of reducing equivalents, reactions (1) to (7) may be summed up as:

$$2CH_2OH \cdot CO_2H + CoASH + NAD \rightarrow$$
$$CH_3 \cdot COSCoA + 2CO_2 + NADH_2 + 2H + H_2O \quad (8)$$

This may seem a complicated way of reducing glycollate to acetate but it should be noted that part of the same sequence (reactions (1) to (4)) also accomplishes the synthesis of oxaloacetate. This is needed as acceptor molecule for the cyclic oxidation of the acetate which is to follow.

Kornberg and Morris found that a similar route, except for reaction (1), was also used for growth on glyoxylate by *M. denitrificans*, although growth on this substrate was much slower than on glycollate.

(c) Glycine

This compound is at a similar oxidation level to glycollate and hence it also would first need to be reduced to acetyl-CoA before it could be oxidized through the tricarboxylic acid cycle. There is evidence that such a mechanism is used in the case of *Arthrobacter globiformis* when growing on glycine as sole carbon source (Jones and Bridgeland, 1966). Three enzyme-catalysed reactions, which are together capable of converting glycine into pyruvate, have been found in extracts of the glycine-grown organism:

$$CH_2NH_2 \cdot CO_2H + THFA \rightarrow \text{methylene–THFA} + CO_2 + NH_3 + 2H \tag{9}$$

$$\text{Methylene–THFA} + CH_2NH_2 \cdot CO_2H + H_2O \rightarrow CH_2OH \cdot CHNH_2 \\ \cdot CO_2H + THFA \tag{10}$$

$$CH_2OH \cdot CHNH_2 \cdot CO_2H \rightarrow CH_3 \cdot CO \cdot CO_2H + NH_3 \tag{11}$$

If acetyl–CoA is formed from pyruvate through the pyruvate dehydrogenase complex of enzymes catalysing reaction (7), the sum of reactions (9), (10), (11) and (7) may be represented by:

$$2CH_2NH_2 \cdot CO_2H + CoASH + NAD + H_2O \rightarrow \\ CH_3 \cdot COSCoA + 2CO_2 + NADH_2 \\ + 2H + 2NH_3 \tag{12}$$

As in the case of glycollate, condensation and decarboxylation reactions serve to effect an indirect net reduction of the C_2-compound to the level of acetate. Total oxidation then follows through the tricarboxylic acid cycle.

2. The dicarboxylic acid cycle

In the previous section it has been pointed out that *M. denitrificans* accomplishes the total oxidation of glycollate or glyoxylate through the tricarboxylic acid cycle, the substrate having first to be reduced to the level of acetate. A different cycle of reactions, the dicarboxylic acid cycle (Figure 2), was discovered in pseudomonads and *Escherichia coli* by Kornberg and Sadler (1960). The C_2-substrate enters this cycle as glyoxylate, being condensed with acetyl-CoA to give malate via the malate synthase reaction:

$$HO_2C \cdot CHO + CH_3 \cdot COSCoA + H_2O \rightarrow$$
$$HO_2C \cdot CHOH \cdot CH_2 \cdot CO_2H + CoASH \quad \textbf{(13)}$$

The malate is then oxidatively decarboxylated to acetyl-CoA which serves as the acceptor molecule for condensation with another molecule of glyoxylate.

It will be noted that in both the tricarboxylic and dicarboxylic acid cycles the port of entry is by way of an aldol condensation reaction between a methyl group and a carbonyl group. In the case of the tricarboxylic acid cycle the acceptor molecule (oxaloacetate) carries the carbonyl group and the substrate to be oxidized (acetate) carries the methyl group. By contrast, these roles are reversed in the dicarboxylic acid cycle where the acceptor molecule (acetate) carries the methyl group and the substrate to be oxidized (glyoxylate) carries the carbonyl group.

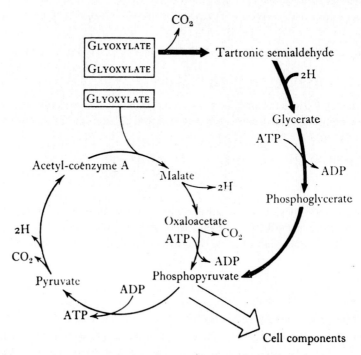

Figure 2. Routes for the provision of energy and of cell components during microbial growth on glyoxylate. The catabolic route (dicarboxylic acid cycle) is shown as light arrows; the anaplerotic sequence (glycerate pathway) as heavy arrows. (Reproduced from *Symp. Soc. Gen. Microbiol.* (1965) **15**, 8, by permission of the Society of General Microbiology)

This simple inversion device, obviating the need for reduction of the substrate prior to its oxidation, may be likened to an attenuator which adjusts a cyclical reaction sequence to work at a different oxidation level.

A further consequence of cyclic oxidation at a higher oxidation level, when fewer electrons have to be abstracted, is that the cycles get smaller. The tricarboxylic acid cycle has a circumference of eight main reaction steps as compared to five main steps in the case of the dicarboxylic acid cycle. This is further exemplified in the case of oxalate oxidation, discussed below.

3. The oxalyl-CoA cycle

The most highly oxidized C_2-substrate is oxalate, in which abstraction of only two electrons results in total oxidation to two molecules of carbon dioxide. This can be accomplished in plant tissue by a single enzyme, oxalic acid oxidase (Datta and Meeuse, 1955; Chiriboa, 1963), which catalyses the reaction:

$$HO_2C \cdot CO_2H + \tfrac{1}{2}O_2 \rightarrow 2CO_2 + H_2O_2 \tag{14}$$

In the case of bacteria growing on oxalate as sole carbon source, a series of reactions, involving acyl–CoA derivatives, has been found to operate (Jakoby, Ohmura and Hayaishi, 1956; Quayle, Keech and Taylor, 1961; Quayle, 1963*a*):

$$HO_2C \cdot CO_2H + H \cdot COSCoA \rightarrow HO_2C \cdot COSCoA + HCO_2H \tag{15}$$
$$HO_2C \cdot COSCoA \rightarrow CO_2 + H \cdot COSCoA \tag{16}$$
$$HCO_2H + NAD \rightarrow CO_2 + NADH_2 \tag{17}$$

Sum: $$HO_2C \cdot CO_2H + NAD \rightarrow 2CO_2 + NADH_2 \tag{18}$$

This is not a cycle of oxidation in the same sense as are the tricarboxylic or dicarboxylic acid cycles. The essence of a true oxidation cycle, as exemplified by the latter two cycles, lies in the substrate being condensed by C–C bonding with an acceptor compound into a chemical framework in which electrons can be moved and abstracted. As the electrons are removed, the resulting fully oxidized carbon atoms are successively expelled as carbon dioxide until the acceptor molecule is regenerated. No such condensation is possible with a molecule at the oxidation level of oxalate, and expulsion of carbon dioxide follows directly on activation of the molecule. The cyclic part of the process is concerned with conservation of the energy required to synthesize an acyl-CoA bond rather than with oxidation *per se*. Thus, oxalate marks the transition between the cyclic oxidation of C_2-compounds and the non-cyclic oxidation of C_1-compounds (see section 4).

4. The oxidation of C_1-compounds

No evidence has yet been found for a cyclic mechanism of oxidation of C_1-compounds in which the substrate is first condensed with an acceptor compound; rather is the C_1-substrate itself oxidized to carbon dioxide by one-step reactions. Despite the simplicity of the substrates, much remains unknown about the detailed enzymology. The following sections will, however, show a pattern of individual oxidation reactions which is common to several different species of organism.

(a) Methane

The available evidence indicates that organisms capable of utilizing methane as sole carbon and energy source oxidize it to carbon dioxide via methanol, formaldehyde and formate. Brown, Strawinski and McCleskey (1964) showed that of a wide variety of organic substrates tested, only methane, methanol, formaldehyde and formate were appreciably oxidized by methane-grown *Methanomonas methanooxidans*. Formic acid was detected in the culture medium after cells had oxidized methane, methanol or formaldehyde; formaldehyde was trapped in the medium after oxidation of methane or methanol.

Although of considerable biochemical interest, nothing is presently known of the enzymology of the first step in the sequence, viz., the oxidation of methane to methanol. However, enzymes capable of oxidizing methanol, formaldehyde and formate have been detected in extracts of *Pseudomonas methanica* (Johnson and Quayle, 1964) and these will be discussed further in the appropriate section below.

(b) Methanol

Anthony and Zatman (1964) discovered in methanol-grown *Pseudomonas* M27 an enzyme which oxidizes methanol to formaldehyde

$$CH_3OH \rightarrow HCHO + 2[H] \tag{19}$$

The enzyme may be coupled to phenazine methosulphate *in vitro*, but the natural electron acceptor is not known. The enzyme-catalysed reaction shows a requirement for either ammonia or methylamine as activator. The authors suggest that the enzyme contains a pteridine compound as prosthetic group (Anthony and Zatman, 1967). Although the enzyme shows a very broad specificity towards oxidation of primary alcohols it is probable that it is of central importance in microbial oxidation of C_1-compounds since it has been detected in several organisms grown on methanol or methane (Johnson and Quayle, 1964), furthermore, mutational loss of the enzyme leads to inability of *Pseudomonas* AM1 to grow on, or oxidize, methanol (Heptinstall and Quayle, 1969).

(c) Methylamine

An enzyme has been discovered by Eady and Large (1968) in methylamine-grown *Pseudomonas* AM1 which oxidizes methylamine to formaldehyde:

$$CH_3NH_2 + H_2O \rightarrow HCHO + NH_3 + 2H \tag{20}$$

The enzyme may be coupled to an artificial electron acceptor, but the natural acceptor is not known. The presence of this enzyme indicates that methylamine is directly oxidized to formaldehyde rather than first being hydrolysed to methanol as an intermediate. This is confirmed by the fact that mutational loss of methanol dehydrogenase in *Pseudomonas* AM1 leads to no impairment of growth on methylamine (Heptinstall and Quayle, 1969).

Eady and Large (1969) have also discovered a mixed-function oxidase in dimethylamine-grown *Pseudomonas aminovorans* which oxidizes one of the methyl groups to formaldehyde:

$$(CH_3)_2 \cdot NH_2Cl + O_2 + NADPH_2 \rightarrow \\ CH_3 \cdot NH_3Cl + HCHO + NADP + H_2O \tag{21}$$

It is not known how the methylamine resulting from this reaction is further oxidized as no methylamine-oxidizing activity has been detected in cell free extracts of the organism.

(d) Formaldehyde

Two distinct formaldehyde dehydrogenases converting formaldehyde to formate have been found in organisms growing on C_1-compounds (see Johnson and Quayle, 1964). Firstly, an NAD-dependent dehydrogenase; secondly, a dehydrogenase which may be linked to 2,6-dichlorophenol-indophenol. It is not yet clear in many organisms which of these enzymes is important physiologically for formaldehyde oxidation. In the case of *Pseudomonas* AM1, the latter enzyme is implicated since this organism does not possess the NAD-dependent dehydrogenase.

(e) Formate

An NAD-linked formate dehydrogenase has been found in several species of C_1-utilizing organisms, including methane-grown *Pseudomonas methanica* (see Johnson and Quayle, 1964). It is assumed that formate is terminally oxidized by this system.

II. BIOSYNTHESIS

The Role of Energy-yielding Cycles in Biosynthesis

1. The need for replenishment [anaplerotic] reactions

As was first clearly emphasized by Krebs and coworkers (1952), the tricarboxylic acid cycle provides not only energy but also the carbon skeletons of many cell components. This biosynthetic function of the cycle becomes particularly important when microorganisms grow on simple carbon compounds, which are not themselves intermediates of the cycle, as their sole source of carbon. Under these circumstances, protein synthesis requires all the members of the 'glutamate family' of amino acids to be made from α-oxoglutarate, and all the members of the 'aspartate family' from oxaloacetate; cytochromes must be assembled in part from succinyl-coenzyme A, and the pyrimidine moieties of nucleic acids must also be derived from oxaloacetate. In the tricarboxylic acid cycle, the oxaloacetate acceptor for C_2-units must be re-formed if the cycle is to continue to function; it follows that the cycle can supply biosynthetic intermediates only if ancillary reactions replace such intermediates as fast as they are removed. These replenishment reactions have been generically termed 'anaplerotic' (Kornberg, 1966a).

Similar considerations apply also to growth on other carbon sources which are catabolized by sequences of lesser complexity. The catabolism of glyoxylate, whether derived from glycollate or glycine, proceeds via a dicarboxylic acid cycle the intermediates of which are also precursors of cell components: indeed, the interrelationship of this smaller cycle with the tricarboxylic acid cycle under these conditions most clearly demonstrates the separation of an energy-supplying from an energy-utilizing cyclic process. Again, reactions must occur which ensure that the C_2-growth substrate can give rise to the net formation of intermediates of either cycle. This applies even to the growth of *A. globiformis* on glycine: although the overall effect of reactions (**9**) to (**11**) is to form one molecular unit of the C_3-compound, pyruvate, from two molecular units of glycine, pyruvate will lose one of its carbons in being oxidized to acetyl-CoA. It is only in *M. denitrificans*, where glyoxylate utilization involves the *net* formation of oxaloacetate [reactions (**2**) to (**4**)], that the energetic and biosynthetic needs of the organism can be met by the same reaction, and no ancillary processes of replenishment need to occur.

Anaplerotic reactions, in the strict sense of the term, must occur only when an energy-supplying cycle serves also as the source of biosynthetic intermediates. The catabolism of oxalate [reactions (**15**) to (**17**)] involves as intermediates oxalyl- and formyl-CoA, and carbon dioxide. None of these compounds is an intermediate of a biosynthetic cycle. Although growth on oxalate clearly requires that reactions occur whereby either oxalate itself or catabolic products of oxalate are transformed to intermediates of the tricarboxylic acid cycle as well as to the precursors of other biosynthetic pathways, such reactions are truly biosynthetic and cannot be considered as being anaplerotic. This argument applies equally to the processes whereby C_1-compounds are utilized for growth.

We propose, in the next section of this article, to discuss the nature of the anaplerotic reactions which enable the tri- and di-carboxylic acid cycles to fulfil their dual purposes during growth on appropriate C_2-compounds.

2. Replenishment of the tricarboxylic acid cycle

(a) Growth on acetate

Two anaplerotic enzymes cooperate to effect the net formation of C_4-acids from acetate, in most microorganisms capable of aerobic growth on this C_2-compound or on substances catabolized to acetyl-CoA. The first of these enzymes is isocitrate lyase, which catalyses the aldol cleavage of L-($+$)-isocitrate to glyoxylate and succinate (Olson, 1954; Saz, 1954; Smith and Gunsalus, 1954):

$$HO_2C \cdot CH_2 \cdot CH \cdot (CO_2H) \cdot CH(OH) \cdot CO_2H \rightleftharpoons HO_2C \cdot CH_2 \cdot CH_2 \cdot CO_2H +$$
$$OCH \cdot CO_2H \qquad (22)$$

In a manner analogous to the condensation of acetyl-CoA with oxaloacetate, which initiates each turn of the tricarboxylic acid cycle, the α-oxo-compound glyoxylate, thus formed, condenses with acetyl-CoA to form L-malate.

$$OCH \cdot CO_2H + CH_3CO \cdot SCoA + H_2O \rightarrow$$
$$HO_2C \cdot CH(OH) \cdot CH_2 \cdot CO_2H + CoASH \qquad (23)$$

The enzyme catalysing this condensation, malate synthase (Wong and Ajl, 1956), is quite distinct from the citrate synthase of the tricarboxylic acid cycle; in E. coli, its formation is specified by a gene located adjacent to that specifying isocitrate lyase synthesis (Brice and Kornberg, 1968) and far from that which specifies citrate synthase (Ashworth, Kornberg and Nothmann, 1965).

It will be apparent that the two anaplerotic reactions (22) and (23) by-pass those reactions of the tricarboxylic acid cycle in which carbon dioxide is lost; for this reason, their cooperative action was first termed the 'glyoxylate bypass of the tricarboxylic acid cycle' (Kornberg and

Madsen, 1957). However, they may also be viewed as a biosynthetic variant of the tricarboxylic acid cycle (Kornberg and Krebs, 1957) if considered together with the other reactions of that cycle which lead to the re-formation of isocitrate from the C_4-acids formed from (22) and (23): this biosynthetic variant has been termed 'the glyoxylate cycle' (see Figure 1).

$$\text{acetyl-SCoA} + \text{oxaloacetate} + H_2O \rightarrow \text{citrate} + \text{CoASH} \quad (24)$$
$$\text{citrate} \rightleftharpoons \text{isocitrate} \quad (25)$$
$$\text{isocitrate} \rightleftharpoons \text{succinate} + \text{glyoxylate} \quad (26)$$
$$\text{acetyl-SCoA} + \text{glyoxylate} + H_2O \rightarrow \text{malate} + \text{CoASH} \quad (27)$$
$$\text{malate} \rightarrow \text{oxaloacetate} + 2H \quad (28)$$

$$\text{Sum: } 2 \text{ acetyl-SCoA} + 2H_2O \rightarrow \text{succinate} + 2 \text{ CoASH} + 2H \quad (29)$$

Of course, the overall reaction (29), which has been arbitrarily written to lead to the net formation of succinate, can equally give rise to any other intermediate of the tricarboxylic acid cycle; the anaplerotic reactions (22) and (23) can thus serve to replenish any intermediate withdrawn from that cycle for synthetic purposes.

Although the anaplerotic enzymes of the glyoxylate cycle play a necessary role in the growth on acetate of a wide variety of aerobic microorganisms (for review, see Kornberg and Elsden, 1961), they are not the only means of facilitating microbial growth on this C_2-compound. For example, certain strains of photosynthetic bacteria grow readily on acetate, aerobically and in the dark, but are devoid of isocitrate lyase activity (Kornberg and Lascelles, 1960): the anaplerotic route in these organisms is still unknown. Furthermore, strictly anaerobic organisms, such as *Clostridium kluyveri*, can effect the reductive carboxylation of acetate to pyruvate (30), using reduced ferredoxin as electron donor (Andrew and Morris, 1965):

$$\text{acetyl-SCoA} + CO_2 + 2FdH \rightarrow \text{pyruvate} + \text{CoASH} + 2Fd \quad (30)$$

Such organisms must then employ a further step to convert the C_3-product to an intermediate of the tricarboxylic acid cycle; the nature of this step will be considered in the following section.

(b) Carboxylation of C_3-compounds

Since the oxidation of pyruvate to acetyl-CoA results in the loss, as carbon dioxide, of the carboxyl-carbon of the C_3-acid, the problems faced by microorganisms growing on precursors of pyruvate are similar in nature to those affecting growth on C_2-units. However, the means whereby the tricarboxylic acid is replenished from C_3-acids is quite different.

It has long been realized (Wood and Werkman, 1938; Krebs, 1943) that carbon dioxide is not solely an end product of metabolism, but can react in a variety of ways with C_3-acids to yield intermediates of the tricarboxylic acid cycle.

Carbon dioxide may be fixed into phosphoenolpyruvate to yield oxaloacetate, either in the absence of other requirements (Bandurski and Greiner, 1953; Large, Peel and Quayle, 1962):

$$CH_2 : C(OPO_3H_2) \cdot CO_2H + CO_2 + H_2O \rightarrow$$
$$HO_2C \cdot CH_2 \cdot CO \cdot CO_2H + H_3PO_4 \quad (31)$$

or with the participation of inorganic phosphate (Lochmüller, Wood and Davis, 1966) in which case pyrophosphate is also produced:

$$CH_2 : C(OPO_3H_2) \cdot CO_2H + CO_2 + H_3PO_4 \rightarrow HO_2C \cdot CH_2 \cdot CO \cdot \quad (32)$$
$$CO_2H + H_4P_2O_7$$

In *Pseudomonas* sp., the PEP-carboxylase reaction (31) operates efficiently as written (Large and coworkers, 1962); in *E. coli*, on the other hand, the enzyme is barely active unless catalytic quantities of acetyl-CoA are also present (Canovas and Kornberg, 1966).

Carbon dioxide may also be fixed on to pyruvate, again to yield oxaloacetate. This process requires ATP and metal ions, and, depending on the nature of the organism studied, may proceed in the absence of other cofactors, as in a species of pseudomonad (Seubert and Remberger, 1961),

$$CH_3 \cdot CO \cdot CO_2H + CO_2 + ATP \rightarrow$$
$$HO_2C \cdot CH_2 \cdot CO \cdot CO_2H + ADP + H_3PO_4 \quad (33)$$

may be stimulated by acetyl-CoA, as in yeasts (Ruiz-Amil, de Torrontegui, Palacán, Catalina and Losada, 1965; Cazzulo and Stoppani, 1965), or may require acetyl-CoA absolutely, as in avian liver (Keech and Utter, 1963): this latter situation holds, for example, for *A. globiformis* (Bridgeland and Jones, 1967; see Section I, 1(c)) and may hold for *Cl. kluyveri* (see Section 11, 2(a)).

There are other enzymes in microorganisms that could catalyse the formation of C_4-dicarboxylic acids from carbon dioxide and C_3-acids, notably the 'malic enzyme',

$$CH_3 \cdot CO \cdot CO_2H + NADPH_2 + CO_2 \rightarrow$$
$$HO_2C \cdot CH_2 \cdot CH(OH) \cdot CO_2H + NADP \quad (34)$$

and PEP-carboxykinase,

$$CH_2 : C(OPO_3H_2) \cdot CO_2H + CO_2 + ADP \rightleftharpoons$$
$$HO_2C \cdot CH_2 \cdot CO \cdot CO_2H + ATP \quad (35)$$

but these do not serve an anaplerotic function: the available evidence (Ashworth and Kornberg, 1966) suggests that their role is to effect the decarboxylation of C_4-acids, either to form PEP (which is the starting material for gluconeogenesis from tricarboxylic acid cycle intermediates, *cf*. Krebs and Kornberg, 1957) or, possibly, to form $NADPH_2$ required for biosynthesis.

(c) *Formation of PEP from pyruvate*

Since organisms such as Enterobacteriaceae do not possess pyruvate carboxylase activity (**33**) and can form C_4-dicarboxylic acids from glycolytic intermediates only via PEP-carboxylase (**31**), the growth of such bacteria on lactate or pyruvate as sole carbon source requires the action of an enzyme capable of effecting the net formation of PEP from pyruvate. This process is catalysed by PEP-synthase (Cooper and Kornberg, 1967a), an enzyme (**37**) quite different from the catabolic pyruvate kinases (Malcovati and Kornberg, 1969); it overcomes the energy barrier associated with a reversal of pyruvate kinase activity (**36**) by utilizing two pyrophosphate bonds of ATP for the synthesis of one molecular unit of PEP:

$$CH_3CO \cdot CO_2H + ATP \rightleftharpoons CH_2 : C(OPO_3H_2) \cdot CO_2H + ADP \quad (36)$$
$$\textit{reversal of pyruvate kinase reaction}$$

$$CH_3CO \cdot CO_2H + ATP \rightleftharpoons CH_2 : C(OPO_3H_2) \cdot CO_2H + AMP + PO_4H_3$$
$$\textit{PEP-synthase reaction} \qquad\qquad\qquad (37)$$

It is interesting to note that Propionibacteria, which carboxylate PEP via an enzyme requiring phosphate and forming pyrophosphate (**32**) use a variation of the PEP-synthase reaction that also requires phosphate and forms pyrophosphate; the enzyme catalysing this reaction has been termed pyruvate phosphate dikinase (Evans and Wood, 1968). Apart from this variation, the mechanism of PEP-formation is strikingly similar in both reactions: in both cases, an enzyme-pyrophosphate is initially formed from ATP and the enzyme (**38**) (Cooper and Kornberg, 1967b) but, whereas in the Propionibacteria this derivative reacts with organic phosphate, to form enzyme-phosphate and inorganic pyrophosphate (**39**), in *E. coli*, enzyme-phosphate is produced apparently by the hydrolysis of the enzyme-PP derivative (**40**) (Cooper and Kornberg, 1967c). The final step of either reaction mechanism is the formation of PEP from enzyme-phosphate and pyruvate (**41**)

$$Enzyme + ATP \rightleftharpoons Enzyme\text{-}PP + AMP \qquad\qquad (38)$$

$$\text{Enzyme-PP} + \text{P}_i \rightleftharpoons \text{Enzyme-P} + \text{PP (Propionibacteria)} \qquad (39)$$
$$\text{Enzyme-PP} + \text{H}_2\text{O} \rightleftharpoons \text{Enzyme-P} + \text{P}_i \ (E.\ coli) \qquad (40)$$
$$\text{Enzyme-P} + \text{pyruvate} \rightleftharpoons \text{PEP} + \text{Enzyme} \qquad (41)$$

3. Replenishment of dicarboxylic acid cycle

Since most of the intermediates of the dicarboxylic acid cycle—particularly oxaloacetate, pyruvate and acetyl-CoA—are themselves the starting materials for biosynthetic sequences, the combustion of glyoxylate via this cycle can occur only if anaplerotic reactions occur which maintain the levels of intermediates of that cycle. The sequence of reactions that serves this anaplerotic function has been termed 'the glycerate pathway' (Kornberg, 1961) (see Figure 2). It has been shown (Kornberg and Gotto, 1959) to consist of three enzymes. Glyoxylate carboligase (42) catalyses the formation of tartronic semialdehyde and carbon dioxide from 2 molecular units of glyoxylate (Krakow and Barkulis, 1956). This C_3-compound is then reduced by either $NADH_2$ or $NADPH_2$ to glycerate, in a reaction catalysed by tartronic semialdehyde reductase (43) (Gotto and Kornberg, 1961), which is then phosphorylated to 3-phosphoglycerate via glycerate kinase (Doughty, Hayashi and Guenther, 1966).

$$2\text{OCH} \cdot \text{CO}_2\text{H} \rightarrow \text{OCH} \cdot \text{CH(OH)} \cdot \text{CO}_2\text{H} + \text{CO}_2 \qquad (42)$$
$$\text{OCH} \cdot \text{CH(OH)} \cdot \text{CO}_2\text{H} + \text{NAD(P)H}_2 \rightarrow$$
$$\text{HO} \cdot \text{CH}_2 \cdot \text{CH(OH)} \cdot \text{CO}_2\text{H} + \text{NAD(P)} \qquad (43)$$
$$\text{HO} \cdot \text{CH}_2 \cdot \text{CH(OH)} \cdot \text{CO}_2\text{H} + \text{ATP} \rightarrow$$
$$\text{H}_2\text{PO}_3 \cdot \text{O} \cdot \text{CH}_2 \cdot \text{CH(OH)} \cdot \text{CO}_2\text{H} + \text{ADP} \qquad (44)$$

The 3-phosphoglycerate thus formed is, of course, an intermediate of glycolysis and can be catabolized, via glycolytic enzymes, to yield PEP and pyruvate (which are intermediates of the dicarboxylic acid cycle).

It should be noted that the same sequence of reactions serves as a major biosynthetic (but not anaplerotic) pathway during growth on oxalate, the glyoxylate being formed from oxalate by reduction of oxalyl-CoA (Quayle, 1963b):

$$\text{HO}_2\text{C} \cdot \text{COSCoA} + \text{NADPH}_2 \rightarrow \text{HO}_2\text{C} \cdot \text{CHO} + \text{CoASH} + \text{NADP}$$
$$(45)$$

Net Biosynthesis from C_1 Compounds

So far, no case has been found in which an organism growing on a C_1-compound oxidizes the growth substrate through a cyclic mechanism which also serves as a source of biosynthetic intermediates. The energy is

either derived from linear sequences of oxidation reactions of the
C_1-compound, or, in the case of autotrophic organisms where the carbon
source is carbon dioxide, from light or inorganic oxidations. Hence, in
growth on C_1-compounds, a clearer distinction may be drawn between
energy-yielding metabolism and biosynthetic metabolism than is commonly encountered in growth on more complex carbon substrates.
Furthermore, the biochemical singularity of a C_1-utilizing organism, able
to synthesize all its cell constituents from C_1 compounds, can be narrowed
down to its ability to synthesize in net fashion a C_3-skeleton from
C_1-compounds. There is no reason to expect in these organisms a fundamental difference in the way the C_3-compound such as pyruvate, phosphopyruvate or triose phosphate thereafter serves as precursor of
carbohydrate, fat and amino acids.

We shall now outline those mechanisms which offer a solution to this
problem of assembling a C_3-skeleton from C_1-units at different oxidation
levels, and at the same time we shall point out the major problems which
still remain unsolved.

1. Growth on methane

It has been mentioned previously that during microbial growth on
methane, the substrate is oxidized to carbon dioxide via methanol,
formaldehyde and formate. Since the oxidation level of the carbon in
cellular material approximates to that of carbohydrate [CH_2O], it might

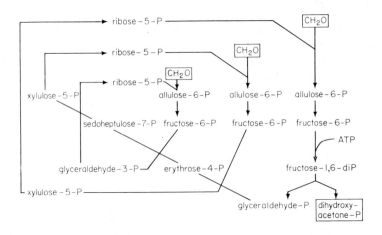

Figure 3.   Ribose phosphate cycle of formaldehyde fixation. (Reproduced from
Process Biochem. (1969) **4**, 25, by permission of the publishers)

be expected that from the range of available C_1-units, CH_4 to CO_2, the greatest economy in intermediary metabolism might be obtained by taking in the C_1-unit at the level of [HCHO] and making therefrom the necessary C_3-skeleton. The ribose phosphate cycle of formaldehyde fixation, discovered in methane or methanol-grown *Pseudomonas methanica*, accomplishes this (Kemp and Quayle, 1967).

The cycle effects a net conversion of formaldehyde units to triose phosphate (Figure 3):

$$3[CH_2O] + ATP \rightarrow \text{triose phosphate} + ADP \qquad (46)$$

The key reactions are the condensation of formaldehyde with ribose-5-phosphate to give allulose-6-phosphate, followed by the epimerization of allulose-6-phosphate to fructose-6-phosphate:

$$
\begin{array}{ccccc}
 & \text{CHO} & \text{CH}_2\text{OH} & \text{CH}_2\text{OH} & \\
 & | & | & | & \\
 & \text{HCOH} & \text{CO} & \text{CO} & \\
 & | & | & | & \\
\text{HCHO} + \text{HCOH} \longrightarrow & \text{HCOH} \longrightarrow & \text{HOCH} & & (47)\\
 & | & | & | & \\
 & \text{HCOH} & \text{HCOH} & \text{HCOH} & \\
 & | & | & | & \\
 & \text{CH}_2\text{OP} & \text{HCOH} & \text{HCOH} & \\
 & & | & | & \\
 & & \text{CH}_2\text{OP} & \text{CH}_2\text{OP} & \\
\end{array}
$$

  ribose-5-phosphate allulose-6-phosphate fructose-6-phosphate

This cycle closely resembles the ribulose diphosphate cycle of carbon dioxide fixation (see Figure 5, section 4), both cycles involve the regeneration of pentose phosphate from hexose phosphates and triose phosphate by means of rearrangements through sedoheptulose and tetrose phosphates. The essential difference between the two cycles lies in the fact that the entering C_1-unit in one case is at the level of formaldehyde and in the other case is at the level of carbon dioxide. Hence, in order to synthesize triose phosphate, net reduction is not necessary with formaldehyde in contrast to carbon dioxide. The cycle of formaldehyde fixation may thus be viewed as a variant of the ribulose diphosphate cycle in which the reductive steps (i.e. phosphoglycerate to phosphoglyceraldehyde) have been eliminated. The economy which results from this may clearly be seen by comparing equation (46) with equation (55). It remains to be seen how general the formaldehyde fixation cycle is amongst organisms capable of growth on methane.

In general methane-utilizing organisms have the remarkable property of only being able to grow on either methane or methanol. This inability to grow on more conventional carbon substrates demands a biochemical explanation.

2. Growth on methanol and methylamine

Elective culture on C_1-substrates (apart from methane), using inocula from a wide range of natural habitats, yields a large number of strains of aerobic C_1-utilizing bacteria which possess similar morphological, cultural and physiological characteristics (see Stocks and McCleskey, 1964). In the past some of these strains have been variously assigned to the genera *Pseudomonas*, *Vibrio* and *Protaminobacter*, but Stocks and McCleskey believe that many of them should be considered as strains of *Vibrio extorquens* (Bassalik). The ubiquity and similarity of these various organisms is such as to suggest that they may be responsible for a great deal of the breakdown of C_1-compounds in nature. It is thus of more than academic importance to know how they grow on these simple substrates. Work with two members of this group, viz. *Pseudomonas* PRL-W4 (Kaneda and Roxburgh, 1959) and *Pseudomonas* AM1 (Large and Quayle, 1963) has shown that serine is one of the earliest compounds to be labelled from [^{14}C]methanol during growth on this substrate. Similar findings have been made by Leadbetter and Gottlieb (1967) in the case of a bacterium growing on methylamine. This suggests that hydroxymethylation of glycine to give serine plays a key role in the synthesis of C_3-compounds from C_2-compounds in such organisms. Work with cell-free extracts indicates that this step is mediated by serine hydroxymethylase (**10**). The methylene tetrahydrofolate is formed from reaction between tetrahydrofolate and formaldehyde, the latter being formed from oxidation of methanol (**19**) or methylamine (**20**). Glycerate may then be formed from serine by the following two steps:

$$HOH_2C \cdot CHNH_2 \cdot CO_2H + R \cdot CO \cdot CO_2H \rightarrow$$
$$HOH_2C \cdot CO \cdot CO_2H + R \cdot CHNH_2 \cdot CO_2H \quad (48)$$
$$HOH_2C \cdot CO \cdot CO_2H + NADH_2 \rightarrow HOH_2C \cdot CHOH \cdot CO_2H + NAD \quad (49)$$

The glycerate thus formed can be phosphorylated to phosphoglycerate by reaction (**44**) and then transformed to phosphopyruvate and pyruvate by established reactions. Confirmation of this general scheme is provided by the finding that mutational loss of hydroxypyruvate reductase, catalysing reaction (**49**), leads to inability to grow on any C_1-compound. Revertants which regain the ability to grow on C_1-compounds are found to be able to synthesize the enzyme (Heptinstall, 1968).

The entire sequence of reactions is dependent on the initial net synthesis of glycine from C_1-units. The mechanism of this seemingly simple reaction remains unknown. It might be thought to proceed by a direct condensation of two C_1-units, or by a cyclic series of reactions as shown in Figure 4. The cyclic system would entail the cleavage of a C_4-compound into two C_2-compounds, one of which would have to be glycine, or a precursor of glycine, in order to regenerate the glycine as acceptor substrate in the cycle. If the other C_2-compound resulting from the cleavage was not glycine or a precursor of glycine, then the problem of net biosynthesis of a C_3-skeleton from this particular C_2-compound would be raised. In the absence of hydroxyaspartate aldolase, isocitrate lyase or glyoxylate carboligase catalysing reactions (3), (22) and (42) respectively, the solution to this problem would not be readily apparent. It should be emphasized that neither a $C_1 + C_1$ condensation nor such a C_4-cleavage reaction has yet been demonstrated in cell-free extracts.

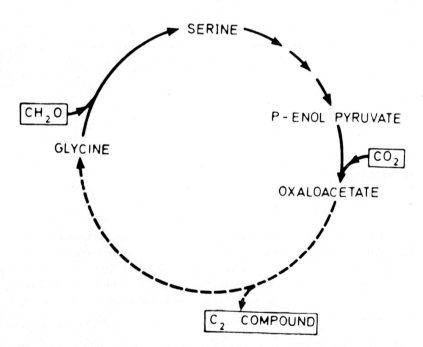

Figure 4. Possible cyclic synthesis of C_2-skeleton from C_1-units by the serine pathway. (Reproduced from *Process Biochem.* (1969) **4**, 25, by permission of the publishers)

Shaw, Tsai and Stadtman (1966) found in pulse labelling experiments that isotope from [^{14}C]methylamine appeared in N-methylglutamate, sarcosine, serine, alanine and aspartate, in that order, during growth of a species of *Pseudomonas* on methylamine. Cell-free extracts of the organism catalysed the formation of N-methylglutamate from methylamine and glutamate by the reaction:

$$CH_3NH_2 + HO_2C \cdot (CH_2)_2 \cdot CHNH_2 \cdot CO_2H \rightarrow$$

$$HO_2C \cdot (CH_2)_2 \cdot CH \cdot CO_2H + NH_3 \quad (50)$$
$$|$$
$$NH \cdot CH_3$$

Similarly, Kung and Wagner (1968) have found early labelling of N-methylglutamate from [^{14}C]methylamine in *Pseudomonas* MS during growth on methylamine. These results contrast with those indicating early labelling of serine in other organisms (see above) as they implicate methylation of the amino groups of glutamate and glycine at an early stage in the assimilation of methylamine into cell constituents. The formation of a C–N bond in this way does not solve the crucial problem of how a C–C bond is made from C_1-units. It may be that N-methyl-glutamate or sarcosine represent carriers of methyl groups in the net biosynthetic process. Should the methyl groups ultimately be used in hydroxymethylation of glycine to give serine, then the N-methylglutamate pathway would be a variant on the serine pathway. It is thus not presently known whether an entirely new pathway of synthesis of cell constituents is involved in those instances in which N-methylglutamate is formed.

Certain of the so-called methane fermenters, for example *Methanosarcina barkerii*, are able to grow anaerobically on methanol in otherwise mineral medium. The overall process of fermentation of the C_1-substrate may be represented by:

$$4CH_3OH \rightarrow 3CH_4 + CO_2 +_2 2H_2O \quad (51)$$

The energy necessary for growth of the organisms is obtained from the above dismutation reaction but nothing is known about the mechanism of coupling. Although considerable advances have been made in elucidating the mechanism of methane formation (Stadtman, 1967) little is known of the way in which cell constituents are made from the C_1-growth substrate.

3. Growth on formate

The carbon in formate is at a more oxidized level than in cell material and hence during growth on this substrate an organism must effect a net reduction. In the case of *Pseudomonas* AM1 it appears that the formate is first reduced to the level of formaldehyde in the form of its tetrahydro-folate derivative (Large and Quayle, 1963):

$$HCO_2H + ATP + THF \rightarrow N^{10}\text{-formyl THF} + ADP + P_i \qquad (52)$$

$$N^{10}\text{-formyl THF} + H^+ \rightarrow N^{5, 10}\text{-methenyl THF} + H_2O \qquad (53)$$

$$N^{5, 10}\text{-methenyl THF} + NADPH_2 \rightarrow N^{5, 10}\text{-methylene THF} + NADP \qquad (54)$$

Thereafter, it is probable that the C_1-unit is assimilated into cell constituents by the same mechanism as is the C_1-unit derived from methanol, namely by reactions (10), (48), (49) and (44). It may be recalled that mutational loss of hydroxypyruvate reductase, catalysing reaction (49), leads to inability to grow on formate.

Throughout this article it has been emphasized that organisms exercise great economy in the number of steps needed to oxidize and assimilate simple carbon substrates. Substrates are not oxidized beyond, and then reduced back to the level appropriate for entry into a cyclic oxidation sequence or a biosynthetic pathway. This would not only involve an unnecessary number of enzymes but would also waste energy in the oxidation and re-reduction processes. Exceptions to this general rule appear in the case of growth on formate by two organisms, *Pseudomonas oxalaticus* (Quayle and Keech, 1959), and *Bacterium formooxydans* (Sorokin, 1961). Both these organisms during growth on formate assimilate more than 90% of their carbon as carbon dioxide. It has been shown by isotopic work with whole cells and enzymatic work with cell-free extracts that *P. oxalaticus* assimilates carbon dioxide by way of the ribulose diphosphate cycle (Quayle and Keech, 1959). The fact that only two cases of autotrophic growth on formate have so far been reported indicates that this may be a rare type of metabolism; considerations of economy may favour the selection of organisms such as *Pseudomonas* AM1 which conserve the reduction level of formate.

The behaviour of *P. oxalaticus* provides a good example of the generalization that in bacterial metabolism maximal growth rate is the guiding principle rather than maximal efficiency (Pardee, 1961). When the organism grows on formate, triose phosphate synthesis from carbon dioxide by the ribulose diphosphate cycle may be expressed by:

$$3CO_2 + 9ATP + 6NADH_2 + 5H_2O \rightarrow \text{triose phosphate} + 9ADP \qquad (55)$$
$$+ 8P_i + 6NAD$$

When the organism grows on oxalate, triose phosphate synthesis by the glycerate pathway may be expressed by:

$$2 \text{ oxalate} + 4ATP + 4NADH_2 \to \text{triose phosphate} + 4ADP$$
$$+ 3P_i + 4NAD + CO_2 \quad (56)$$

Therefore, heterotrophic growth on oxalate is more economical of energy to the extent of $2NADH_2 + 5ATP$ per mole of triose phosphate formed than is growth on carbon dioxide (Blackmore, Walker and Quayle, 1968). It should be remembered that the energy source is the same for growth on both substrates, i.e. NAD-linked dehydrogenation of formate to carbon dioxide (reaction (**42**)). It is thus surprising to find that the growth rate on formate is faster by 38% as compared to growth on oxalate (Blackmore and Quayle, 1968). Furthermore, in an equimolar mixture of formate and oxalate, the organism adopts a metabolism in which autotrophic metabolism of formate predominates. In this case, oxalate is used as an ancillary energy source, being decarboxylated to formate by reactions (**15**) to (**17**) but it is not used as a carbon source. The biosynthetic enzyme, oxalyl-CoA reductase (**45**) is only formed to the extent of 2–3% of its value during growth on oxalate. The control mechanisms in this organism thus produce an enzymic make-up which would not seem ideal for this particular set of circumstances. It is reminiscent of the rather more stark situation brought about when the facultative autotroph *Hydrogenomonas* H16 is placed in a fructose growth medium under a gas mixture of hydrogen and oxygen (Gottschalk, 1965); slow linear growth results due to the hydrogen repressing heterotrophic growth on fructose, and the fructose repressing lithotrophic utilization of hydrogen. Rittenberg (1969) has eloquently described this as 'paralysis in the midst of plenty'.

Formate also can serve as growth substrate for the anaerobes *Methanobacterium formicicum* and *Methanococcus vannielii*, which ferment the formate to methane and carbon dioxide:

$$4HCO_2H \to CH_4 + 3CO_2 + 2H_2O \quad (57)$$

As is the case with the fermentation of methanol little is known about the synthesis of cell constituents from the C_1-substrates or the mechanism of energy coupling from the dismutation reaction.

4. Growth on carbon dioxide

Carbon dioxide is a unique carbon source; it is unique because it represents the ultimate state of biochemical oxidation of carbon and hence no organism can grow on it as a combined carbon and energy source. Energy must be obtained from elsewhere, for example from light in the case of photosynthetic organisms, from inorganic oxidation in the case of chemolithotrophs, or from organic oxidation in the case of an organism such as *P. oxalaticus* growing on formate. The mechanisms of energy coupling which operate are complex and have been fully reviewed elsewhere (Vernon, 1968; Peck, 1968).

The carbon metabolism of autotrophic bacteria growing on carbon dioxide as the sole carbon source is largely accounted for by operation of the ribulose diphosphate cycle (Figure 5). This cycle of reactions was

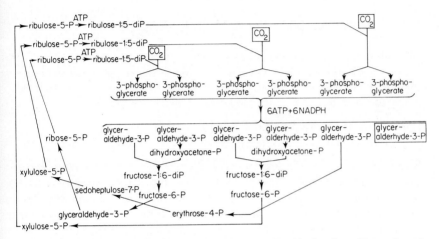

Figure 5. Ribulose diphosphate cycle of carbon dioxide fixation. (Reproduced from *Process Biochem.* (1969) **4**, 25, by permission of the publishers)

discovered in plant tissue mainly by the work of Calvin and his colleagues (see Bassham and Calvin, 1960). The two key reactions of the cycle which are unique to it are ribulose diphosphate carboxylase catalysing the carboxylation and dismutation of ribulose-1, 5-diphosphate:

$$
\begin{array}{cccc}
\text{CH}_2\text{OP} & & & \\
| & & & \\
\text{CO} & & \text{CO}_2\text{H} & \\
| & & | & \\
\text{HCOH} & + \text{CO}_2 + \text{H}_2\text{O} \rightarrow 2 & \text{HCOH} & \quad (58) \\
| & & | & \\
\text{HCOH} & & \text{CH}_2\text{OP} & \\
| & & & \\
\text{CH}_2\text{OP} & & &
\end{array}
$$

and, phosphoribulokinase catalysing the phosphorylation of ribulose-5-phosphate:

$$
\begin{array}{ccc}
\begin{array}{l}
\text{CH}_2\text{OH} \\
| \\
\text{CO} \\
| \\
\text{HCOH} + \text{ATP} \\
| \\
\text{HCOH} \\
| \\
\text{CH}_2\text{OP}
\end{array}
& \rightarrow &
\begin{array}{l}
\text{CH}_2\text{OP} \\
| \\
\text{CO} \\
| \\
\text{HCOH} + \text{ADP} \qquad (59) \\
| \\
\text{HCOH} \\
| \\
\text{CH}_2\text{OP}
\end{array}
\end{array}
$$

The input of carbon into the cycle occurs by way of reaction (58), the necessary net reduction of carbon from the level of carbon dioxide to that of [CH$_2$O] is then effected by reduction of the carboxyl group of phosphoglycerate to the aldehyde group of phosphoglyceraldehyde:

$$H_2PO_3 \cdot O \cdot CH_2 \cdot CH(OH) \cdot CO_2H + ATP + NADPH_2 \rightarrow$$
$$H_3PO_3 \cdot O \cdot CH_2 \cdot CH(OH) \cdot CHO + ADP + H_3PO_4 + NADP \quad (60)$$

Regeneration of the ribulose skeleton then takes place through a series of rearrangements and the cycle is finally completed by the resynthesis of the acceptor compound ribulose-1,5-diphosphate by reaction (59). The overall operation of the cycle results in the net synthesis of triose phosphate from three molecules of carbon dioxide according to reaction (55).

An alternative cycle of net carbon dioxide fixation involving reversal of a large part of the tricarboxylic acid cycle has been proposed by Arnon and his colleagues. They suggest that it may operate alongside the ribulose diphosphate cycle during photosynthetic growth of *Chlorobium thiosulphatophilum* (Evans, Buchanan and Arnon, 1966) and *Rhodospirillum rubrum* (Buchanan, Evans and Arnon, 1967).

The concomitant utilization of organic compounds and carbon dioxide by chemosynthetic and photosynthetic autotrophs gives rise to complicated intermediary metabolism. This topic lies outside the scope of this article but has been covered in recent reviews (Gibbs, 1967; Rittenberg, 1969).

III. CO-ORDINATION OF METABOLIC ROUTES

The operation of the various metabolic routes that we have described does not occur in a random and uncontrolled fashion but is precisely adjusted to the needs of the organism. These needs are largely determined by the nature of the carbon source for growth. Clearly, if no restrictions are placed in growth, the rate at which microorganisms double will be dictated by the balance between the rates of inflow of metabolites into the energy-yielding pathways, the rates of outflow into anabolic routes, and (where appropriate) the rates of replenishment of cyclic sequences that serve a catabolic as well as an anabolic function. Two types of mechanisms ensure that these various metabolic processes are coordinated one with another.

The first of these, which may be loosely termed 'fine' control, affects the rate at which key enzymes *already present in a cell* act. This type of control is often mediated via metabolites that are not themselves transformed in the catalytic process but are produced by a neighbouring pathway, or are either a distant precursor or product of the pathway in which the enzyme plays a necessary role; the controlling metabolite exerts its effect by causing conformational changes in the sensitive enzyme that profoundly affect the rate of its catalytic activity. Since the controlling metabolite usually bears no structural similarity to the reactants or products of the reaction catalysed by the key enzyme, it is termed an 'allosteric' effector (Monod and Jacob, 1961).

Allosteric effectors either accelerate or decelerate enzymic processes. Examples of the former, taken from the pathways we have described, are the effect of acetyl-CoA on the carboxylation of C_3-compounds (see section II, 2(b)): neither the carboxylation of pyruvate (reaction (33)) in for example *A. globiformis* (Bridgeland and Jones, 1967) or thermophilic bacilli (Sundaram, Cazzulo and Kornberg, 1969) nor the carboxylation of PEP in the Enterobacteriaceae (Canovas and Kornberg, 1966) proceed at rates physiologically sufficient in the absence of acetyl-CoA. Similarly, the need for high activity of PEP carboxylation during glycolysis, both via PEP-carboxylase and via pyruvate kinase is 'signalled' by the potentiating effect exerted by fructose-1,6-diphosphate, on PEP-carboxylase (Sanwal and Maeba, 1966) and on *one* of the two types of pyruvate kinase found in *E. coli* (Malcovati and Kornberg, 1969).

Deceleration of enzyme activity by allosteric effectors was first observed by Umbarger (1956) in an anabolic pathway, who referred to this process as 'end product' or 'feedback' inhibition. Neither term is strictly applicable to the pathways we described in this article: as previously emphasized (Kornberg, 1965), the metabolic reactions we discuss have no unambiguously identifiable end product. However, the allosteric inhibition of enzyme activity that plays so important a role in the coordination of these pathways can often be loosely described in the same terms more aptly applied to anabolic routes. Thus, if the tricarboxylic acid cycle can be said to have end products, these are CO_2, $NADH_2$ and (ultimately) ATP. It is thus suggestive that the citrate synthases, the action of which initiate each turn of the cycle, are subject to allosteric inhibition by either $NADH_2$ or ATP. The enzyme from Gram-positive bacteria is inhibited by ATP but not by $NADH_2$; the converse applies to the citrate synthases of Gram-negative organisms (Weitzman, 1966; Weitzman and Jones, 1968). This difference is reflected also in the molecular size of the enzymes: those citrate synthases not inhibited by $NADH_2$ were found to be much smaller (i.e. to be composed of fewer sub-units) than those sensitive to $NADH_2$ (Weitzman and Dunmore, 1969).

It is of interest to compare this behaviour with the action of ATP and AMP on phosphoribulokinase (reaction (59)). This enzyme catalyses the formation of ribulose-1,5-diphosphate, the acceptor molecule for carbon dioxide in the ribulose diphosphate cycle of carbon dioxide fixation. Hence, one way in which the input of carbon dioxide into the cycle might be controlled is by regulation of the rate at which ribulose-1,5-diphosphate is formed. It has been found that the phosphoribulokinase from several different types of autotrophic organisms, for example *Thiobacillus thioparus*, *Chromatium* D and spinach is inhibited by AMP (Johnson, 1966). Furthermore, at low concentrations of ATP the activity of the enzyme is increased in a cooperative fashion by increasing concentrations of the ATP (McElroy, Johnson and Johnson, 1968). The activity of the enzyme can thus be regulated by the ratio of the relative concentrations of ATP and AMP, the activity being greatest when ATP > AMP and lowest when AMP > ATP. This could of course be in accord with the need of a cell to increase the input of carbon into an anabolic cycle when the energy status is high, and *vice versa*.

Similar arguments apply to the allosteric control of anaplerotic reactions. The physiological function of the carboxylases that act on C_3-compounds is to form C_4-acid intermediates of the tricarboxylic acid cycle; it is therefore reasonable that the potentiating effect of acetyl-CoA on these enzymes can be overcome by sufficiently high concentrations of C_4-acids, such as aspartate (Izui, Iwatani, Nishikido, Katsuki and Tanaka, 1967; Smith, 1968; Cazzulo, Sundaram and Kornberg, 1969). By the same token the glyoxylate cycle ensures that, during microbial growth on acetate, the tricarboxylic acid cycle is not drained of its biosynthetic precursors. One of the quantitatively most important drains on these intermediates is the synthesis of carbohydrate: these carbohydrates form the glycerol moieties of membrane lipids, components of the cell wall, storage polysaccharides, and the pentoses of DNA and RNA. In addition, the aromatic amino acids, and others such as histidine, alanine, isoleucine and serine, are derived from intermediates of glycolysis. The synthesis of all these substances from the C_4-dicarboxylic acids of the tricarboxylic acid cycle requires, as the first step, the formation of phospho*enol*pyruvate through the action of PEP-carboxykinase (35) or, possibly (in mutants lacking this enzyme), through the combined action of the 'malic enzyme' (reaction (34)) and PEP-synthase reaction (37). Phospho*enol*pyruvate may thus be regarded as a major end product of the glyoxylate cycle, and it is thus not surprising that, by analogy with the end product inhibition of other metabolic pathways (Umbarger, 1964), both phospho*enol*-pyruvate (Ashworth and Kornberg, 1963) and pyruvate (Kornberg, 1966b) inhibit the activity of isocitrate lyase. Since this enzyme is considerably more sensitive to inhibition by PEP than by pyruvate at pH $< 8 \cdot 5$, but more sensitive to pyruvate than to PEP at higher pH values (Ashworth, 1965; Syrett and John, 1968), the possibility of regulating the activity of this enzyme by either C_3-compound may be of advantage to an organism growing in an unbuffered environment.

In addition to these two main types of allosteric effects on enzyme activity, a possible allosteric control of the *formation* of an active enzyme from its apo-enzyme has been indicated by the observation that cell-free extracts of a thermophilic bacillus convert apo-pyruvate carboxylase and biotin to the active pyruvate carboxylase only slowly, but do so rapidly if acetyl-CoA is also present; this stimulating effect of acetyl-CoA is largely overcome by aspartate (Cazzulo and coworkers, 1969). However, the physiological significance of this effect, and its implications for other enzymic processes, remain to be clarified.

The regulatory reactions so far discussed act on enzymes already present in the cell and, as implied by their description as 'fine control' processes, are immediate in their effect. In addition to them, microorganisms possess the striking ability to 'select' the metabolic routes most appropriate to the utilization of their carbon sources, by regulating the rate at which key enzymes of these pathways are *synthesized*. This type of control through 'enzymic adaptation' (Karström, 1938), which may be viewed as a 'coarse' control process, is inevitably less immediately responsive to environmental changes than 'fine' controls; it is achieved by regulating the activity not of enzymes, but of genes.

The conclusion that a certain metabolic pathway plays a necessary as well as a sufficient role in the utilization of a particular carbon compound usually rest on two types of experimental observation (not necessarily in the order here listed). One depends on the isolation of mutants deficient in a component enzyme of that pathway: if such mutants fail to grow on the carbon source believed to be utilized via that pathway, and 'revertants' able again to utilize that carbon source also regain the activity of the defective enzyme, the physiological role of the pathway may be regarded as being, if not established, at least strongly indicated. The use of this type of evidence in establishing the importance of the tricarboxylic acid cycle in providing both energy and biosynthetic intermediates is perhaps most clearly illustrated by the work of Gilvarg and Davis (1956), who were first to show that an *E. coli* mutant devoid of citrate synthase activity not only failed to oxidize acetate but also required glutamate for growth. Similar evidence has been obtained in elucidating other biosynthetic and anaplerotic pathways, and this has been already referred to in previous sections.

Another type of evidence is provided by measurement of the rates of 'preferential synthesis' (Monod, 1956) of key enzymes of the pathway under consideration, compared with the rates of growth of the organism as a whole. (This, indeed, is a means of quantifying the process of 'enzymic adaptation'.) This type of experimental test has been applied to discern the role of virtually all the metabolic routes discussed in this article. Thus, the unique nature of the biosynthetic routes for growth on C_1-compounds is illustrated by the preferential synthesis of hydroxypyruvate reductase when organisms are transferred from media containing for example succinate as sole carbon source to media containing only the C_1-compound methanol (Large and Quayle, 1963); the interrelationship of the pathways required for the utilization of formate and oxalate is suggested by the observations that phosphoribulokinase and ribulose diphosphate carboxylase are synthesized during growth on formate but not appreciably synthesized during growth on oxalate (Quayle and Keech, 1960; Blackmore and Quayle, 1968), whereas oxalyl-CoA decarboxylase and oxalyl-CoA reductase are synthesized during growth on oxalate but not appreciably during growth on formate (Quayle and coworkers, 1961; Quayle, 1963a). The role of the glyoxylate cycle during growth on acetate is suggested by the finding that its key enzymes are preferentially synthesized as succinate or lactate-grown cells are transferred to media containing acetate (Kornberg, Gotto and Lund, 1958; Kornberg, 1966b); the change-over from the tricarboxylic to the dicarboxylic acid cycle as main energy yielding pathway is indicated by the alteration in the ratio of malate to citrate-synthase activity as cells adapt to glycollate utilization (Kornberg, 1961); and the operation of the glycerate pathway is reflected in the high rates of preferential synthesis of glyoxylate carboligase and tartronic semialdehyde reductase under these circumstances (Kornberg, 1961; Sadler, 1961).

Although these types of study provide good evidence for the physiological role of metabolic pathways, they do not provide more than anecdotal evidence on the mechanisms of operation of these 'coarse' controls.

This is because, as stated earlier, these controls are symptomatic of the selective expression of genetic potential, and can be fully understood only in the knowledge of that potential. Unfortunately, genetic analysis is feasible only with microorganisms in which the recombination of hereditary material from a donor cell with that of a recipient can be demonstrated: this, at present limits the range of test organisms to fungi and to a few species of bacteria. For lack of other data, we shall consider in detail the analysis of the mechanism of 'coarse' control processes with only one pathway: the glyoxylate cycle.

Physiological studies (Kornberg, 1966b) indicated that, in addition to the 'fine' control of isocitrate lyase activity, pyruvate and/or PEP act also as metabolite repressors, and thus exert also a 'coarse' control over the cycle. Genetic analysis of mutants of *E. coli* further indicates that the synthesis of the anaplerotic enzymes of the glyoxylate cycle is regulated in a manner similar to that governing the expression of the *lac* operon (Jacob and Monod, 1961). The evidence for this view may be summarized as follows:

(a) Isocitrate lyase and malate synthase are coordinately induced and repressed (Kornberg, 1966b).

(b) Mutants that form isocitrate lyase constitutively also form malate synthase constitutively (Vanderwinkel, Liard, Ramos and Wiame, 1963).

(c) The structural genes for the (anaplerotic) malate synthase (Vanderwinkel and de Vlieghere, 1968) and isocitrate lyase (Kornberg and Smith, 1966) are situated in close proximity to each other and to a regulator gene (Brice and Kornberg, 1968) that specifies the inducibility of both enzymes, on the *E. coli* genome.

(d) In merodiploids, inducibility of isocitrate lyase (and malate synthase) synthesis is *trans*-dominant to constitutivity (Kornberg, 1969).

These observations suggest that the regulator gene specifies the synthesis of a repressor, activated by pyruvate or PEP; the activated repressor prevents the transcription of the genetic information for the synthesis of the two anaplerotic enzymes of the glyoxylate cycle. 'Constitutive' mutants would either produce no repressor, or (more likely) a repressor altered in its ability to interact with the genome or with the C_3-acid co-repressor; the introduction, via an F′ particle, of a normal regulator gene restores the inducibility of the enzymes since the episomal gene specifies the synthesis of a normal repressor.

F

References

Andrew, I. G., and Morris, J. G. (1965). *Biochem. Biophys. Acta*, **97**, 176.

Anthony, C., and Zatman, L. J. (1964). *Biochem. J.*, **92**, 614.

Anthony, C., and Zatman, L. J. (1967). *Biochem. J.*, **104**, 960.

Ashworth, J. M. (1965). Ph.D. Thesis, University of Leicester.

Ashworth, J. M., and Kornberg, H. L. (1963). *Biochim. Biophys. Acta*, **73**, 519.

Ashworth, J. M., and Kornberg, H. L. (1966). *Proc. Roy. Soc., B.*, **165**, 179.

Ashworth, J. M., Kornberg, H. L., and Nothmann, D. L. (1965). *J. Mol. Biol.*, **11**, 654.

Bandurski, R. S., and Greiner, C. M. (1953). *J. Biol. Chem.*, **204**, 781.

Bassham, J. A., and Calvin, M. In *Encyclopedia of Plant Physiology*, V. Pt. 1, p. 884. Ruhland, W. Ed., Springer Verlag, 1960.

Blackmore, M. A., and Quayle, J. R. (1968). *Biochem. J.*, **107**, 705.

Blackmore, M. A., Walker, I. O., and Quayle, J. R. (1968). *Biochem. J.*, **107**, 699.

Brice, C. B., and Kornberg, H. L. (1968). *J. Bact.*, **96**, 2185.

Bridgeland, E. S., and Jones, K. M. (1967). *Biochem. J.*, **104**, 9P.

Brown, L. R., Strawinski, R. J., and McCleskey, C. S. (1964). *Can. J. Microbiol.*, **10**, 791.

Buchanan, B. B., Evans, M. C. W., and Arnon, D. I. (1967). *Arch. Microbiol.*, **59**, 32.

Canovas, J. L., and Kornberg, H. L. (1966). *Proc. Roy. Soc., B.*, **165**, 189.

Cazzulo, J. J., and Stoppani, A. O. M. (1965). *Biochim. Biophys. Acta*, **100**, 276.

Cazzulo, J. J., Sundaram, T. K., and Kornberg, H. L. (1969). *Nature*, Lond., **223**, 1137.

Chiriboa, J. (1963). *Biochem. Biophys. Res. Commun.*, **11**, 277.

Cooper, R. A., and Kornberg, H. L. (1967a). *Proc. Roy. Soc., B.*, **168**, 263.

Cooper, R. A., and Kornberg, H. L. (1967b). *Biochim. Biophys. Acta*, **141**, 211.

Cooper, R. A., and Kornberg, H. L. (1967c). *Biochem. J.*, **105**, 49C.

Datta, P. K., and Meeuse, B. J. D. (1955). *Biochim. Biophys. Acta*, **17**, 602.

den Dooren de Jong, L. E. (1926). Dissertation, Rotterdam (seen in Stephenson, M. (1960). *Bacterial Metabolism*, 3rd ed., p. 183. London: Longmans, Green & Co.).

Doughty, C. C., Hayashi, J. A., and Guenther, H. L. (1966). *J. Biol. Chem.*, **241**, 568.

Eady, R. R., and Large, P. J. (1968). *Biochem. J.*, **106**, 245.

Eady, R. R., and Large, P. J. (1969). *Biochem. J.*, **111**, 37P.

Evans, H. J., and Wood, H. G. (1968). *Proc. Nat. Acad. Sci.*, Wash., **61**, 1448.

Evans, M. C. W., Buchanan, B. B., and Arnon, D. I. (1966). *Proc. Nat. Acad. Sci.*, Wash., **55**, 928.

Gibbs, M. (1967). *Ann. Rev. Biochem.*, **36**, 757.

Gilvarg, C., and Davis, B. D. (1956). *J. Biol. Chem.*, **222**, 307.

Gotto, A. M., and Kornberg, H. L. (1961). *Biochem. J.*, **81**, 273.

Gottschalk, G. (1965). *Biochem. Z.*, **341**, 260.

Heptinstall, J. (1968). Ph.D. Thesis, University of Sheffield.

Heptinstall, J., and Quayle, J. R. (1969). *J. Gen. Microbiol.*, **55**, xvi.

Izui, K., Iwatani, A., Nishikido, T., Katsuki, H., and Tanaka, S. (1967). *Biochim. Biophys. Acta*, **139**, 188.

Jacob, F., and Monod, J. (1961). *J. Mol. Biol.*, **3**, 318.
Jakoby, W. B., Ohmura, E., and Hayaishi, O. (1956). *J. Biol. Chem.*, **222**, 435.
Johnson, E. J. (1966). *Arch. Biochem. Biophys.*, **114**, 179.
Johnson, P. A., and Quayle, J. R. (1964). *Biochem. J.*, **93**, 281.
Jones, K. M., and Bridgeland, E. S. (1966). *Biochem. J.*, **99**, 25P.
Kaneda, T., and Roxburgh, J. M. (1959). *Can. J. Microbiol.*, **5**, 87.
Karström, H. (1938). *Ergebn. Enzymforsch.*, **7**, 350.
Keech, D. B., and Utter, M. F. (1963). *J. Biol. Chem.*, **238**, 2609.
Kemp, M. B., and Quayle, J. R. (1967). *Biochem. J.*, **102**, 94.
Kornberg, H. L. (1959). *Ann. Rev. Microbiol.*, **13**, 49.
Kornberg, H. L. (1961). *Cold Spr. Harb. Symp. Quant. Biol.*, **26**, 257.
Kornberg, H. L. (1965). *Symp. Soc. Gen. Microbiol.*, **15**, 8.
Kornberg, H. L. (1966a). *Essays in Biochemistry*, **2**, 1.
Kornberg, H. L. (1966b). *Biochem. J.*, **99**, 1.
Kornberg, H. L. (1969). *Symp. 6th FEBS Meeting, Madrid*, **19**, 5.
Kornberg, H. L., and Elsden, S. R. (1961). *Advanc. Enzymol.*, **23**, 401.
Kornberg, H. L., and Gotto, A. M. (1959). *Nature, Lond.*, **183**, 1791.
Kornberg, H. L., Gotto, A. M., and Lund, P. (1958). *Nature, Lond.*, **182**, 1430.
Kornberg, H. L., and Krebs, H. A. (1957). *Nature, Lond.*, **179**, 988.
Kornberg, H. L., and Lascelles, J. (1960). *J. Gen. Microbiol.*, **23**, 511.
Kornberg, H. L., and Madsen, N. B. (1957). *Biochim. Biophys. Acta*, **24**, 651.
Kornberg, H. L., and Morris, J. G. (1965). *Biochem. J.*, **95**, 577.
Kornberg, H. L., and Sadler, J. R. (1960). *Nature, Lond.*, **185**, 153.
Kornberg, H. L., and Smith, J. (1966). *Biochim. Biophys. Acta*, **123**, 654.
Krakow, G., and Barkulis, S. S. (1956). *Biochim. Biophys. Acta*, **21**, 593.
Krebs, H. A. (1943). *Ann. Rev. Biochem.*, **12**, 529.
Krebs, H. A., Gurin, S., and Eggleston, L. V. (1952). *Biochem. J.*, **51**, 614.
Krebs, H. A., and Johnson, W. A. (1937). *Enzymologia*, **4**, 148.
Krebs, H. A., and Kornberg, H. L. (1957). *Ergebn. Physiol.*, **49**, 212.
Krebs, H. A., and Lowenstein, J. M. In *Metabolic Pathways*, vol. 1, p. 129, Greenberg, D. M., Ed., Academic Press, 1960.
Kung, H., and Wagner, C. (1968). *Bact. Proc.*, 115.
Large, P. J., Peel, D., and Quayle, J. R. (1962). *Biochem. J.*, **85**, 243.
Large, P. J., and Quayle, J. R. (1963). *Biochem. J.*, **87**, 386.
Leadbetter, E. R., and Gottlieb, J. A. (1967). *Arch. Microbiol.*, **59**, 211.
Lochmüller, H., Wood, H. G., and Davis, J. J. (1966). *J. Biol. Chem.*, **241**, 5678.
Malcovati, M., and Kornberg, H. L. (1969). *Biochim. biophys. Acta*, **178**, 420.
McElroy, R. D., Johnson, E. J., and Johnson, M. K. (1968). *Biochem. Biophys. Res. Commun.*, **30**, 678.
Monod, J. In *Enzymes: Units of biological structure and function*, p .7, Gaebler O. H., Ed., Academic Press, 1956.
Monod, J., and Jacob, F. (1961). *Cold Spr. Harb. Symp. Quant. Biol.*, **26**, 389.
Olson, J. A. (1954). *Nature, Lond.*, **194**, 695.
Pardee, A. B. (1961). *Symp. Soc. Gen. Microbiol.*, **11**, 19.
Peck, H. D. (1968). *Ann. Rev. Microbiol.*, **22**, 489.
Quayle, J. R. (1963a). *Biochem. J.*, **89**, 492.
Quayle, J. R. (1963b). *Biochem. J.*, **87**, 368.
Quayle, J. R., and Keech, D. B. (1959). *Biochem. J.*, **72**, 631.
Quayle, J. R., and Keech, D. B. (1960). *Biochem. J.*, **75**, 515.

Quayle, J. R., Keech, D. B., and Taylor, G. A. (1961). *Biochem. J.*, **78**, 225.
Rittenberg, S. C. (1969). *Advanc. Microbiol. Physiol.*, **3**, 159.
Ruiz-Amil, M., de Torrontegui, G., Palacián, E., Catalina, L., and Losada, M. (1965). *J. Biol. Chem.*, **240**, 3485.
Sadler, J. R. (1961). D.Phil. Thesis, University of Oxford.
Sanwal, B. D., and Maeba, P. (1966). *Biochem. Biophys. Res. Commun.*, **22**, 194.
Saz, H. J. (1954). *Biochem. J.*, **58**, xx.
Seubert, W., and Remberger, V. (1961). *Biochem. Z.*, **334**, 401.
Shaw, W. V., Tsai, L., and Stadtman, E. R. (1966). *J. Biol. Chem.*, **241**, 935.
Smith, T. E. (1968). *Arch. Biochem. Biophys.*, **128**, 611.
Smith, R. A., and Gunsalus, I. C. (1954). *J. Amer. Chem. Soc.*, **76**, 5002.
Sorokin, Y. I. (1961). *Microbiol. (U.S.S.R.) Eng. Trans.*, **30**, 337.
Stadtman, T. C. (1967). *Ann. Rev. Microbiol.*, **21**, 121.
Stocks, P. K., and McCleskey, C. S. (1964). *J. Bact.*, **88**, 1065.
Sundaram, T. K., Cazzulo, J. J., and Kornberg, H. L. (1969). *Biochim. Biophys. Acta*, **192**, 355.
Syrett, P. J., and John, P. C. L. (1968). *Biochem. Biophys. Acta*, **151**, 295.
Umbarger, H. E. (1956). *Science*, **123**, 848.
Umbarger, H. E. (1964). *Science*, **145**, 674.
Vanderwinkel, E., and de Vlieghere, M. (1968). *European J. Biochem.*, **5**, 81.
Vanderwinkel, E., Liard, P., Ramos, F., and Wiame, J. M. (1963). *Biochem. Biophys. Res. Commun.*, **12**, 157.
Vernon, L. P. (1968). *Bact. Rev.*, **32**, 243.
Weitzman, P. D. J. (1966). *Biochim. Biophys. Acta*, **128**, 213.
Weitzman, P. D. J., and Jones, D. (1968). *Nature*, Lond., **219**, 270.
Weitzman, P. D. J., and Dunmore, P. (1969). *Biochim. Biophys. Acta*, **171**, 198.
Wong, D. T. O., and Ajl, S. J. (1956). *J. Amer. Chem. Soc.*, **78**, 3230.
Wood, H. G., and Werkman, C. H. (1938). *Biochem. J.*, **32**, 1262.

EXPERIMENTS WITH (−)-HYDROXYCITRATE

John M. Lowenstein

Graduate Department of Biochemistry, Brandeis University,
Waltham, Massachusetts 02154

INTRODUCTION

Hydroxycitrate was first reported to occur as a minor constituent of sugar beets by E. von Lippman (1883). The first biochemical investigation of the stereoisomers of hydroxycitrate was conducted by Martius and Maué (1941). Using the methylene blue test for dehydrogenase activity, these authors demonstrated that racemic hydroxycitrate is attacked by what was presumed to be isocitrate dehydrogenase from various sources. On the other hand, racemic *allo*-hydroxycitrate is not attacked. Racemic hydroxycitrate was resolved, and it was shown that only the (+)-isomer is attacked. These results have recently been confirmed in my laboratory by Jean White. She found that highly purified preparations of isocitrate dehydrogenase from beef heart and beef liver catalyse the reduction of TPN to TPNH when the (+) but not the (−)-isomer of hydroxycitrate is tested as substrate.

The (−)-isomer of hydroxycitrate was first isolated from *Garcinia cambogia* by Lewis and Neelakantan (1964, 1965). The (+)-*allo*-isomer was first isolated from *Hibiscus sabdariffa* by Griebel (1939, 1942). Isolation procedures for both isomers have recently been described in detail by Lewis (1969). The absolute configurations of the lactones of these compounds have been determined by X-ray crystallography (Glusker, 1969). This work confirms the predictions of the absolute configurations made earlier by Lewis.

The steric relation of citrate and 'natural' isocitrate to the four stereoisomers of hydroxycitrate is shown in Scheme 1. The absolute configuration of citrate derived from oxaloacetate and acetyl CoA via the citrate synthase reaction are shown in Scheme 1a, as are the absolute configurations of *cis*-aconitate and D_s-isocitrate derived from such citrate via the aconitase reaction (Lowenstein, 1967). Scheme 1b shows that the stereochemistry of (+)-hydroxycitrate corresponds to that of D_s-isocitrate, the

* Publication number 705 of the Graduate Department of Biochemistry, Brandeis University.

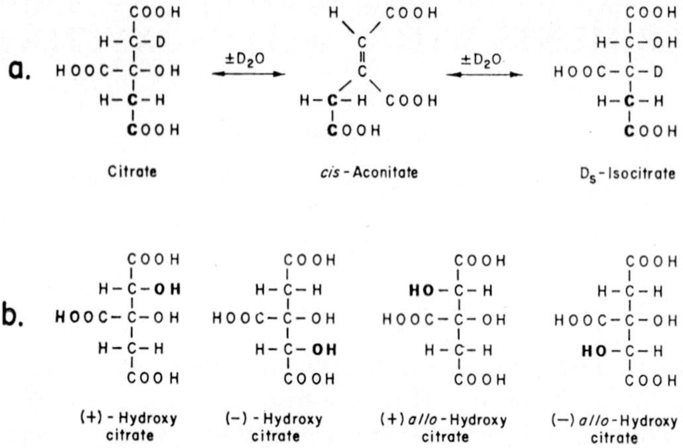

Scheme 1. Fischer projection formulas of the absolute configuration of the stereoisomers of hydroxycitrate in relation to the absolute configuration of citrate, *cis*-aconitate and D_s-isocitrate. In a, the carbon atoms from the acetyl group of acetyl–CoA which become citrate in the citrate synthase reaction are shown in heavy outline. The stereochemistry of the aconitase reaction is shown by depicting the reaction as it occurs in D_2O. In b, the hydroxyl group shown in heavy outline is unique to the particular stereoisomer of hydroxycitrate. The configuration of (+)-hydroxycitrate corresponds to that of D_s-isocitrate. (Note that in the projection formulas the horizontal bonds point from the vertical bonds towards the reader)

'natural' substrate of isocitrate dehydrogenases from animal sources. This is in harmony with the finding that (+)-hydroxycitrate is a substrate for isocitrate dehydrogenase.

In the reaction catalysed by citrate cleavage enzyme (reaction **1**), the carbon atoms of citrate which become the acetyl group of acetyl CoA are the same stereochemically as the carbon atoms of the acetyl group of acetyl CoA which become citrate in the reaction catalysed by citrate synthase (reaction **2**)

$$\text{citrate} + \text{ATP} + \text{CoA} \rightarrow \text{acetyl CoA} + \text{oxaloacetate} + \text{ADP} + P_i \quad (1)$$
$$\text{acetyl CoA} + \text{oxaloacetate} + H_2O \rightarrow \text{citrate} + \text{CoA} \quad (2)$$

(Spencer and Lowenstein, 1962). This finding has been confirmed (Bhaduri and Srere, 1963). The carbon atoms of citrate in question are shown in heavy outline in Scheme 1a. Comparison with the four compounds in Scheme 1b shows that (−)-hydroxycitrate and (−)-*allo*-hydroxycitrate carry a hydroxyl group on the carbon atom of citrate which normally becomes the methyl group of acetyl CoA in the citrate cleavage reaction.

It might be mentioned that from the mechanistic view, the presence of an additional hydroxyl group in the 2-position of citrate would be expected to facilitate cleavage of the carbon–carbon bond between the two hydroxyl-carrying carbons. However, (−)-hydroxycitrate does not appear to be cleaved by citrate cleavage enzyme, at least not as far as can be ascertained through hydroxamate assays. Instead, we have found that (−)-hydroxycitrate is a potent inhibitor of citrate cleavage enzyme (Watson, Fang and Lowenstein, 1969). Apparently the steric positioning of the additional hydroxyl group enhances binding to the enzyme but prevents a subsequent step in the catalytic sequence. The other stereo-isomer, (−)-*allo*-hydroxycitrate, has not so far been available for testing in the citrate cleavage reaction.

INHIBITION OF CITRATE CLEAVAGE ENZYME*
BY HYDROXYCITRATE

(−)-Hydroxycitrate is a powerful inhibitor of the reaction catalysed by citrate cleavage enzyme (reaction 1). The inhibition is competitive with respect to citrate. At a KCl concentration of 300 mM, the K_m for citrate is about 200 μM, while the K_i for (−)-hydroxycitrate is about 0·57 μM (Figure 1). At a KCl concentration of 85 mM the K_m and K_i values are 70 and 0·15 μM respectively (Watson, Fang and Lowenstein, 1969). Under similar conditions, (+)-*allo*-hydroxycitrate has little inhibitory effect on the enzyme.

FATTY ACID SYNTHESIS IN NON-RUMINANT MAMMALS

In the breakdown of foodstuffs, pyruvate derived from carbohydrate and fatty acids derived from fat are converted to acetyl-CoA by intra-mitochondrial enzyme systems. Under normal conditions of carbohydrate utilization, the rate of oxidation of the acetyl group of acetyl-CoA via the citric acid cycle is determined by the energy demands of the tissue, or its equivalent, the availability of ADP. When the carbohydrate intake of an animal is in excess of its energy requirements the glycogen stores become filled. Thereafter excess carbohydrate is broken down to pyruvate. The reactions of glycolysis occur in the extramitochondrial space of the cell. However, the oxidation of pyruvate to acetyl-CoA occurs in the mito-chondria. Acetyl groups not required for energy production are converted into fatty acids. In the rat, fatty acid synthesis occurs predominantly in the extramitochondrial space of the cell. The transfer of the acetyl group of acetyl-CoA from the intramitochondrial space into the cytoplasm is thus

---

* ATP: citrate–oxaloacetatelyase (CoA-acetylating and ATP-dephosphorylat-ing), EC 4.1.3.8.

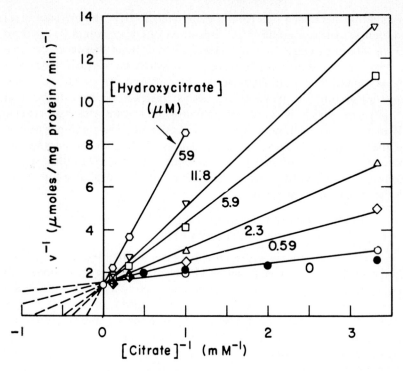

Figure 1. Inhibition of citrate cleavage by $(-)$-hydroxycitrate. The reaction mixture contained 20 mM $MgCl_2$, 300 mM KCl, 0·34 mM CoA, 93 mM Tris–HCl buffer, pH 8·2, 10 mM dithiothreitol, 3·33 mM ATP, 0·16 mM DPNH, malate dehydrogenase (0·33 unit/ml) citrate cleavage enzyme (1·7 milliunits/ml, specific activity about 2), and citrate and $(-)$-hydroxycitrate as indicated. The final volume was 3·0 ml and the temperature was 23° C. The assay was started by addition of ATP, and the reaction was followed by measuring the decrease in absorbance at 340 mμ (Watson, Fang and Lowenstein, 1969)

an important step in the conversion of carbohydrate into fat by non-ruminant mammals (Lowenstein, 1968).

Various ways in which the acetyl group of intramitochondrial acetyl-CoA might be transferred into the extramitochondrial space of the cell are summarized in Scheme 2 (Spencer and Lowenstein, 1962; Lowenstein, 1963). Each of the possible pathways shown in the Scheme was examined in terms of rates of diffusion of metabolites and of intra- and extramito-chondrial enzyme levels. On this basis it was concluded that *citrate is the major source of the acetyl group of acetyl CoA which is used for the extramitochondrial synthesis of fatty acids* in non-ruminant mammals

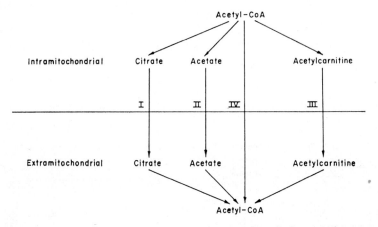

Scheme 2. Four possible pathways for the transfer of the acetyl group of acetyl-CoA from the intra- to the extramitochondrial space of the cell. In I, citrate is formed from acetyl-CoA by the citrate synthase reaction. Citrate is then transferred into the extramitochondrial space before being converted back to acetyl-CoA by the citrate cleavage enzyme reaction. In II, acetyl-CoA is hydrolysed to acetate which is transferred into the extramitochondrial space and is converted back to acetyl-CoA by the acetate thiokinase reaction. In III, acetyl-CoA is converted to acetyl carnitine, which after diffusing from the mitochondria is converted back to acetyl-CoA. The enzyme which catalyses both reactions is acetyl-CoA–carnitine acetyl transferase. In IV, acetyl-CoA is depicted as leaving the mitochondria by direct diffusion of the intact molecule.
(From Kornacker and Lowenstein, 1965)

(Lowenstein, 1968). Scheme 3 shows an elaboration of the citrate pathway indicated in outline in Scheme 2. Starting with intramitochondrial acetyl-CoA this pathway involves the formation of citrate via the citrate synthase reaction, the diffusion of intramitochondrial citrate into the extramitochondrial space (possibly as a magnesium citrate chelate), and the formation of acetyl-CoA via the citrate cleavage reaction. Oxaloacetate formed in the citrate cleavage reaction must be returned to the intramitochondrial space. Mitochondria are exceedingly impermeable to oxaloacetate at the low concentrations of this substance which prevail in the cell (Lardy, 1966). The extramitochondrial conversion of oxaloacetate to malate, and the intramitochondrial conversion of malate to oxaloacetate are shown in Scheme 3 as a possible way to overcome the permeability barrier presented to oxaloacetate. This proposal is based on the ubiquitous occurrence of both intra- and extramitochondrial malate dehydrogenases. However, other means of returning the carbon skeleton of oxaloacetate into the mitochondria are not ruled out. For example,

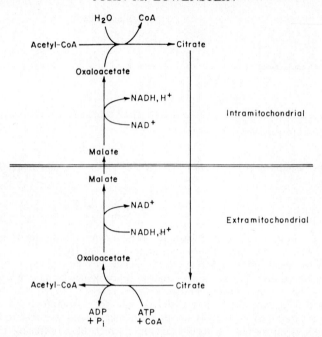

Scheme 3. Transfer of the acetyl group of acetyl-CoA from the intra- to the extramitochondrial space of the cell via citrate. The 'carrier' in this scheme is oxaloacetate, which is used up in the mitochondria and is regenerated in the extramitochondrial space. Unless the carrier is returned to the mitochondria, it will accumulate in the extramitochondrial space. The return of oxaloacetate is shown to proceed through the intermediate formation of malate, but other intermediate reactions are not ruled out

oxaloacetate may be converted into aspartate, which may diffuse into the mitochondria and then be converted back to oxaloacetate. This pathway is feasible because of the ubiquitous occurrence of extra- and intramitochondrial glutamate–aspartate transaminase (Borst, 1961; Lardy, 1966; Chappell and Robinson, 1968). Another possibility is the conversion of malate to pyruvate. The pyruvate may diffuse into the mitochondria and then be converted back to oxaloacetate. This pathway is feasible because of the occurrence of malic enzyme in the extramitochondrial space of the cell, particularly under conditions when fatty acid synthesis is high (Lowenstein 1961; Wood and Utter, 1965; Ballard and Hanson, 1967). Much material has been published in the last five years that is pertinent to the entry and egress from mitochondria of citric acid cycle compounds and of reducing equivalents. A comprehensive treatment of various facets of these topics is given in the recent reviews by Greville (1969), Utter (1969), and Tager, de Haan and Slater (1969).

The role of the citrate cleavage reaction in the formation of extramito-chondrial acetyl-CoA was also investigated by Daikuhara, Tsunemi, and Takeda (1968). A reconstructed system was used which consisted of mitochondria and particle-free supernatant prepared from rat liver. The acetylation of either sulfanilamide or p-toluidine was studied using either ^{14}C-labelled or unlabelled pyruvate as the source of carbon. Treatment of the supernatant with antiserum to pure citrate cleavage enzyme (Inoue, Suzuki, Fukunishi, Adachi and Takeda, 1966) reduced the acetylation of sulfanilamide and p-toluidine to about 15% of the amounts observed in controls. Neither L- nor D-carnitine affected the rates of acetylation in the presence or absence of antiserum. The authors concluded that more than 80% of the extramitochondrial acetyl-CoA derived from pyruvate is supplied through the citrate cleavage pathway.

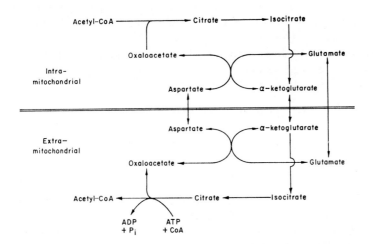

Scheme 4.   Transfer of the acetyl group of acetyl-CoA from the intra- to the extramitochondrial space of the cell via α-ketoglutarate and glutamate. Acetyl-CoA is converted to α-ketoglutarate through the intermediate formation of citrate and isocitrate. The scheme is intended to show that α-ketoglutarate can diffuse into the extramitochondrial space as such or after conversion to glutamate via transamination. Either glutamate or α-ketoglutarate or both are then converted back to citrate, which is converted to acetyl-CoA and oxalo-acetate by the citrate cleavage reaction (adapted from D'Adamo and Haft, 1962). The return of oxaloacetate into the mitochondria is shown to proceed through the intermediate formation of aspartate, but other intermediate reactions are not ruled out

In 1962 D'Adamo and Haft reported experiments which showed that the radioactive carbon of [5-^{14}C]glutamate, but not that of [2-^{14}C]glutamate, is incorporated into fatty acids (see also Abraham, Madsen and Chaikoff, 1964; Madsen, Abraham, and Chaikoff, 1964; D'Adamo and Haft, 1965; Leveille and Hanson, 1966a, 1966b). On the basis of these observations, and of the presumed impermeability of mitochondria to polyanions such as citrate, it was proposed that extramitochondrial citrate is derived from intramitochondrial citrate via the intermediate formation of α-ketoglutarate or glutamate, as shown in Scheme 4. According to this view intramitochondrial citrate is converted to α-ketoglutarate or glutamate or both. α-Ketoglutarate or glutamate or both then diffuse into the extramitochondrial space where they are converted back to citrate by a reversal of the intramitochondrial reactions. Oxaloacetate formed in the citrate cleavage reaction must then be returned into the mitochondria by one of the pathways discussed above. Scheme 4 shows this to take place via transamination reactions, but other pathways are not ruled out. The enzymes necessary for the pathway proposed by D'Adamo and Haft are found both in the intra- and extramitochondrial space of the cell. However, a *de novo* synthesis of fatty acids from glutamate was not demonstrated in the experiments referred to above, and caution must be exercised in interpreting isotope incorporation experiments in terms of net synthesis along a pathway.

A NEW ASSESSMENT OF THE CITRATE PATHWAY OF FATTY ACID SYNTHESIS IN RAT LIVER

The finding that (−)-hydroxycitrate is a powerful inhibitor of citrate cleavage enzyme has made it possible to test in a new way the hypothesis that citrate is the major precursor of the acetyl groups used for the extramitochondrial synthesis of fatty acids when the major source of carbon is pyruvate. The experiments presented below involved the use of a reconstituted system consisting of mitochondria and high speed supernatant (cytoplasmic protein) prepared from rat liver. In initial experiments we used [2-^{14}C]pyruvate to generate intramitochondrial acetyl-CoA. Subsequently we used [^{14}C]alanine for this purpose, since it is much stabler than pyruvate and can be stored readily in a state of purity.

Figure 2 shows that fatty acid synthesis from [^{14}C]alanine requires the presence of both mitochondria and high speed supernatant. In the reconstituted system employed by us, *fatty acid synthesis can be severely depressed by the addition of a low concentration of (−)-hydroxycitrate* (Figure 3). As little as 3·5 μM hydroxycitrate suppresses fatty acid synthesis by 44%; 14 μM suppresses it by 88%; and 48 μM suppresses it

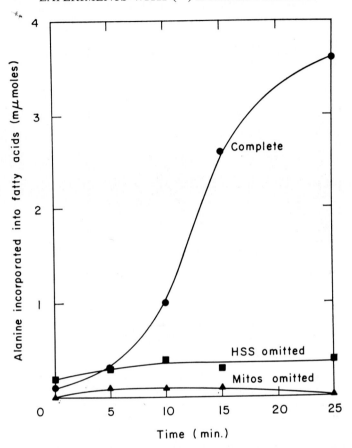

Figure 2. Requirement for mitochondria and high speed supernatant for fatty acid synthesis from [¹⁴C]alanine. The complete system contained mitochondria, 2·3 mg protein per ml and activated high speed supernatant, 3·0 mg protein per ml, prepared from rat liver. The high speed supernatant was activated by incubation with 20 mM $MgCl_2$ 10 mM dithiothreitol, and 50 mM glycylglycine buffer, pH 7·4, at 38° C for 20 minutes, just before use (Fang and Lowenstein, 1967). In addition the complete system contained 22 mM $KHCO_3$, 4 mM L-malate, 4 mM α-ketoglutarate, about 0·13 mM CoA, 2 mM ATP, 4 mM $MgCl_2$, about 0·13 mM NAD, about 0·5 mM NADP, 4 mM glucose-6-phosphate, 4 mM potassium phosphate, pH 7·3, and 1 mM [U-¹⁴C]alanine (200 cpm per mμ mole). The mixture had a final pH of 7·3. The initial volume was 6 ml, and the incubations were carried out in conical flasks which were shaken at 125 strokes per minute in a water bath at 38° C. Aliquots of 1·0 ml were removed at the times indicated, pipetted into 2·0 ml 5N NaOH and analysed as described previously (Fang and Lowenstein, 1967; Watson and Lowenstein, unpublished)

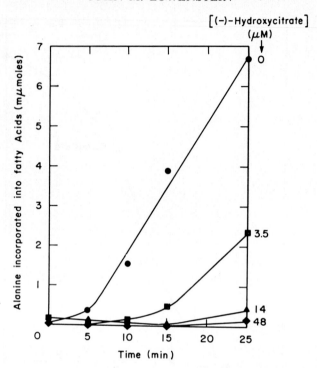

Figure 3. Effect of (−)-hydroxycitrate on fatty acid synthesis from [^{14}C]alanine. The complete system described in the legend to Figure 2 was used, except that (−)-hydroxycitrate was added to the reaction mixture as indicated (Watson and Lowenstein, unpublished)

by over 95%. By comparison, 100 μM (−)-hydroxycitrate has been found to be without effect on two key enzymes which catalyse reactions in pathways 2 and 3 of Scheme 2, namely acetate thiokinase and acetyl-CoA–carnitine acetyl transferase. A possible alternative explanation for the inhibition of fatty acid synthesis in the presence of (−)-hydroxycitrate is that this substance inhibits some vital part of intramitochondrial metabolism. This possibility may be ruled out on the basis of the observation that 75 μM (−)-hydroxycitrate has no effect on mitochondrial respiration (Table 1). Moreover, this amount of hydroxycitrate does not affect the rate of $^{14}CO_2$ production from [2-^{14}C]pyruvate. The experiment shown in Figure 3 therefore provides new evidence that the acetyl group of acetyl-CoA is transferred from the intra- into the extramitochondrial space in the form of citrate, or a near relative of citrate, and not in the form of either acetyl-CoA, acetyl carnitine, or free acetate.

Table 1. Lack of effect of (−)-hydroxycitrate on mitochondrial respiration. The suspending medium consisted of a solution containing 0·245 M sucrose, 20 mM Tris-HCl buffer, pH 7·3, 2·5 mM MgCl$_2$, and 2 mM potassium phosphate. It was saturated with air and stored at 25° while experiments were in progress. Suspending medium (1·8 ml) was added to the reaction chamber and was allowed to equilibrate. Mitochondria (0·1 ml, about 3·0 mg protein) were added to the medium. After the endogenous rate of oxygen consumption was established this was followed by either 20 μmoles pyruvate plus 10 mM malate, or 5 μmoles succinate, or 8 mM citrate (with and without 10 μmoles malate). All substrates were added in the form of their potassium salts which had been neutralized to pH 7·3. Where indicated, 0·2 to 1·0 μmoles ADP was added with the substrates. Oxygen consumption was measured at 28° with a Clark electrode in a magnetically stirred chamber with a total capacity of 2·2ml

Substrate	ADP	[(−)-Hydroxycitrate]	
		None	75 μM
		Oxygen uptake (mμ atoms/mg protein/minute)	
Pyruvate plus malate	absent	13·9	13·9
	present	31·2	31·2
Succinate	absent	30	30
	present	95	95
Citrate	absent	13·3	13·2
	present	53·7	53·7
Citrate plus malate	absent	16·6	13·3
	present	53·7	53·7

The question of whether the transfer of the acetyl group occurs via a tricarboxylic acid such as citrate itself, or via glutamate or α-ketoglutarate, was put to experimental test. If the pathway of acetyl group transfer involves α-ketoglutarate then the addition of a pool of unlabelled α-ketoglutarate should lead to a trapping of [4,5-14C]α-ketoglutarate formed from [U-14C]alanine via the reactions: alanine → pyruvate → acetyl-CoA → citrate → isocitrate → α-ketoglutarate.* Such a trapping should be reflected in a reduction of 14C incorporated into fatty acids. The results in Figure 4 show that addition of α-ketoglutarate does not

---

* [U-14C]Alanine gives rise via pyruvate to [1,2-14C]acetyl labelled acetyl-CoA. The latter gives rise via the citrate synthase reaction to stereospecifically-labelled [1,2-14C]citrate, which in turn gives rise to [4,5-14C]α-ketoglutarate. These steric interrelations have been discussed fully elsewhere (Lowenstein, 1967).

diminish the formation of labelled fatty acids. At the highest concentration of α-ketoglutarate added (12 mM), the total amount of α-ketoglutarate present exceeded the amount of acetyl group incorporated into fatty acids by a factor of about 1200. Some of the α-ketoglutarate added was converted to glutamate by transamination with alanine; this probably accounts for the increase in fatty acid synthesis from [¹⁴C]alanine which occurred as the concentration of α-ketoglutarate was increased. Even so, α-ketoglutarate was present in great excess. Since it failed to dilute the radioactive carbon pool which serves to supply precursors for the synthesis

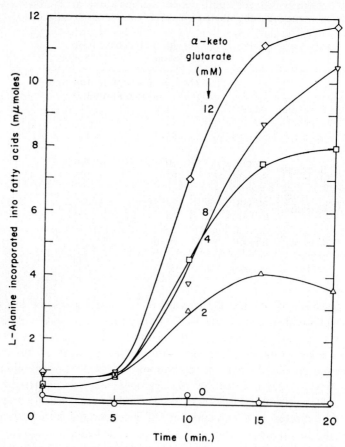

Figure 4. Effect of α-ketoglutarate on fatty acid synthesis from [¹⁴C]alanine. The complete system described in the legend to Figure 2 was used, except that α-ketoglutarate was added to the reaction mixture as indicated, and the alanine concentration was 6 mM (Watson and Lowenstein, unpublished)

of fatty acids, it is concluded that the acetyl group of intramitochondrial acetyl-CoA is most probably not exported from the mitochondria as α-ketoglutarate or glutamate but as citrate.*

It is possible that in the *in vitro* system employed by us the reductive carboxylation of α-ketoglutarate by isocitrate dehydrogenase does not occur, whereas in the intact cell conditions for this reaction are more favourable. The *in vitro* system described here contained a NADPH regenerating system, which makes it unlikely that the reductive decarboxylation did not occur for lack of NADPH.

In conclusion, the experiments presented here provide new evidence that the citrate cleavage pathway is the major source of carbon for the synthesis of fatty acids in rat. Transfer of citrate carbon from the mitochondria into the cytoplasm probably occurs in the form of tricarboxylic acids, and not via α-ketoglutarate or glutamate.

References

Abraham, S., Madsen, J., and Chaikoff, I. L. (1964). *J. Biol. Chem.*, **239**, 855.

Ballard, F. J., and Hanson, R. W. (1967). *J. Lipid Res.*, **8**, 73.

Bhaduri, A., and Srere, P. A. (1963). *Biochim. Biophys. Acta*, **70**, 221.

Borst, P. (1961). *Proc. 5th Intern. Congr. Biochem.*, Moscow, **2**, 233.

Chappell, J. B., and Robinson, B. H. (1968). *Biochem. Soc. Symp.*, **27**, 123.

D'Adamo, A. F., Jr., and Haft, D. E. (1962). *Federation Proc.*, **21**, 6.

D'Adamo, A. F., Jr., and Haft, D. E. (1965). *J. Biol. Chem.*, **240**, 613.

Daikuhara, Y., Tsunemi, T., and Takeda, Y. (1968). *Biochim. Biophys. Acta*, **158**, 51.

Fang, M., and Lowenstein, J. M. (1967). *Biochem. J.*, **105**, 803.

Glusker, J. P., Minkin, J. A., Casciato, C. A., and Soul, F. B. (1969). *Arch. Biochem. Biophys.*, **132**, 573.

Greville, G. C., in *Citric Acid Cycle: Control and Compartmentation.* Ed. by J. M. Lowenstein, New York: Marcel Dekker, p. 1, 1969.

Griebel, C. (1939). *Z. Lebensm. Untersuch.-Forsch.*, **77**, 560. *Chem. Abstr.*, **33**, 7491.

Griebel, C. (1942). *Z. Lebensm. Untersuch.-Forsch.*, **83**, 481. *Chem. Abstr.*, **37**, 4704.

Inoue, H., Suzuki, F., Fukunishi, K., Adachi, K., and Takeda, Y. (1966). *J. Biochem. Tokyo*, **60**, 543.

Kornacker, M. S., and Lowenstein, J. M. (1965). *Biochem. J.*, **94**, 209.

Krebs, H. A. (1953). *Biochem. J.*, **54**, 78.

Lardy, H. A. (1966). *Harvey Lectures*, **60**, 261.

Leveille, G. A., and Hanson, R. W. (1966a). *J. Lipid Res.* **7**, 46.

Leveille, G. A., and Hanson, R. W. (1966b). *Can. J. Physiol. Pharmacol.* **44**, 275.

* The egress from the mitochondria of *cis*-aconitate and isocitrate is not excluded by these experiments. The equilibrium mixture of these tricarboxylic acids contains about 91% of citrate (Krebs, 1953).

Lewis, S. Y., in *Methods in Enzymology*, Vol. 13. Ed. by J. M. Lowenstein, New York: Academic Press, p. 613, 1969.

Lewis, Y. S., and Neelakantan, S. (1964). *Current Sci. India*, **33**, 82.

Lewis, Y. S., and Neelakantan, S. (1965). *Phytochemistry*, **4**, 619.

von Lippmann, E. (1883). *Ber. chem. Ges.*, **16**, 1078.

Lowenstein, J. M. (1961). *J. Biol. Chem.*, **236**, 1213.

Lowenstein, J. M. (1963). *Biochem. Soc. Symp.*, **24**, 57.

Lowenstein, J. M., in *Metabolic Pathways*, Vol. 1, 3rd ed. Ed. by D. M. Greenberg, New York: Academic Press, p. 146, 1967.

Lowenstein, J. M. (1968). *Biochem. Soc. Symp.*, **27**, 61.

Madsen, J., Abraham, S., and Chaikoff, I. L. (1964). *J. Biol. Chem.*, **239**, 1305.

Martius, C., and Maué, R. (1941). *Z. physiol. Chem.*, **269**, 33.

Spencer, A. F., and Lowenstein, J. M. (1962). *J. Biol. Chem.*, **237**, 3640.

Tager, J. M., de Haan, E. J., and Slater, E. J., in *Citric Acid Cycle: Control and Compartmentation*. Ed. by J. M. Lowenstein, New York: Marcel Dekker, p. 213, 1969.

Utter, M. F., in *Citric Acid Cycle: Control and Compartmentation*. Ed. by J. M. Lowenstein, New York: Marcel Dekker, p. 249, 1969.

Watson, J., Fang M., and Lowenstein, J. M. (1969). *Arch. Biochem. Biophys.*, **130**, 209.

Wood, H. G., and Utter, M. F., in *Essays in Biochemistry.*, Vol. 1. p. 1., Ed. by P. N. Campbell and G. D. Greville. New York: Academic Press, 1965.

THE REGULATION OF AMMONIA METABOLISM IN MAMMALIAN TISSUES

Patricia Lund, J. T. Brosnan and L. V. Eggleston

Metabolic Research Laboratory, Nuffield Department of Clinical Medicine, Radcliffe Infirmary, Oxford

Introduction

The definition of ammonia given by Dr. Johnson (1755) is ascribed to Pliny and Dioscorides: 'a native salt, generated . . . where the crouds of pilgrims, coming from the temple of Jupiter Ammon, used to lodge; who, in those parts, travelling upon camels . . . urining in the stables, or, say some, in the parched sands, out of this urine, which is remarkably strong, arose a kind of salt, denominated from the temple, Ammoniac.' Even as recently as 1935 ammonia was described in Harrow and Sherwin's 'Textbook of Biochemistry' as 'essentially an excretory product'. It is to a large extent due to the work of Hans Krebs that ammonia is now recognized as an important cellular constituent.

This essay is concerned with the important positive functions of ammonia in metabolism, which include its role in the regulation of the mitochondrial redox state, in the maintenance of acid–base balance, and in biosynthetic reactions. The regulation of the ammonia concentrations of blood, brain, liver and kidney in normal conditions and in conditions of increased ammonia, such as hepatic failure or after administration of an ammonia load, is discussed.

Difficulties inherent in the study of ammonia metabolism

The study of ammonia metabolism *in vivo* has been hampered by limitations of the methods available. There are no suitable radioactive isotopes of nitrogen, so that labelling experiments are restricted to the use of the stable [^{15}N], which requires a mass spectrometer and relatively large amounts of [^{15}N], making 'tracer' experiments very difficult.

Early micromethods for determining ammonia involved microdistillation under reduced pressure (Parnas and Heller, 1924) or microdiffusion followed by colourimetric measurement or titration (Conway and Byrne, 1933; Seligson and Hirahara, 1957). The risk of non-specificity is the main limitation of these methods. More recently a specific enzymatic assay employing glutamate dehydrogenase (E.C. 1.4.1.2) has been developed

167

(Kirsten, Gerez and Kirsten, 1963). This, together with the tissue 'freeze-clamping' technique of Wollenberger, Ristau and Schoffa (1960) which minimizes the post-mortem increases in ammonia that occur, has made *in vivo* studies more meaningful.

Blood ammonia

Early investigators doubted whether ammonia was present in blood. This is hardly surprising as its concentration is very low except in portal venous blood (Table 1), which contains ammonia largely derived from

Table 1. Ammonia concentrations in arterial and venous blood in rat and man
Concentrations are expressed as μmoles/ml of whole blood

Species	Arterial	Portal venous	Hepatic venous	Renal venous	Reference
Rat	0·02	0·261	0·031	0·116	Brosnan, unpublished
Man (fasted)	0·036	0·178	0·057	0·071	McDermott, Adams and Riddell (1954)

bacterial degradation of amino acids and urea in the gut. Administration of bacteriostatic agents such as Neomycin decreases the ammonia concentration (Silen, Harper, Mawdsley and Weirich, 1955). The difference in concentration between portal and hepatic venous ammonia shows that it is largely removed by the liver; thus the liver is responsible for the low levels circulating ammonia. This is confirmed by perfusion of the isolated rat of liver. If ammonium chloride (0·5–1·0 mM) is added to the perfusion medium, it is rapidly removed until the concentration approaches the normal *in vivo* hepatic venous level (Brosnan and Lund, unpublished). Under pathological conditions (liver failure, or injection of an ammonia load) brain and muscle can also play a part in removing circulating ammonia (Bessman and Bessman, 1955; Flock and coworkers. 1953; Rosado, Flores, Mora and Soberon, 1962).

Ammonia metabolism in the liver

(i) The urea cycle

By far the most important fate of the large amounts of ammonia formed and taken up by the liver is synthesis to urea. The amounts synthesized and excreted per day (30 g for man; 0·65 g for rat) require a considerable amount of energy (4 moles~P/mole urea). In mammals synthesis occurs entirely in the liver. Other tissues possessing arginase activity are capable of forming urea from arginine, but the complete pathway is virtually confined to the liver. Ammonium carbamate and ammonium cyanate were originally discussed as possible precursors of urea. These theories were discarded with the discovery by Krebs and Henseleit (1932) that ornithine or citrulline in catalytic amounts stimulated urea synthesis from ammonia in liver slices. They proposed that urea is formed via the cyclic interconversion of these amino acids. At that time the concept of a metabolic 'cycle' was completely original, and was forerunner to the elucidation of other cyclic processes.

Present knowledge of the individual steps of the urea cycle is given in Figure 1. It is essentially the scheme proposed by Krebs and Henseleit in

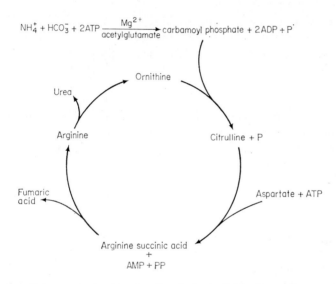

Figure 1. The urea cycle. For details of the individual reactions, see Cohen and Sallach (1961)

1932. The involvement of aspartate was shown by Ratner and Pappas (1949) and carbamoyl phosphate was identified as an intermediate in citrulline synthesis by Jones, Spector and Lipmann (1955).

(ii) *Other biosynthetic reactions of ammonia*

Whilst synthesis to urea is quantitatively the most important fate of ammonia, glutamate dehydrogenase in particular,

α-oxoglutarate $+$ NAD(P)H $+$ NH$_4^+$ $+$ H$^+$ $\rightleftharpoons$

$$\text{L-glutamate} + \text{NAD(P)}^+ + \text{H}_2\text{O}$$

and glutamine synthetase (E.C. 6.3.1.2)

L-glutamate $+$ NH$_3$ $+$ ATP $\rightleftharpoons$ L-glutamine $+$ ADP $+$ orthophosphate

are two 'biosynthetic' enzymes of importance in the regulation of intracellular ammonia levels. Other reactions of ammonia which will not be considered are its involvement in the *de novo* synthesis of amino acids, amino sugars, purines, pyrimidines, nucleotides etc. In many instances the involvement of ammonia is indirect, and glutamine (or in some cases another amino acid) is the immediate nitrogen donor; in fact glutamine may be regarded as an active form of ammonia.

(iii) *Compartmentation of the enzymes of the urea cycle*

The enzymes of the cycle are not confined to any one subcellular compartment; carbamoyl phosphate synthase (E.C. 2.7.2.5) and ornithine carbamoyl transferase (E.C. 2.1.3.3) occur in the mitochondria (Grisolia and Cohen, 1953; Charles, Tager and Slater, 1967); argininosuccinate synthetase (E.C. 6.3.4.5), argininosuccinate lyase (E.C. 4.3.2.1.) and arginase (E.C. 3.5.3.1) are extramitochondrial (Ratner, 1954; Rosenthal, Gottlieb, Gorry and Vars, 1956). On the basis of this distribution the operation of the urea cycle within the cell requires the transfer of ornithine into the mitochondrion and the transfer of citrulline out. Assuming no energy requirement for the transfer processes, the complete oxidation of 11 gram glucose would be required to provide the ATP necessary for the synthesis of the 30 gram urea excreted per day by a 70 kilogram man in normal nitrogen balance.

(iv) *Regulation of the urea cycle*

The individual enzymes of the urea cycle show adaptive increases in activity to conditions demanding increased urea production. The phenomenon has been studied in rats when urea synthesis has been stimulated by an increased protein intake (Schimke, 1962a), starvation (Schimke, 1962b), cortisone treatment (Schimke, 1963), glucagon treatment or alloxan diabetes (McLean and Novello, 1965). After showing increases in the enzymes leading to arginine on feeding rats on an arginine-free diet, Schimke (1963) has suggested feedback by arginine as a control mechanism. The arginine synthetase system (argininosuccinate synthetase $+$ argininosuccinate lyase) has been discussed as the rate limiting step of the cycle, because it has the lowest activity *in vitro* (Freedland and Sodikoff, 1962; McLean and Novello, 1965). In all cases these adaptive enzyme increases have been measured in livers from animals treated for several days, and the time course of the enzyme changes has not been correlated with the early stages of increased urea excretion. However, it is well established that increased flux through the pathway of urea synthesis can be achieved before any adaptation by enzyme synthesis could have occurred. This has been shown *in vivo* after administration of ammonia or amino acids (Kamin and Handler, 1951), *in vitro* in liver slices (Krebs and Henseleit, 1932) and in the isolated perfused liver by ammonia (Hems, Ross, Berry and Krebs, 1966) or glucagon (Miller, 1960). The rates of urea synthesis from ammonia are further increased in slices and perfused liver by addition of ornithine. The explanation of the ornithine effect is that ornithine carbamoyl transferase, in reacting rapidly with its substrates (ornithine and carbamoyl phosphate), brings about an increase in the rate of synthesis of carbamoyl phosphate. Thus a strong argument can be made for regulation at the first step. Under normal conditions *in vivo* availability of ammonia might well be the major rate limiting factor. The K_m for ammonia of rat liver carbamoyl phosphate synthase ($7 \cdot 1 \times 10^{-4}$M; Caravaca and Grisolia, 1960) is close to the tissue content ($0 \cdot 7$ μmoles/g fresh wt) which means that the enzyme would be very responsive to small changes in ammonia concentration.

(v) *Ammonia and the redox state of the intramitochondrial pyridine nucleotides.*

The steady state concentration of ammonia in the liver is regulated by glutamate dehydrogenase in combination with glutamate–pyruvate aminotransferase (E.C. 2.6.1.2) and glutamate–oxaloacetate aminotransferase (E.C. 2.6.1.1) because these enzymes have been shown to be close to equilibrium under many conditions (Williamson, Lund and Krebs, 1967; Williamson, Lopes-Vieira and Walker, 1967). The urea cycle may be regarded as being responsible for the removal of 'excess' ammonia under normal conditions. The location of glutamate dehydrogenase exclusively in the mitochondrial matrix means that ammonia is intimately linked to the mitochondrial free NAD(P)/free NAD(P)H ratio, and plays an important role in the control of the mitochondrial redox state. A sudden increase in the ammonia concentration drives the mitochondrial pyridine nucleotide ratios in favour of oxidation. Ammonia would play the same important regulatory role in any other tissue in which glutamate dehydrogenase is sufficiently active to maintain equilibrium. Thus the 'toxic' effects associated with raised ammonia could be primarily due to disturbance either of the redox-state or of the tissue concentrations of the other reactants in the glutamate dehydrogenase system, which might have other secondary effects. This is illustrated by the inhibition of the tricarboxylic acid cycle and the ketogenesis caused by ammonia *in vitro* (Recknagel and Potter, 1951). Here the primary effect is depletion of α-oxoglutarate through reaction with glutamate dehydrogenase, which results in an inhibition of the tricarboxylic acid cycle. Ketogenesis is the secondary effect.

(vi) *The fate of an ammonia load in vivo.*

Schoenheimer and his collaborators (see Schoenheimer, 1942), by administration of [^{15}N] labelled ammonium compounds, demonstrated that label appeared not only in urea, but also in amino acids and tissue proteins. Of the amino acids, glutamate, aspartate, glutamine and asparagine were most heavily labelled, especially in the amide groups of the latter. Later experiments by Duda and Handler (1958) confirmed that label preferentially appeared in glutamine after injection into rats of a small dose (0·17 mMoles/kg body wt) of [^{15}N]-ammonium lactate. Within 5 minutes the specific activity of the amide-N of glutamine was three times higher than that of the amino-N of glutamate. The specific activity of the amide-N reached a peak at seven times the glutamate specific activity. However, it can be calculated that the actual glutamine concentration increased by only 8 μmoles/liver (approximately 0·5 μmoles/g) Experiments with larger doses of unlabelled ammonia by du Ruisseau, Greenstein, Winitz and Birnbaum (1957) (10·8 mMoles ammonium acetate/kg body wt) and Brosnan (1968) (2·5 mMoles ammonium chloride/kg body wt) gave large increases in aspartate and alanine with only small increases in glutamine. The time course of these changes in frozen-clamped liver from fed and starved rats is given in Figures 2 and 3 (Brosnan, 1968). In the starved rats there was actually a *decrease* in glutamine after administration of ammonia.

The above experiments do not exclude the possibility that glutamine is synthesized and rapidly released into the circulation. Perfusion of the isolated rat liver, however, supports the view that glutamine synthetase plays a minor role in disposal of ammonia (Lund, unpublished). No substrate, or combination of substrates, giving rise to high intracellular concentrations of glutamate and ammonia (histidine, asparagine, proline plus alanine, etc.) significantly increased the rate of synthesis of glutamine over the endogenous level. The maximum rate of glutamine synthesis by the perfused liver was less than one-thirtieth of the capacity of glutamine synthetase *in vitro*.

Thus the data of du Ruisseau and coworkers (1957), Brosnan (1968) and these perfusion experiments show that glutamine synthesis is of less sig-

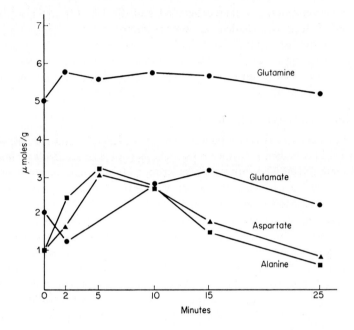

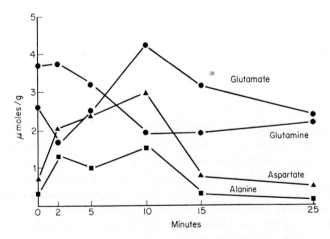

Figures 2 and 3. Liver content of glutamine, glutamate, alanine and aspartate after administration of NH_4Cl (2·5 mMoles/kg body wt; i.p.). Figure 2 = fed rats. Figure 3 = 48 h starved rats. Data from Brosnan (1968)

nificance than glutamate dehydrogenase and the aminotransferases when the urea cycle is overloaded, as after administration of ammonia. The reason for the discrepancy between these findings and those of Schoenheimer (1942) and Duda and Handler (1958), or the recent experiments of Addae and Lotspeich (1968), which provide evidence that glutamine synthesis is an active process in rat liver, is not clear.

Ammonia metabolism in the brain

Nervous activity is accompanied by a liberation of ammonia (see Weil-Malherbe, 1962), but it is not known whether the overall result of normal brain metabolism is an uptake or an output of ammonia. A rapid release of ammonia occurs when brain slices are incubated in a glucose-free medium (Weil-Malherbe and Green, 1955). The production of ammonia is inhibited by anaerobiosis. Glutamine, glutamate and adenine nucleotides were ruled out as precursors and protein breakdown was suggested as a partial explanation. The reason for the energy requirement is not clear, nor has the *in vivo* significance of the process been established.

It is a well-documented fact that glucose carbon appears rapidly in brain amino acids; in the rat, 20 minutes after injection of a small dose of [U-^{14}C] glucose, 42–59% of the label appeared in the amino acid fraction (Gaitonde and Richter, 1966). The extent of *de novo* synthesis of amino acids (and hence ammonia incorporation) cannot be calculated from such data because exchange reactions are largely responsible for the rapid incorporation of the glucose carbon (Haslam and Krebs, 1963). In conditions where blood ammonia is abnormally high, such as in hepatic failure or after an ammonia load, there is uptake of ammonia by the brain which causes severe neurological disturbances that may be followed by convulsions and coma.

(i) *Possible explanations for the toxic effects of ammonia on the brain:* (a) α-oxoglutarate depletion

Bessman and Bessman (1955) postulated that the removal of ammonia by the sequential action of glutamate dehydrogenase and glutamine synthetase depletes the pool of α-oxoglutarate available to the tricarboxylic acid cycle. This would decrease the concentration of other intermediates of the cycle and could result in a disturbance of energy metabolism with consequent coma. Bessman (1959) has suggested that the brain may be particularly sensitive to depletion of Krebs' cycle intermediates because (a) the blood–brain barrier effectively prevents replenishment of intermediates from the blood, and (b) a deficiency of CO_2-fixing enzymes in brain prevents intracellular replenishment. More recently Berl, Takagaki,

Clarke and Waelsch (1962a) have demonstrated fixation of CO_2 into aspartate, glutamate and glutamine in cat cerebral cortex. The amount of CO_2 fixed increases with increasing ammonia levels (Berl and coworkers, 1962b) and is quantitatively significant (Waelsch and coworkers, 1964).

However, there is direct support for the Bessman hypothesis in the experiments of Warren and Schenker (1964). The synthesis of glutamine in mice was inhibited by treatment with methionine sulphoximine (a competitive inhibitor of glutamine synthetase). Large doses of ammonium chloride were then injected into these mice and into a control group. Methionine sulphoximine had a protective effect. Whereas 50% of the control mice were killed by 6·6 mMoles NH_4Cl/kg body wt, the treated group survived even though the level of ammonia in the brain was greater than in the untreated group. Only at a concentration of 10 mMoles NH_4Cl/kg body wt were 50% of the methionine sulphoximine treated animals killed. Methionine sulphoximine prevented the decrease in brain α-oxoglutarate that follows administration of ammonia.

(b) Acetylcholine depletion

Ulshafer (1958) has shown that administration of sufficient ammonium carbonate to produce convulsions in rats causes a decrease in the brain content of acetylcholine. It is also known that ammonia inhibits the synthesis of acetylcholine by brain cortex slices, and that the inhibition is relieved by addition of glutamine synthetase inhibitors (Braganca, Faulkner and Quastel, 1953).

(c) ATP and creatine phosphate depletion

After administration of ammonium acetate to produce coma in rats, the concentrations of ATP and creatine phosphate were unaltered in brain cortex but had decreased significantly in the base of the brain (Schenker, McCandle, Brophy and Lewis, 1967). The authors point out that many of the symptoms of hepatic coma (and hence of ammonia toxicity) may be produced in this region.

The above effects can be interpreted as evidence that ammonia *per se* is not the immediate toxic agent in 'ammonia intoxication'; they point only to its possible multiple biochemical effects. It is conceivable that its primary effect is a disturbance of the oxidoreduction state of the pyridine nucleotides, as has already been discussed for liver, or that it replaces K^+ (Tower, Wherrett and McKhann, 1961), a cation essential for nervous function.

(ii) *Glutamine synthesis in brain*

There is no doubt that the brain synthesizes an appreciable amount of glutamine after an ammonia load (du Ruisseau and coworkers, 1957; Berl and coworkers, 1962a) or after hepatectomy (Flock and coworkers, 1953; Flock and Bollman, 1962). After administration of a large dose of ammonium acetate there was a 4-fold increase in cerebral glutamine in the rat (du Ruisseau and coworkers, 1957) before death occurred at 15 minutes. The *in vivo* synthesis of glutamine in brain has been studied by Berl and coworkers (1962a) by infusion of [^{15}N] ammonium acetate into the carotid arteries of anaesthetized cats. A high concentration of [^{15}N] appeared in the amide group of glutamine, with lower concentrations in glutamate and aspartate. The α-amino group of glutamine was more heavily labelled than that of glutamate. Since glutamate is the direct precursor of glutamine the data are difficult to explain. Berl and coworkers (1962a) postulate the existence of two distinct pools of glutamate, a small rapidly metabolizing pool which supplies glutamate for glutamine synthesis and a larger less active pool. Analogous results and conclusions were obtained in guinea pig brain cortex slices (Berl, Nicklas and Clarke, 1968). The existence of two pools of glutamate appears unlikely on consideration of the sub-cellular distribution of the enzymes responsible for glutamine formation from α-oxoglutarate. Glutamate dehydrogenase is located in the mito-chondria of rat brain (Balazs, Dahl and Harwood, 1966) whereas gluta-mine synthetase is associated with the microsomal fraction (Sellinger and de Balbian Verster, 1962). Thus, the synthesis of glutamine appears to involve reductive amination of α-oxoglutarate in the mitochondria and transfer of the newly synthesized glutamate to the endoplasmic reticulum for amidation. Presumably during the transfer the newly synthesized gluta-mate will have mixed with, and been diluted by, glutamate in the mito-chondria and cytoplasm. As these compartments account for the major portion of the cell volume it is difficult to visualize another separate pool of unlabelled glutamate.

Alternatively, the existence of different cell types having different gluta-mate concentrations must be invoked. Considerable variation in the glutamate and glutamine content of different layers of rabbit brain has been shown (Young and Lowry, 1966).

Ammonia metabolism in the kidney

The non-volatile acids produced during normal metabolism cannot be excreted as Na^+, K^+, Mg^{2+} or Ca^{2+} salts without depletion of the cation reserves of the body, nor can they be excreted as the free acid within the limits of urinary pH. In fact they are largely excreted as ammonium salts.

Renal tubular cells exchange H^+ for Na^+, then NH_3 diffuses into the tubular fluid at the sites of acidification and is 'trapped' as NH_4^+. In man 30–50 mEquivalents of acid, produced during normal metabolism, are excreted per day as ammonium salts (Pitts, 1964); the quantity may increase 5–10 fold in metabolic acidosis. Thus ammonia is directly involved in the kidney in the regulation of acid-base balance.

(i) *Origin of urinary ammonia*

The problem of the origin of urinary ammonia and its relation to the acid–base balance of the organism has long been of interest to physiologists. In the normal animal the arterial ammonia concentration is too low to account for the urinary ammonia; in fact the kidney adds ammonia to the circulation (Nash and Benedict, 1921; see also Table 1). Van Slyke and coworkers (1943) found that glutamine is the major precursor. This work has been extended by Pitts and coworkers to measure amino–acid arterio-venous differences across the kidneys of acidotic and alkalotic dogs. The amounts of amino acid extracted from (or added to) the blood have been correlated with the quantity of ammonia excreted (Shalhoub and co-workers, 1963; Pitts, de Haas and Klein, 1963). Glutamine is the major precursor under all conditions. Pitts (1964) has calculated that 37–38% of urinary ammonia is derived from the amide nitrogen of glutamine.

Glutamine has also been shown to be the major precursor of urinary ammonia in man (Owen and Robinson, 1963), but there is little information on the rat. It is likely that glutamine is important in acidosis. However, in the normal rat it is possible that the kidney adds glutamine to the circulation, because of a species difference in the capacity to synthesize glutamine. Kidney cortex from rat, sheep, guinea-pig and rabbit possesses glutamine synthetase activity, whereas that from pig, dog, cat or mink does not (Krebs, 1935; Wu, 1963). A rapid synthesis of glutamine from glutamate has been shown in the isolated perfused rat kidney (Nishiitsut-suji-Uwo, Ross and Krebs, 1967) which does not occur in perfused kidneys of acidotic rats (D. A. Hems, personal communication).

(ii) *Pathways of ammonia formation from glutamine in the kidney*

Ammonia can be formed directly from glutamine by the following enzyme systems

glutaminase (E.C. 3.5.1.2)

$$\text{L-glutamine} + H_2O \rightarrow \text{L-glutamate} + NH_3 \qquad \textbf{(1)}$$

L-glutamine-oxoacid aminotransferase

$$\text{L-glutamine} + \alpha\text{-oxoacid} \rightarrow \alpha\text{-oxoglutaramate} + \text{amino acid} \qquad \textbf{(2)}$$

The α-oxoglutaramate formed in (2) is immediately hydrolysed by an omegaoxidase to α-oxoglutarate and ammonia.

Reaction (2) has been shown to predominate in dog kidney by Stone and Pitts (1967) on the basis of [^{15}N] glutamine infusion experiments. On the other hand, glutaminase is considered to be predominant in the rat (Goldstein, 1967).

(iii) *The control of glutamine hydrolysis*

The factors that regulate glutamine hydrolysis in normal animals and allow increased hydrolysis in acidosis suggest two types of control mechanism: (*a*) enzyme induction, and (*b*) regulation of the activity of the existing enzymes by intracellular conditions.

Metabolic acidosis in the dog is not associated with an increase in the activity of either glutaminase or the glutamine aminotransferase (Rector and Orloff, 1959; Pollak, Mattenheimer, de Bruin and Weinman, 1965) so that intracellular control mechanisms alone must be responsible for the increased ammonia excretion. Adaptation of the ammonia-producing enzyme does occur in response to acidosis in the guinea-pig (Goldstein and Kensler, 1960) and the rat (Rector, Seldin and Copenhaver, 1955).

The time course of increased ammonia excretion is not exactly paralleled by induction of glutaminase (Leonard and Orloff, 1965): a 4-fold increase in ammonia excretion occurred 24 hours after administration of NH$_4$Cl without a demonstrable increase in glutaminase activity. Here again is an example of increased flux occurring prior to enzyme induction. A small dose of actinomycin can prevent the increase in glutaminase demonstrable after 2 days of feeding NH$_4$Cl (Bignall, Elebute and Lotspeich, 1968), yet produces only a small (but significant) decrease in ammonia excretion compared with control acidotic animals. It therefore appears that induction of glutaminase is not of primary importance in adaptation to acidosis.

The properties of glutaminase *per se* are probably of more regulatory significance. It has long been known to be inhibited by glutamate (Krebs, 1935) and activated by phosphate, arsenate or sulphate (Carter and Greenstein, 1947). Recently Katunuma, Tomino and Nishino (1966) have separated glutaminase from various tissues into two isoenzymes: a phosphate-dependent and a phosphate-independent form. The allosteric properties of the glutaminase described by Kvamme, Tveit and Svenneby (1965) are those of the phosphate-independent kidney enzyme (Katsunuma, Temma and Katunuma, 1968). The adaptive changes in response to increased urea excretion are associated with the phosphate-dependent isoenzyme in the kidney. The kinetic and adaptive characteristics are different for other tissues (Katunuma, Huzino and Tomino, 1967). From the kinetic properties of the phosphate-dependent enzyme of kidney it would appear to be a poor candidate for a regulatory role, its requirements suggesting rather that it catalyses the reversal of glutamine synthetase. It has a high K_m for both glutamine (4 $\times$ 10^{-2}M) and phosphate (10^{-1}M) and a pH optimum at 8·5 (Katunuma and coworkers, 1967). The only likely regulatory property of this isoenzyme is its inhibition by glutamate. Goldstein (1966) has suggested feed-back as a control mechanism on the basis of his studies on *total* glutaminase of rat kidney. At pH 7·0, the activity is inhibited 55% by 2mM glutamate with 20mM glutamine as substrate. The glutamate concentration of rat kidney is lower than normal in acidosis, and higher in alkalosis (Goldstein, 1966). Feed-back by glutamate could therefore be a factor in the regulation of ammonia production both in the rat and in the dog, as Goldstein (1966) has pointed out. The glutaminase story is by no means clear cut. A more recent paper gives the K_m for glutamine of the phosphate-dependent glutaminase as 2 $\times$ 10^{-3}M (Goldstein, 1967). Furthermore, studies of ammonia production by intact kidney mitochondria suggest that ammonia may be formed from glutamine other than via glutaminase or glutamine aminotransferase (Hird and Marginson, 1968).

The evidence that renal glutaminase may be controlled by feedback by glutamate is strengthened by the close relationship that exists between ammoniagenesis and gluconeogenesis. The deamination of glutamine is not accompanied by release of glutamate or α-oxoglutarate into the renal venous blood; it is now apparent that the carbon skeleton of glutamine is used for gluconeogenesis. Goodman, Fuisz and Cahill (1966) found that gluconeogenesis from glutamine, glutamate and α-oxoglutarate is increased in kidney slices from acidotic or K^+-depleted rats. Both states are associated with increased ammonia excretion and adaptation of the ammonia-producing enzymes. In alkalosis, when ammonia excretion is lower than normal, gluconeogenesis is decreased. The rate of gluconeogenesis is related to pH (see Cahill, 1967). Thus the regulation of ammonia excretion may be brought about by the following sequence of events. Acidosis produces a lower intracellular pH which stimulates gluconeogenesis from glutamate, and the resulting decrease in glutamate concentration releases the inhibition of glutaminase. As yet, the pH sensitive step in gluconeogenesis has not been identified. Phosphoenolpyruvate carboxykinase has been suggested (Alleyne, 1968).

The concentrations of ammonia in blood and tissues

In the previous sections the term 'ammonia' has been used to include both the non-ionized, lipid soluble NH_3 and the ionized NH_4^+ which are in the equilibrium determined by the equation

$$NH_4^+ \rightleftharpoons NH_3 + H^+$$

The pK of NH_4^+ is 9·02, and the relative proportions of NH_3 and NH_4^+ can be calculated from the Henderson–Hasselbalch equation

$$pH = pK + \log \frac{[NH_3]}{[NH_4^+]}$$

It is clear that, within the range of physiological pH, ammonia exists largely as NH_4^+—about 1% is in the form of NH_3 at pH 7·0.

Living cells are generally assumed to be relatively permeable to NH_3 and impermeable to NH_4^+, so that theoretically no concentration gradients should exist provided the pH is constant throughout the body. The gradient for ammonia between kidney tubular cells and tubular fluid can be explained on the basis of a pH gradient. NH_3 continuously diffuses into the more acidic tubular fluid and is trapped as NH_4^+ (for a full discussion, see Pitts, 1968). Recently, concentration gradients for ammonia have been confirmed between tissues (Table 2) and blood (Table 1) in the normal rat

Table 2. Ammonia content of various rat tissues

Tissue	μmole/g fresh tissue
Liver	0·71
Abdominal muscle	0·87
Kidney	0·88
Brain	0·34
Thigh muscle	0·26
Spleen	0·20
Heart	0·20

Tissue was freeze-clamped as described by Wollenberger and coworkers (1960). Ammonia was determined enzymatically (Kirsten and coworkers, 1963). Data from Brosnan (1968)

which a pH gradient does not satisfactorily explain in all cases. Other possible mechanisms for maintenance of these gradients are (a), distribution of NH_4^+ in response to a membrane potential, or (b), active transport of NH_4^+ across cell membranes.

Energy would be required for both processes. Alternative (a) requires that the cell membrane should be permeable to NH_4^+ and impermeable to NH_3. Back-diffusion of NH_3 would counteract the effect of the membrane potential. Mechanism (b) would also demand that diffusion of NH_3 out of the cell should be absent or very small. The mechanism for maintenance of the gradient has been investigated in rat liver in this laboratory.

(i) *The concentration gradient of ammonia between rat liver and blood*

Comparison of the data in Tables 1 and 2 shows that the gradient for ammonia between the liver and the venous outflow *in vivo* is 23-fold. The actual concentration gradient must be higher. Assuming that ammonia ($0 \cdot 71$ μmole/g) is confined to the tissue water, which represents 73% of the tissue weight, the gradient must be at least 31-fold. No correction is made for the blood content of the tissue. If the concentration of ammonia in rat erythrocytes is higher than in plasma, as is true for human blood (Seligson and Hirahara, 1957), the gradient would be still greater. To explain even a 31-fold gradient on the basis of pH alone would require an intracellular pH of $5 \cdot 89$ (assuming a blood pH of $7 \cdot 4$), using the formula of Milne, Scribner and Crawford (1958).

The ammonia gradient is maintained during perfusion of the isolated liver, and ammonium chloride ($0 \cdot 5$ mM) added to the medium is rapidly removed against a concentration gradient until the concentration in the medium approaches that of the normal venous outflow. Anaerobiosis (95% N_2: 5% CO_2 in the gas phase, with 2 mM cyanide in the medium) reduced the gradient to $3 \cdot 3$. The ATP concentration in the liver at the time was very low ($0 \cdot 06$ μmole/g). The data suggest that energy from oxidative metabolism maintains the normal ammonia gradient in rat liver.

Of the possible mechanisms (b) seems more likely. A consideration of (a) shows that a membrane potential of $-91 \cdot 3$ mV would be required to maintain a $31 \cdot 4$-fold gradient, which would be unlikely to exist in a non-excitable tissue such as liver. It is conceivable that NH_4^+ could be actively pumped across the membrane. NH_4^+ has the same hydration diameter as K^+ (Kielland, 1937), and can replace K^+ in Na^+, K^+-activated ATP-ase *in vitro* (Skou, 1960; Rendi and Uhr, 1964). That NH_4^+ can compete with K^+ for inward transport has been shown in erythrocytes by Post and Jolly (1957). A similar mechanism has been suggested to explain the gradient in brain (Tower and coworkers, 1961), and in muscle after an ammonia load (Rosado and coworkers, 1962).

On the whole, the evidence favours active transport of NH_4^+, but does not exclude the involvement of the other possible mechanisms in maintaining the ammonia gradient.

G

Concluding remarks

The fact that tissues maintain a gradient for ammonia, and can only do so at the expense of energy, emphasizes its importance as a cellular constituent. Its primary function, as a reactant of glutamate dehydrogenase, lies in the regulation of the mitochondrial redox state in those tissues in which the enzyme is active enough to maintain equilibrium (Williamson and coworkers, 1967). Ammonia might also play a role in the regulation of glutamine synthetase and glutaminase, since the presence of both enzymes in the same cell in some tissues demands control mechanisms to prevent wasteful 'cycling' of glutamate and glutamine. A good deal of work remains to be done on the *in vivo* significance of the various effectors and inhibitors of the two enzymes, particularly in animal tissues. Another property of NH_4^+ is that it can replace K^+ as activator of certain important regulatory enzymes, for example phosphofructokinase (Muntz and Hurwitz, 1951; Passonneau and Lowry, 1964) and pyruvate kinase (Kachmar and Boyer, 1953). Under normal conditions this is unlikely to be of any significance because the intracellular concentrations of K^+ are much higher than of NH_4^+. However the functions of ammonia will be accentuated when it accumulates in blood and tissues as in pathological states associated with disorders of the urea cycle, such as inborn errors of the urea cycle, viral hepatitis and cirrhosis. The metabolic acidoses of diabetes or of severe exercise provide another example of a stress situation in which ammonia is directly involved in order to maintain acid–base balance. Insight into the response of individual tissues to metabolic stress has been gained from experimentally induced hyperammonaemia or acidosis; these pathological conditions in turn have provided information on the regulatory mechanisms that operate normally *in vivo*. The three tissues, liver, brain and kidney, discussed in detail in this essay were chosen because they have been studied most intensively from the point of view of ammonia metabolism.

APPENDIX

Recollections of ammonia metabolism in Sheffield (1936–54)

When one of us (L.V.E.) joined H. A. Krebs in January 1936 he was concentrating on two main lines of research. One was on intermediary stages of carbohydrate metabolism with the collaboration of W. A. Johnson, and later with E. A. Evans, Jr., A. Kleinzeller, and D. H. Smyth. These studies resulted in the 'citric acid cycle' and an eventual Nobel Prize. His other line of work, extending that done earlier in Germany and

Cambridge, continued to be on ammonia and amino acid metabolism. This was a period of very high productivity for H.A.K. and until his marriage in 1938 he was usually the first to arrive and the last to leave. He seemed to spend almost no time at all over lunch, and one day we (secretary Irene Millis and L.V.E.) decided to time him with a stop clock. From the time he disappeared across the quadrangle to the Refectory below Firth Hall and then reappeared, fed, took just eleven minutes.

In this period before the war Åke Örström and his wife Margot collaborated with H.A.K. in work which culminated in the publication of papers on the micro determination of hypoxanthine and xanthine, and proved that hypoxanthine and not xanthine is the purine base formed in pigeon liver and requires one molecule of oxygen for its quantitative conversion to uric acid. Also, the rates of hypoxanthine formation were increased particularly by glutamine, and by pyruvate and NH_3, or oxaloacetate and NH_3 (Krebs and Örström, 1939; Örström, Örström and Krebs, 1939). This was followed by the demonstration that liver slices of pigeon, fowl and duck form glutamine from ammonium pyruvate, equivalent to 40–50% of the total NH_3 removed, and about 20% appeared as hypoxanthine (Örström, Örström, Krebs and Eggleston, 1939). The experimental work of this period was especially enjoyed because after a neat incision to remove the hen or duck liver, the virtually intact birds were taken home and eaten. With pre-war salaries, this was luxury.

It is perhaps not appreciated these days how much of this early work was carried out with relatively simple equipment and techniques. The animal tissue experiments were almost invariably carried out on slices, cut by hand with a saline moistened razor, and incubated in Warburg cups in a tank heated by Bunsen burners with a gas thermo-regulator of erratic efficiency. In 1936, there were two of these primitive looking baths on an island bench, with a single $\frac{1}{4}$ horsepower electric motor to operate the stirrers and shakers by a system of pulleys and leather belts. These belts had the nasty habit of breaking in the middle of the most vital experiments, but with practice they could be replaced with hastily tied string belts as a temporary makeshift, and, provided that the worker was young and agile, it was possible (but slightly nerve-racking) to do 24-cup experiments at a time (i.e. 22 experimental cups with 2 thermobarometers). The sides of these Warburg tanks were decorated with the more humorous advertisements for beer (although H.A.K. is almost a non-drinker), and for several of the pre-war years the equipment and shelves were decorated with feather-dressed dolls and small lead animals, and a celluloid swan floated round and round in a Warburg tank. During the war, one of our group (R. Hems) was in the army in Egypt and he called in the University of

Alexandria one day to see one of H.A.K.'s former colleagues (M. M. Hafez), and was amused to find there a small toy pig which Hafez had 'borrowed' from the lab. on leaving Sheffield.

During the winter of 1940–41, when air-raids caused a disruption of Sheffield's gas supply, the Warburg tanks were heated by 'spirit bottles' (glass bottles containing methylated spirits with several thicknesses of cotton bandages as a wick). After a cold night if one lighted these burners at nine o'clock, then round about noon the bath water had reached 38°– 40° and could be 'controlled' by inserting or removing one or more bottles.

Ammonia was determined colourimetrically after steam distillation *in vacuo* in a Parnas–Heller apparatus which at first sight appeared dilapidated, rusty, and most insecure. It was located on one end of a lead-topped bench, the boiler heated by an enormous Bunsen, and long lengths of glass tubing and rubber joints led to a water pump round the corner on another bench. The only thing about it which impressed the novice favourably was the knowledge that the long metal tube through both condensers was 'solid silver'. Hissing, rattling and wobbling, the whole apparatus worked astonishingly well and provided accurate NH_3 determinations for over 20 years. During the 1950's however, it was replaced by other methods of NH_3 determination, such as the Conway unit technique and nowadays by spectophotometry with purified commercial enzymes. In 1967 when H.A.K. retired from the Oxford Chair, the old Parnas–Heller was disinterred from its resting place under a sink, some glass parts already broken, so after salvaging the silver tube the rest was finally discarded, but not too sadly.

To the NH_3 obtained from the Parnas–Heller was added Nessler's reagent which we had to make ourselves from metallic mercury and iodine. The yellow colours were then examined in a visual colourimeter in which the observer adjusted the depth of the coloured solution he was looking through to match a standard, preferably with the instrument facing light from the north, and an average of several depth readings was taken. With practice the accuracy was quite good. Colourimeters with photo-electric cells and coloured glass filters did not arrive in the laboratory until after the war.

Urea determinations were carried out in Warburg manometers using urease obtained by soaking jack bean meal in water for several hours. During the war when this American product was not readily available, iron hard jack beans were individually cracked open with a hammer and then ground in a coffee mill. Many compounds, easily obtained now from commercial firms, we had to prepare ourselves. These included glutamine isolated from mangel-wurzels, xanthine oxidase from milk, mixed 'co-factors' from boiled muscle extracts, and a 'nucleotide-mixture' from chilled rabbit muscle.

Also with H.A.K. in 1938–9 was Philip P. Cohen, who, during his stay in Sheffield, devised a method for the determination of glutamic acid involving its conversion by means of chloramine-T and acid hydrolysis to succinic acid, which was then extracted with ether and determined manometrically with succinic dehydrogenase from washed pigeon breast muscle. It is interesting now to compare this day-long determination with the variety of present-day methods of a few minutes' duration using a spectrophotometer with purified enzymes and nucleotides. Nevertheless with Cohen's method it was then possible to do quantitative experiments on glutamic acid synthesis, '. . . when ammonia salts catalytically increase the rate of oxidation of α-ketoglutarate' in sliced kidney cortex and minced heart muscle (Krebs and Cohen, 1939):

$$2 \text{ α-ketoglutarate} + 1 \text{ NH}_3 \rightarrow \text{glutamate} + \text{succinate} + CO_2$$

During the war years H.A.K. was partly occupied with nutritional biochemistry, but he also found time to do additional experiments on urea synthesis from NH_3 because of some criticisms of the Krebs–Henseleit urea cycle put forward by F. Leuthardt, by S. J. Bach, and by O. A. Trowell. These experiments (see Krebs, 1942; Krebs, 1943) provided extra evidence against the critics' own theories of urea synthesis.

After the war H.A.K. developed a simpler manometric method for the determination of glutamic acid and glutamine utilizing a decarboxylase and glutaminase in *Clostridium welchii* and this method was extensively made use of during further studies on NH_3 metabolism and urea formation (Krebs, Eggleston and Hems, 1947; Krebs and Eggleston, 1948; Krebs, 1948; Krebs, Eggleston and Hems, 1948; Krebs, Eggleston and Hems, 1949). Instead of using slices of tissue, most of the work involved homogenized tissue as it had been shown by Cohen and Hayano (1946) that, in the presence of added ATP, homogenates also would synthesize urea at a substantial rate from NH_3. Great interest was aroused about this time (1948–56) by the inclusion in the Krebs–Henseleit urea cycle of carbamyl phosphate (by P. P. Cohen and his associates) and argininosuccinate (by Sarah Ratner's group) and the important roles played by acetyl glutamate, aspartate and ATP. Visitors and members of the Department of Biochemistry in Sheffield who joined in the work on amino acid metabolism included Arnold E. Bender and Kenneth Burton (amino acid oxidases), Joseph R. Stern (accumulation of glutamic acid in isolated brain tissue), Charles Terner (role of glutamic acid in the transport of K^+ in brain and retina), and Victor A. Knivett (citrulline degradation). The publications of this period (1949–55) can be found in the Biochemical Journal.

During his tenure of the Whitley Chair of Biochemistry in Oxford

(1954–67) H.A.K. spent less time on NH_3 and amino acid metabolism than on other fields of biochemistry, but an occasional publication from him showed his continued interest. With Dennis Bellamy he studied the interconversion of glutamate and aspartate in respiring tissues (Krebs and Bellamy, 1960), and with Richard J. Haslam the metabolism of glutamate in brain cortex slices and homogenate (Haslam and Krebs, 1963).

Since his 'retirement' into his new laboratory in the Radcliffe Infirmary, Oxford, H.A.K. has pursued his many research interests with renewed vigour and enthusiasm, and we are all hoping this will continue for many years to come.

References

Addae, S. K., and Lotspeich, W. D. (1968). *Am. J. Physiol.*, **215**, 269.

Alleyne, G. A. O. (1968). *Nature*, **217**, 847.

Balazs, R., Dahl, D., and Harwood, J. R. (1966). *J. Neurochem.*, **13**, 897.

Berl, S., Takagaki, G., Clarke, D. D., and Waelsch, H. (1962a). *J. Biol. Chem.*, **237**, 2570.

Berl, S., Takagaki, G., Clarke, D. D., and Waelsch, H. (1962b). *J. Biol. Chem.*, **237**, 2562.

Berl, S., Nicklas, W. J., and Clarke, D. D. (1968). *J. Neurochem.*, **15**, 131.

Bessman, S. P. (1959). In *Proceedings of the Fourth International Congress of Biochemistry. Vol. III*, p. 141. Ed. by Brucke, F. New York: Pergamon Press.

Bessman, S. P., and Bessman, A. N. (1955). *J. Clin. Invest.*, **34**, 622.

Bignall, M. C., Elebute, O., and Lotspeich, W. D. (1968). *Am. J. Physiol.*, **215**, 289.

Braganca, B. M., Faulkner, P., and Quastel, J. H. (1953). *Biochim. Biophys. Acta*, **10**, 83.

Brosnan, J. T. (1968). D.Phil. Thesis: Oxford University.

Cahill, G. F. (1967). *Adv. Enz. Reg.*, **5**, 87.

Caravaca, J., and Grisolia, S. (1960). *J. Biol. Chem.*, **235**, 684.

Carter, C. E., and Greenstein, J. P. (1947). *J. Natl. Cancer. Inst.*, **7**, 433.

Charles, R., Tager, J. M., and Slater, E. C. (1967). *Biochem. Biophys. Acta.*, **131** 29.

Cohen, P. P., and Hayano, M. (1946). *J. Biol. Chem.*, **166**, 239.

Cohen, P. P., and Sallach, H. J. (1961). In *Metabolic Pathways*, vol. II, p. 1. Ed. by Greenberg, D. M. Academic Press: New York.

Conway, E. J., and Byrne, A. (1933). *Biochem. J.*, **27**, 419.

Duda, G. D., and Handler, P. (1958). *J. Biol. Chem.*, **232**, 303.

du Ruisseau, J. P., Greenstein, J. P., Winitz, M., and Birnbaum, S. M. (1957). *Arch. Biochem. Biophys.*, **68**, 161.

Flock, E. V., Block, M. A., Grindlay, J. H., Mann, F. C., and Bollman, J. L (1953). *J. Biol. Chem.*, **200**, 529.

Flock, E. V., and Bollman, J. L. (1962). In *Amino Acid Pools*, p. 449, Ed. by Holden, J. T. Amsterdam: Elsevier.

Freedland, R. A., and Sodikoff, C. H. (1962). *Proc. Soc. Exp. Biol., Med.*, **109**, 394.

Gaitonde, M. K., and Richter, D. (1966). *J. Neurochem.*, **13**, 1309.

Goldstein, L. (1966). *Am. J. Physiol.*, **210**, 661.

Goldstein, L. (1967). *Am. J. Physiol.*, **213**, 983.

Goldstein, L., and Kensler, C. J. (1960). *J. Biol. Chem.*, **235**, 1086.

Goodman, A. D., Fuisz, R. E., and Cahill, G. F. (1966). *J. Clin. Invest.*, **45**, 612.

Grisolia, S., and Cohen, P. P. (1953). *J. Biol. Chem.*, **204**, 753.

Haslam, R. J., and Krebs, H. A. (1963). *Biochem. J.*, **86**, 432.

Hems, R., Ross, B. D., Berry, M. N., and Krebs, H. A. (1966). *Biochem. J.*, **101**, 284.

Hird, F. J. R., and Marginson, M. A. (1968). *Arch. Biochem. Biophys.*, **127**, 718.

Johnson, S. (1755). 'A Dictionary of the English Language', London.

Jones, M. E., Spector, L., and Lipmann, F. (1955). *J. Amer. Chem. Soc.*, **77**, 819.

Kachmar, J. F., and Boyer, P. D. (1953). *J. Biol. Chem.*, **200**, 669.

Kamin, H., and Handler, P. (1951). *J. Biol. Chem.*, **188**, 193.

Katsunuma, T., Temma, M., and Katunuma, N. (1968). *Biochem. Biophys. Res. Communs.*, **32**, 433.

Katunuma, N., Huzino, A., and Tomino, I. (1967). *Adv. Enz. Reg.*, **5**, 55.

Katunuma, N., Tomino, I., and Nishino, H. (1966). *Biochem. Biophys. Res. Communs.*, **22**, 321.

Kielland, J. (1937). *J. Amer. Chem. Soc.*, **59**, 1675.

Kirsten, E., Gerez, C., and Kirsten, R. (1963). *Biochem. Z.*, **337**, 312.

Krebs, H. A. (1935). *Biochem. J.*, **29**, 1951.

Krebs, H. A. (1942). *Biochem. J.*, **36**, 758.

Krebs, H. A. (1943). *Nature, Lond.*, **151**, 23.

Krebs, H. A. (1948). *Biochem. J.*, **43**, 51.

Krebs, H. A., and Bellamy, D. (1960). *Biochem. J.*, **75**, 523.

Krebs, H. A., and Cohen, P. P. (1939). *Biochem. J.*, **33**, 1895.

Krebs, H. A., and Eggleston, L. V. (1948). *Biochim. Biophys. Acta*, **2**, 319.

Krebs, H. A., and Henseleit, K. (1932). *Hoppe-Seyl. Z.*, **210**, 33.

Krebs, H. A., and Örström, Å. (1939). *Biochem. J.*, **33**, 984.

Krebs, H. A., Eggleston, L. V., and Hems, R. (1947). *Nature, Lond.*, **159**, 808.

Krebs, H. A., Eggleston, L. V., and Hems, R. (1948). *Biochem. J.*, **43**, 406.

Krebs, H. A., Eggleston, L. V., and Hems, R. (1949). *Biochem. J.*, **44**, 159.

Kvamme, E., Tveit, B., and Svenneby, G. (1965). *Biochem. Biophys. Res. Communs.*, **20**, 566.

Leonard, E., and Orloff, J. (1965). *Am. J. Physiol.*, **182**, 131.

McDermott, W. V. Jr., Adams, R. D., and Riddell, A. G. (1954). *Ann. Surg.*, **140**, 539.

McLean, P., and Novello, F. (1965). *Biochem. J.*, **94**, 410.

Miller, L. L. (1960). *Nature, Lond.*, **185**, 248.

Milne, M. D., Scribner, B. H., and Crawford, M. A. (1958). *Am. J. Med.*, **24**, 709.

Muntz, J. A., and Hurwitz, J. (1951). *Arch. Biochem. Biophys.*, **32**, 137.

Nash, T. P., and Benedict, S. R. (1921). *J. Biol. Chem.*, **48**, 463.

Nishiitsutsuji-Uwo, J., Ross, B. D., and Krebs, H. A. (1967). *Biochem. J.*, **103**, 852.

Örström, Å., Örström, M., and Krebs, H. A. (1939). *Biochem. J.*, **33**, 990.

Örström, Å., Örström, M., Krebs, H. A., and Eggleston, L. V. (1939). *Biochem. J.*, **33**, 995.

Owen, E. E., and Robinson, R. R. (1963). *J. Clin. Invest.*, 42, 263.

Parnas, J. K., and Heller, J. (1924). *Biochem. Z.*, **152**, 1.

Passonneau, J. V., and Lowry, O. H. (1964). *Adv. Enz. Reg.*, **2**, 265.

Pitts, R. F. (1964). *Am. J. Med.*, **36**, 720.
Pitts, R. F. (1968). In *The Physiology of the Kidney and Body Fluids*, 2nd. Ed. Chicago: Yearbook Medical Publishers Inc.
Pitts, R. F., De Haas, J. C. M., and Klein, J. (1963). *Am. J. Physiol.*, **204**, 187.
Pollak, V. E., Mattenheimer, H., De Bruin, H., and Weinman, K. J. (1965). *J. Clin. Invest.*, **44**, 169.
Post, R. L., and Jolly, P. C. (1957). *Biochim. Biophys. Acta*, **25**, 118.
Ratner, S. (1954). *Adv. Enzymol.*, **15**, 319.
Ratner, S., and Pappas, A. (1949). *J. Biol. Chem.*, **179**, 1183.
Recknagel, R. O., and Potter, V. R. (1951). *J. Biol. Chem.*, **191**, 263.
Rector, F. C. Jr., and Orloff, J. (1959). *J. Clin. Invest.*, **38**, 366.
Rector, F. C. Jr., Seldin, D. W., and Copenhaver, J. H. (1955). *J. Clin. Invest.*, **34**, 20.
Rendi, R., and Uhr, M. L. (1964). *Biochim. Biophys. Acta*, **89**, 520.
Rosado, A., Flores, G., Mora, J., and Soberon, G. (1962). *Am. J. Physiol.*, **203**, 37.
Rosenthal, O., Gottlieb, B., Gorry, J. D., and Vars, H. M. (1956). *J. Biol. Chem.*, **223**, 469.
Schenker, S., McCandless, D. W., Brophy, E., and Lewis, M. S. (1967). *J. Clin. Invest.*, **46**, 838.
Schimke, R. T. (1962a). *J. Biol. Chem.*, **237**, 459.
Schimke, R. T. (1962b). *J. Biol. Chem.*, **237**, 1921.
Schimke, R. T. (1963). *J. Biol. Chem.*, **238**, 1012.
Schoenheimer, R. (1942). *The Dynamic State of Body Constituents*, Harvard University Press, Cambridge, Mass.
Seligson, D., and Hirahara, K. (1957). *J. Lab. Clin. Med.*, **49**, 962.
Sellinger, O. Z., and de Balbian Verster, F. (1962). *J. Biol. Chem.*, **237**, 2836.
Shalhoub, R., Webber, W., Glabman, S., Canessa-Fischer, M., Klein, J., De Haas, J., and Pitts, R. F. (1963). *Am. J. Physiol.*, **204**, 181.
Silen, W., Harper, H. A., Mawdsley, D. L., and Weirich, W. L. (1955). *Proc. Soc. Exp. Biol. Med.*, **88**, 138.
Skou, J. C. (1960). *Biochim. Biophys. Acta*, **42**, 6.
Stone, W. J., and Pitts, R. F. (1967). *J. Clin. Invest.*, **46**, 1141.
Tower, D. B., Wherrett, J. R., and McKhann, G. M. (1961). In *Regional Neurochemistry*, p. 65. Ed. by Kety, S. S., and Elkes, J. Oxford: Pergamon Press.
Ulshafer, T. R. (1958). *J. Lab. Clin. Med.*, **52**, 718.
Van Slyke, D. D., Phillips, R. A., Hamilton, P. B., Archibald, R. M., Futcher, P. H., and Hiller, A. (1943). *J. Biol. Chem.*, **150**, 481.
Waelsch, H., Berl, S., Rossi, C. A., Clarke, D. D., and Purpura, D. P. (1964). *J. Neurochem.*, **11**, 717.
Warren, K. S., and Schenker, S. (1964). *J. Lab. and Clin. Med.*, **64**, 442.
Weil-Malherbe, H. (1962). In *Neurochemistry*. Ed. by Elliott, K. A. C., Page, I. H., and Quastel, J. H. (2nd Ed.), p. 321. Springfield: Thomas.
Weil-Malherbe, H., and Green, R. H. (1955). *Biochem. J.*, **61**, 218.
Williamson, D. H., Lund, P., and Krebs, H. A. (1967). *Biochem. J.*, **103**, 514.
Williamson, D. H., Lopes-Vieira, O., and Walker, B. (1967). *Biochem. J.*, **104**, 497.
Wollenberger, A., Ristau, O., and Schoffa, G. (1960). *Pflüg. Arch. Ges. Physiol.*, **270**, 399.
Wu, C., (1963). *Comp. Biochem. Physiol.*, **8**, 335.
Young, R. L., and Lowry, O. H. (1966). *J. Neurochem.*, **13**, 785.

THEORETICAL AND EXPERIMENTAL CONSIDERATIONS ON THE CONTROL OF GLYCOLYSIS IN MUSCLE

E. A. Newsholme

Agricultural Research Council Unit of Muscle Mechanisms and Insect Physiology, Department of Zoology, University of Oxford

I joined the Department of Biochemistry, Oxford, in October 1962 having just finished my Ph.D. studies at Cambridge, and I was exceedingly fortunate to find that I was to work in one of the huts that housed the Medical Research Council Unit for Research in Cell Metabolism. Later in 1964 I became a member of this unit and continued in that position until I joined the Agricultural Research Council Unit in the Department of Zoology, Oxford, in 1967. Thus for almost five years I worked in very close contact with Sir Hans Krebs and his research group. The most important lesson which I think I learned from this contact was that of simplicity and directness of experimental approach to biochemical and physiological problems. This simplicity applies to design of experiments as well as to experimental technique. But let it be quite clear, such simplicity is in no way synonymous with ease or speed of scientific progress; the simplest approach is sometimes the most arduous and time consuming process. For example, if in the interpretation of some metabolic process it was important to know the direction of changes in the concentration of a particular metabolite, the most direct approach would be to measure the concentration of it in the tissue. However, if it was present at very low concentrations, or if it was relatively unstable, such a direct approach might be extremely difficult, and an indirect method for detecting changes might be more attractive from the point of view of rate of progress of the work. The advantage of the simple, direct approach is that it provides the minimum number of possible interpretations of experimental data. The fewer the assumptions, either in the experimental technique or in the logic of the experimental design, the more reliance can be placed on interpretations based on the results of these experiments. Moreover, if the result of such an experiment is unexpected, it is less likely that it is due to a false premise or an error in the experimental technique or design, and therefore the more likely that the original theory, on which the experiments were based, requires modification. Thus, complementary to

189

such a straightforward approach is a readiness to reject or substantially modify a theory in order to comply with some new experimental finding. The mental agility which is necessary to use this approach is one of the greatest attributes of Sir Hans Krebs; he has used it so successfully so many times.

As the control of metabolic processes has been of great interest to him for many years I should like to honour this occasion by discussing a problem which has intrigued me since the beginning of my research career—the control of glycolysis in muscle.

I. INTRODUCTION TO CONTROL OF GLYCOLYSIS

In his classical experiments on yeast (1876) Pasteur observed that the presence of oxygen decreased fermentation. He suggested that the decreased appearance of alcohol under aerobic conditions could be explained either by oxidation of alcohol as soon as it was produced, or by inhibition of the process of production. He did not, however, attempt to explain the phenomenon apart from pointing out that the energy derived from fermentation was less than that from oxidation, and consequently the fermentation rate might be expected to be greater. However, most of the later workers in this field attempted to explain the phenomenon, and at one stage, as Burk (1939) has pointed out, there were nearly as many theories as there were investigators. Consequently it is impossible to review the early work on this problem in the present essay.

Work on the Pasteur effect up to about 1950 had established that the inhibition of glycolysis by the presence of oxygen was intimately associated with aerobic phosphorylation. The work of Meyerhof and Fiala (1950) with sonically disrupted yeast showed that a Pasteur effect could be obtained with what was essentially a cell-free preparation. This opened up a new field for investigating the control of glycolysis, as now it could be studied in a system which allowed chemical manipulations, direct chemical analysis and a simple experimental approach. Thus between 1950 and 1959 a large number of investigations into the mechanism of the Pasteur effect in cell free systems were carried out. However, the results from such studies provided neither a consistent nor a generally acceptable theory for the control of glycolysis. The reason for this was that glycolysis and aerobic respiration have a number of reactions where metabolic overlap occurs, and any one of these reactions might provide favourable conditions for glycolysis to be inhibited by aerobic respiration. Thus the position and the mechanism of control could be changed by small variations in the experimental conditions presented to the cell-free extract. Towards the end of the nineteen-fifties it was realized that experiments with cell free systems would not provide unequivocal evidence as to which reactions controlled glycolysis in the intact cell. It was therefore necessary to return to investigations using intact cell or tissue preparations, for example ascites tumour cells, yeast cells, the *in vitro* preparations of the rat diaphragm, and the perfused isolated rat heart.

Moreover at about this time a theoretical approach to the problem of identifying control reactions in living cells was being established by H. A. Krebs (1957); Chance, Holmes, Higgins and Connelly (1958); and Bücher and Rüssmann (1964); this theoretical basis, together with the availability of commercial enzymes for the measurement of most of the glycolytic intermediates, provided favourable conditions for the rapid advance in knowledge of glycolytic regulation which has taken place from about 1960 to the present time. Thus the regulatory enzymes of glycolysis have been identified and the properties of these enzymes studied in detail, so that a general theory of the control of glycolysis, and therefore an explanation of the Pasteur effect, can be provided. It is interesting that an explanation of the Pasteur effect at a biochemical level furnishes a theory of control that explains many physiological phenomena concerning glucose metabolism and energy utilization. Thus the reason it has taken almost a hundred years to provide a satisfactory explanation for this effect is that the effect was dependent on a fundamental cellular control mechanism and it required detailed knowledge of the reactions involved in energy production in the cell.

With the establishment of different techniques for investigating various aspects of metabolic control it became possible to synthesize a general systematic approach to the problem of metabolic control and this has been discussed in detail by Newsholme and Gevers (1967). However this review left some points unanswered in regard to the problems of identification of regulatory enzymes and these are discussed in Section II of this essay; Section III comprises a discussion of properties of the regulatory enzymes of glycolysis and describes in detail how the currently accepted theory of control of glycolysis is developed from the *in vitro* properties of these enzymes. In Section IV I have described some of the recent work in my laboratory on comparative enzymology of muscle.

II. SOME THEORETICAL CONSIDERATIONS CONCERNING METABOLIC CONTROL

In this section I shall endeavour to explain new ideas or clarifications in the theoretical approach to metabolic control that have developed since the review (Newsholme and Gevers, 1967) was written; this will be restricted to the problems of definition and identification of regulatory enzymes. One of the major problems in metabolic control is the definition of a regulatory enzyme, because, to some extent, the activities of all enzymes that constitute a metabolic pathway are regulated; and I consider that this problem of definition is responsible for much of the present confusion about metabolic regulation. It is possible to distinguish both theoretically and experimentally between two classes of regulatory enzyme and two types of regulation, and I believe this may clarify some of the current misunderstandings in this subject. Most of the central ideas which I shall discuss have been either described or foreshadowed by two eminent biochemists in this field, Th. Bücher and H. A. Krebs; and I recommend two excellent reviews of metabolic control written by these workers, H. A. Krebs (1957) and Bücher and Rüssmann (1964). My understanding of this subject owes much to the intelligent review and appraisal of the literature carried out by one of my research students, F. S. Rolleston, in 1966, and the subsequent discussions which we had on these problems; the subject was reviewed by Rolleston in his D.Phil. thesis (Oxford University 1966).

A. Regulation at non-equilibrium reactions

With remarkable foresight H. A. Krebs in 1946 stated that reversible reactions cannot result in any major changes within living tissue, and that irreversible ones must control the rate and direction of metabolism; this point, which has been stressed many times since, is the theme of this sub-section. With the development of knowledge of metabolic regulation over the last few years the significance of non-equilibrium reactions in control has emerged; it is the means by which specific feedback inhibition in a metabolic pathway is established. In such a system the rate of the metabolic pathway is measured by some factor and the information which this factor receives about the pathway is used to regulate the activity of the 'non-equilibrium' enzyme; in a simple example, the concentration of the end product of a metabolic pathway can measure its rate and, if this compound inhibits the regulatory enzyme of that pathway, a feedback inhibition mechanism is established. However, the important point for the present discussion is that the factor, which measures the rate of the metabolic pathway, may have no connection with the reaction catalysed by the regulatory enzyme. Therefore, in order to regulate the flux through this reaction, this factor must modify the catalytic activity of the enzyme (and not the concentrations of substrate, product, cofactor, competitive inhibitor, etc.). This implies that the catalytic activity of the enzyme must limit the rate of the reaction, and consequently the reaction must be non-equilibrium.

However, identification of a non-equilibrium reaction does not necessarily indicate a regulatory enzyme; it depends on the definition of a regulatory enzyme. The definition used by Rolleston and Newsholme (1967) is as follows: a regulatory enzyme is one whose activity controls the rate of flux through a metabolic pathway (i.e. a non-equilibrium reaction), and whose activity is regulated by factors other than the substrate concentration. This is an operational definition and indicates experimentally how a regulatory enzyme can be identified; thus the rate of flux through the pathway is changed (using intact tissue preparations) and the steady state concentration of the substrate of the non-equilibrium enzyme is measured in the two conditions of flux. If the flux rate is increased and the substrate decreased, or vice versa, this indicates a regulatory enzyme. The rationale behind this approach is very simple: if the flux through the pathway increases, the catalytic activity of the 'non-equilibrium' enzyme must increase and this cannot be due to an increase in the substrate, if, experimentally, it has been shown to decrease. Consequently, it must be due to some other factor which is designated as the specific regulator. If such evidence for a regulatory enzyme is obtained it suggests that an investigation into the properties of the enzyme in search of a possible regulator molecule is worthwhile. This, then, is the particular virtue of the experimental approach and of the above definition of a regulatory enzyme. The measurement of steady state concentrations of intermediates under various states of flux of a pathway in order to locate regulatory reactions was first suggested by H. A. Krebs in 1957. It was developed in terms of the crossover theorem by Chance, Holmes, Higgins and Connelly (1958) for study of the electron transport in the respiratory chain, but this is only a special case of the more general approach given above and first suggested by H. A. Krebs (see Bücher, 1965; Rolleston and Newsholme, 1967). The adherence to such an approach, and the availability of specific and precise enzymatic methods for measuring many of the metabolic intermediates, have been largely responsible for the rapid advance in knowledge of metabolic regulation over the last few years.

B. Regulation at equilibrium reactions

If an enzyme catalyses an equilibrium reaction (or a reaction close to equilibrium), the catalytic activity cannot regulate the flux through the reaction (unless it is so strongly inhibited that it becomes a non-equilibrium reaction). However, the rate of flux in one direction can be limited by the concentration of substrate or cofactor; in this condition it is possible to consider situations where an equilibrium reaction might control the flux through a pathway.

An enzyme catalyses the following equilibrium reaction $A + X \rightleftharpoons B + Y$ that initiates a metabolic pathway, $A \rightleftharpoons B \rightleftharpoons C \rightleftharpoons O \rightleftharpoons P$, in which all the other reactions are single substrate equilibrium reactions and are regulated by their substrate concentrations. If the assumptions are made that the rate of production of A and the rate of removal of P are dependent upon their concentrations, then the reaction $A + X \rightleftharpoons B + Y$ could regulate the pathway by means of the cofactor levels X and Y. If the concentration of X increased and Y decreased this would raise the concentration of B, and as the concentration of A would remain fairly constant, due to its increased supply, the rate of the forward reaction $A \rightarrow B$ would also remain constant. The increased concentration of B would increase the conversion of B to C, etc., and the increased concentration of P would stimulate its removal from the pathway. Thus the control of the pathway is achieved by the concentration ratio X/Y, which may have no direct relationship to the rate of production of the end product of the pathway (i.e. P); for this reason it may be termed an open loop system of control by analogy to controls in engineering systems; this is in contrast to the control by a specific regulator at a non-equilibrium reaction which is perhaps analogous to a closed loop control mechanism in engineering systems (see Wilkins, 1966).

An example of an equilibrium system of control may be the mitochondrial electron transport system, which is normally coupled to oxidative phosphorylation. In the transference of electrons along the system of carriers from $NADH_2$ to oxygen there are three phosphorylation sites at which ADP and P_i are converted into ATP. There is now an accumulation of evidence to support the idea that at least the first two reactions that couple electron transport to oxidative phosphorylation are reversible, and therefore that the same mechanism (which is, of course, unknown at present) is involved in both the forward and reverse directions (see Klingenberg, 1964). This has led Klingenberg to propose that control of electron transport (cell respiration) is brought about by the concentration ratio of ATP/ADP (or more correctly $ATP/ADP + P_i$). We can now analyse this in terms of the scheme proposed above; if discussion is limited to the first phosphorylation reaction then we know that:

$$NADH_2 + ADP + P_i + FP_{oxid} \rightleftharpoons NAD + ATP + FP_{red} \qquad (1)$$

and

$$FP_{red} \rightarrow \rightarrow \rightarrow \rightarrow O_2 \qquad (2)$$

It is known that the supply of $NADH_2$ is increased when cellular respiration is increased (i.e. an increase in glycolysis and TCA cycle) so that the concentration of mitochondrial $NADH_2$ will remain constant. It seems likely that there is a non-equilibrium reaction somewhere towards the end of electron transport chain (possibly the last phosphorylation step), which may be controlled simply by the concentration of reduced substrate; and the assumption is made that the concentration of FP_{red} regulates the next stage in the transport process (reaction (2)). Then the conditions for the equilibrium control system (as described above) are satisfied, so that the rate of electron transport will be controlled at the first and perhaps the second phosphorylation sites by the concentration ratio of ATP/ADP.

This control therefore may be described as an open loop system, although to some extent ATP is an end product of the reaction. Nevertheless ATP cannot be described as a specific regulator of the reaction as its effect will depend upon the concentrations of all the participants of the reaction and, in particular, the equilibrium constant of the reaction. It is interesting to note that the equilibrium control cannot function without it is limited on both sides by non-equilibrium reactions, and the control of substrate supply (e.g. $NADH_2$) for such an equilibrium reaction will be a metabolic closed loop system as discussed in Section II(A).

There is an important fundamental difference between control at equilibrium and non-equilibrium reactions which should be stressed. At equilibrium reactions and those close to equilibrium there is a minimum change in free energy (AF is close to zero), so that if energy transference is taking place in the reaction this can proceed with a minimum loss of energy as heat—in other words maximum efficiency. This is of particular importance in oxidative phosphorylation, in which the chemical energy released from electron transfer along the redox gradient is transferred to the molecule ATP, as it ensures that maximum efficiency of energy transfer is obtained; and this may explain why mitochondrial respiration is controlled by an equilibrium rather than a non-equilibrium system. However a price is paid for such energy transfer efficiency; the control is restricted to the participants of the coupling reactions and no specific regulation for the pathway as a whole is possible. At non-equilibrium reactions the free energy change is large and some of the chemical energy involved in the reaction is lost as heat; but the pathway can be regulated by factors that are unrelated to any reaction in the pathway. This characteristic of non-equilibrium control is of importance in evolutionary development of regulation of metabolic pathways. Thus there need be no restrictions placed on the regulatory mechanism by the nature of the metabolic pathway, so that the selection of regulators for a given pathway could be based on consideration for the metabolism of the cell as a whole, rather than the individual pathway *per se*. The significance of this property for the development of an integrated metabolic control system is obvious, and the loss of energy as heat which is incurred in these reactions, is an example, in biological systems, where energy has to be expended to provide the potential for metabolic control. Examples of such controls are given in the next section and the relationship between the mechanism of control and the metabolism of the cell as a whole is discussed in detail.

III. THE DEVELOPMENT OF A THEORY FOR THE REGULATION OF GLYCOLYSIS IN MUSCLE

One major fuel for the provision of energy in muscle is glucose (and/or glycogen—see Section IV), and the series of enzyme-catalysed reactions which break down this fuel is known as glycolysis. In muscles which normally function aerobically the end product of glycolysis, pyruvate, is oxidized within the mitochondria by the TCA cycle and the respiratory chain to provide ATP; whereas in the more anaerobic muscle, pyruvate is converted to lactate and most of the ATP is produced by glycolysis. In the present discussion it will be assumed that the main role of glycolysis is the production of pyruvate (or lactate) for the formation of ATP (either aerobically or anaerobically). In order to provide a straightforward account of control in glycolysis, the discussion will emphasize generalities and similarities between different muscles and other tissues; enzymatic differences resulting from diversity of function will be deferred until Section IV.

Evidence has been obtained that membrane transport of glucose, hexokinase, phosphorylase, phosphofructokinase, glyceraldehyde-3-phosphate dehydrogenase and pyruvate kinase may all play a role in the regulation of glycolysis (Randle, 1963; Williamson, 1965), but the first four 'systems' appear to play the major role in regulation of the overall flux through glycolysis. However, as almost nothing is known about the molecular details of either transport or its regulation, discussion will be limited to the three enzymes.

A. Evidence for regulatory enzymes in glycolysis

Evidence has been obtained that hexokinase, phosphorylase and phosphofructokinase are regulatory enzymes for glycolysis (see Section II for definition).

1. *Hexokinase*

The low activity of hexokinase in muscle and the fact that the mass action ratio is very much smaller than the apparent equilibrium constant suggest that this reaction is non-equilibrium. However, the precise measurement of intracellular glucose is the main drawback in calculation of the mass action ratio for this reaction. Intracellular glucose is usually measured by subtracting the extracellular volume (e.g. sorbitol or inulin volume) from the total glucose volume (extra-plus intracellular volume) in the muscle, and if the total volume exceeds the extracellular by only a small amount, the value for the intracellular glucose will not be accurate. Under certain experimental conditions (e.g. perfused heart preparation in the presence of insulin) intracellular glucose is sufficiently large to be measured precisely and the mass action ratio of the reaction is much lower than the equilibrium constant for hexokinase reaction. Under these conditions it can be shown that if the flux rate through glycolysis is increased (e.g. anaerobic conditions, respiratory poisons) the intracellular concentration of glucose is decreased, and vice versa if the rate of glycolysis is decreased (e.g. perfusion with fatty acids; Newsholme and Randle, 1964); thus the enzyme is regulatory for glycolysis. However, because of the difficulties discussed above, it is possible under some conditions that hexokinase catalyses an equilibrium reaction.

2. Phosphorylase

Although the standard free energy change of the phosphorylase reaction is small (i.e. apparent equilibrium constant is close to unity), the enzyme appears to catalyse a non-equilibrium reaction in the muscle; this is because the intracellular concentration of G-1-P (about 0.05 mM) is maintained much lower than that of P_i (about 10 mM). Moreover, when glycogen breakdown is increased the glycogen concentration is decreased (in comparison to the control condition), and vice versa; thus phosphorylase is a regulatory enzyme for glycogenolysis.

3. Phosphofructokinase

Measurements of mass action ratios or of total enzyme activity strongly suggest that this enzyme catalyses a non-equilibrium reaction. In experiments with the perfused rat heart and isolated diaphragm preparations it has been shown to be a regulatory enzyme (i.e. the concentration of F-6-P changes in opposite direction to change in flux rates; (Newsholme and Randle, 1961, 1964)). However, experiments with skeletal muscle preparations do not provide positive evidence for a regulatory enzyme, as the concentration of F-6-P increases with an increased flux rate. It is generally accepted that phosphofructokinase is a regulatory enzyme for glycolysis in skeletal muscle because its properties are very similar to those of the enzyme from rat heart (cf. Passonneau and Lowry, 1962, with

Mansour, 1963). An explanation for the above phenomenon is that the conditions which increase the glycolytic rate stimulate phosphorylase activity to a greater extent than that of phosphofructokinase.

B. Properties of regulatory enzymes

In this section the properties of phosphofructokinase, hexokinase and phosphorylase will be described briefly, but the theory of control of glycolysis, which is based on these properties, will be discussed in some detail. It is my opinion that although the properties of these enzymes have been adequately described in the literature, the basis for the current theory of the control of glycolysis has not been satisfactorily explained.

Phosphofructokinase catalyses the following reaction:

$$F\text{-}6\text{-}P + ATP \rightarrow FDP + ADP.$$

Plots of the activity of this enzyme against ATP and F-6-P concentrations are shown in Figure 1: above an optimum concentration ATP inhibits the enzyme, and this inhibition is potentiated by citrate but is relieved by AMP, FDP and P_i (Figure 1a); it is stressed that in the absence of ATP

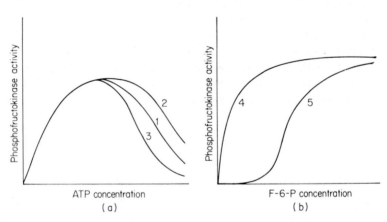

Figure 1. Diagrammatic representations of the effects of changes in the substrate concentrations on the catalytic activity of phosphofructokinase. (*a*) At a fixed concentration of F-6-P, the effect of changes in the concentration of ATP (1), in the presence of FDP, AMP or P_i (2), and in the presence of citrate (3). (*b*) The effect of changes in the concentration of F-6-P on the activity of phosphofructokinase at a non-inhibitory concentration of ATP (4) and at an inhibitory concentration of ATP (5)

inhibition there is no effect of AMP, citrate, etc., on phosphofructokinase activity. It can be seen from the plot of activity against F-6-P concentration (Figure (1b)) that ATP appears to cause inhibition by raising the apparent K_m of the enzyme for F-6-P; and in a limited sense it could be described as competitive inhibition.

Phosphorylase catalyses the following reaction

$$(G\text{-}G\text{-}G)_n + P_i \rightarrow G\text{-}1\text{-}P + (G\text{-}G\text{-}G)_{n-1}$$

This enzyme exists in two forms, phosphorylase a and b; the significance of the two forms will be discussed later. Phosphorylase b is activated by AMP or P_i and these effects are reduced by ATP or G-6-P (i.e. deactivators); thus the enzyme has a very low activity in the absence of AMP and in the presence of low concentrations of P_i (Morgan and Parmeggiani, 1964).

Hexokinase catalyses the following reaction:

$$G + ATP \rightarrow G\text{-}6\text{-}P + ADP.$$

This enzyme is inhibited by G-6-P in a non-competitive manner with respect to the substrate glucose: the significance of this non-competitive inhibition will be discussed later. In heart muscle the G-6-P inhibition is relieved by P_i (England and Randle, 1967).

C. A mechanism for the regulation of glycolysis in muscle

In this essay I have chosen to discuss in detail the regulation of glycolysis at the phosphofructokinase reaction for a number of reasons: the properties of this enzyme from a variety of tissues and organisms are very similar; the properties serve to illustrate a number of fundamental principles in regulation of energy metabolism; and the regulation at this reaction can be simply extended to produce an integrated mechanism of control of all three enzymes, phosphofructokinase, hexokinase and phosphorylase.

1. The problems associated with control of phosphofructokinase by ATP

The important end product of glycolysis and aerobic oxidation in muscle is biological energy, ATP, and this compound, when it is hydrolysed to ADP, provides energy for most if not all of the major energy requiring reactions of the muscle (e.g. muscular contraction, ion transport, biosyntheses). Therefore the ATP inhibition of phosphofructokinase could provide a closed loop system of feedback control of glycolysis in relation to the balance between the reactions producing ATP and those utilizing ATP. An increase in the rate of ATP utilization would lower the concentration of this compound and this would stimulate phosphofructokinase and therefore glycolysis; thus the rate of ATP production would be increased and the balance between utilization and production of this compound would be restored. Although, superficially, this simple ATP control mechanism appears satisfactory, it suffers from the disadvantage that, in order to regulate glycolysis, the concentration of ATP must change inversely with the rate of utilization (i.e. ATP concentration should be higher in resting than in mechanically active muscle). Such a feedback mechanism may be satisfactory for the control of the concentration of amino acids in bacteria, in which the regulatory enzyme of the biosynthetic pathway is inhibited by the end product amino acid (e.g. isoleucine inhinits threonine deaminase). Changes in the concentration of an amino acid of sufficient magnitude to control a regulatory enzyme (approximately 4–10-fold, see below) may be acceptable to a cell. However, variations in the concentration of ATP raise a problem in energetics because of the relationship between the ATP concentration and the free energy of ATP hydrolysis. The amount of free energy that is available from this hydrolysis depends upon the concentrations (or more correctly the thermodynamic activities) of ATP and ADP; some indication of the variation in free energy of hydrolysis with changes in nucleotide concentrations is shown in Table 1. Assuming a reasonably physiological

Table 1. The effect of changes in the ATP/ADP concentration ratio on the free energy of hydrolysis of ATP. The change in free energy was calculated from $\Delta F = \Delta F_0 + RT \ln \dfrac{[ADP][P_i]}{[ATP]}$; ΔF_0 was taken to be -7000 cal; by convention the concentration of water was taken to be unity. In A the changes in the concentrations of ATP and ADP are in accord with an adenylate kinase equilibrium and a total nucleotide concentration of 5 mM (see Table 2). In B the changes in concentrations of ATP and ADP are not related to adenylate kinase and the total nucleotide concentration is 12 mM

| | Concn. (mM) | | | |
	ATP	ADP	P_i	ΔF for ATP hydrolysis (cal)
A.	4·95	0·05	8·0	12,834
	3·90	1·0	8·0	10,849
	2·20	2·0	8·0	10,047
	1·42	2·15	8·0	9,734
B.	11·0	1·0	8·0	11,475
	10·0	2·0	8·0	10,986
	6·0	6·0	8·0	9,990
	2·0	10·0	8·0	8,993
	1·0	11·0	8·0	8,505

concentration of ATP, a 10-fold change in concentration (with the corresponding change in ADP) results in a change in free energy of hydrolysis of 20–30%. If a 10-fold decrease in the concentration of ATP was necessary to stimulate phosphofructokinase maximally (and this might be the case—see below), this would mean that many (perhaps all) energy utilizing processes (including muscular contraction) would have to function with a loss in energy transfer efficiency of at least 20–30%. This is because these processes would function at both the maximum and minimum concentrations of ATP, and, in order to release sufficient free energy for the particular reaction at the minimum ATP concentration, these reactions would have to function inefficiently at the maximum concentration of ATP. Moreover a similar situation would pertain to oxidative phosphorylation: in order for the energy of electron transfer to be converted into 'phosphate bond' energy (i.e. ATP formation) at the maximum concentration, the process would be inefficient at the minimum concentration. Inefficiency means that during reactions involving ATP–ADP interconversions some of the available energy would be lost as heat rather than being conserved as chemical energy (i.e. a non-equilibrium reaction). In order to overcome such inefficiency an organism would require to ingest some 20–30% more food than a more efficient competitor. Obviously any changes in the control process which tended to stabilize the ATP concentration would be selectively advantageous. It could be argued that perhaps the ATP inhibition of phosphofructokinase represents an early control mechanism during evolutionary development, which has been modified according to pressures of natural selection to produce a more efficient control mechanism.

So far it has been assumed that a 10-fold change in ATP was necessary to control phosphofructokinase; it might be expected that natural selection would have allowed phosphofructokinase to develop an exceedingly sensitive response to small changes in ATP concentration above and below the physiological normal concentration. However, it can be shown that there are limits to the degree of sensitivity of an enzyme to a regulator molecule; these limits are defined by the physical chemistry of the interaction between a protein and small molecule (ligand). The particular characteristics of a regulatory enzyme have been described in physico-chemical terms by Monod, Wyman and Changeux (1965), and it is possible using this as a model to describe the maximum theoretical sensitivity of phosphofructokinase to changes in ATP. This is shown in Table 2. The change in concentration of the ligand (e.g. ATP) to produce a change in the fractional saturation from 0·1 (i.e. 10% inhibition) to 0·9 (i.e. 90% inhibition) varies with the extent of the sigmoid nature of the

Table 2. The change in ATP concentration necessary to change the fractional saturation of an allosteric enzyme from $0 \cdot 1$ to $0 \cdot 9$, according to the Monod, Wyman and Changeux model (1965). It is assumed that ATP is a ligand for a tetrameric enzyme which binds four molecules of ATP per molecule of enzyme (i.e. $n = 4$), and that of the two states of the enzyme (R and T), ATP only binds to one state (R) and then inhibits the enzyme. The allosteric constant (L) is ratio T/R. It is assumed that fractional saturation of the enzyme with ATP is equivalent to percentage inhibition (i.e. fractional saturation of $0 \cdot 1 \equiv 10\%$ inhibition). The simplified model of Monod and coworkers (1965) has been used to calculate the fractional saturation, i.e.

$$\bar{Y} = \frac{\alpha(1 + \alpha)^{n-1}}{L + (1 + \alpha)^n}$$

| Allosteric constant (L) | Concn. of ATP providing: | |
	10% inhibition	90% inhibition
1	$0 \cdot 18$	$8 \cdot 0$
100	$1 \cdot 2$	$9 \cdot 8$
500	$2 \cdot 0$	$11 \cdot 5$
1,000	$2 \cdot 6$	$12 \cdot 6$
10,000	$5 \cdot 0$	$19 \cdot 6$

response (i.e. with the allosteric constant); if the value of the allosteric constant is 10^2, a 10-fold change in the concentration of ATP is required whereas if the value is 10^4 a 4-fold change is required. In other words, the response of an enzyme to a regulatory molecule cannot be excessively sharp, as it is dependent upon the binding of the regulator molecule to the protein. Thus the cooperative effect of an allosteric protein does not solve the problem of the unsatisfactory ATP feedback signal for glycolytic control. It is interesting that Garland (1968) has observed that almost a 10-fold decrease in the mitochondrial content of ATP was necessary to stimulate citrate synthase in experiments with isolated mitochondria; this enzyme has been shown to be inhibited by ATP *in vitro*, which is considered to be of regulatory significance, but no other modifiers of this enzyme are known.

2. *AMP as an amplification signal for changes in ATP*

As the ability of an enzyme to respond to changes in a concentration of a ligand is limited by the physical chemistry of interaction between a protein and a ligand, Nature has sought another means to increase the sensitivity of phosphofructokinase to changes in ATP; an amplification system has been developed. The clue to the nature of the amplification system is provided by the properties of phosphofructokinase: the ATP inhibition can be removed by AMP. In the cell there is an enzyme, adenylate kinase, which appears to maintain an equilibrium between ATP, ADP and AMP as follows:

$$ATP + AMP \rightleftharpoons 2ADP.$$

The normal balance between ATP formation and utilization in the cell ensures that the concentration of ATP is maintained higher than that of ADP, and, because of the equilibrium catalysed by adenylate kinase, AMP is maintained at a very low concentration (e.g. approximate concentrations in resting muscle may be: ATP 5·0 mM, ADP 0·8 mM, AMP 0·05 mM). The equilibrium constant for the reaction catalysed by adenylate kinase is 0·44, and it can be shown from a simple theoretical calculation that if the ATP concentration is decreased slightly (and therefore ADP is increased slightly) the proportional increase in the concentration of AMP is very much greater (see Table 3). Therefore it is

Table 3. Variations in adenine nucleotide concentrations based on the equilibrium of the reaction catalysed by adenylate kinase. The concentrations are calculated from the equilibrium constant for the adenylate kinase reaction,

$$K = \frac{[AMP][ATP]}{[ADP^2]} = 0·44 \text{ assuming a constant total nucleotide concentration}$$

of 5 mM. The algebraic equation for calculation is

$$x = \sqrt{\left[\left(\frac{c-a}{2}\right)^2 - 0·44a^2\right]} + \frac{c-a}{2},$$

where c is total nucleotide concentration, a is ADP concentration, and x is AMP concentration. This is a simple extension of H. A. Krebs (1964)

	Concn. (mM)		
ADP	ATP	AMP	$\frac{ATP}{ADP}$
0·1	4·899	0·001	49·0
0·2	4·796	0·004	24·0
0·3	4·691	0·009	15·6
0·5	4·48	0·02	8·9
1·0	3·89	0·11	3·9
1·5	3·19	0·31	2·1
2·0	2·2	0·80	1·1

suggested that in the cell the role of AMP is to act as an amplification signal for changes in the concentration of ATP, so that a small change in ATP, which would elicit little response from the regulatory enzyme, causes a greater change in AMP concentration which is sufficient to change significantly the catalytic activity of the regulatory enzyme.

3. Another amplification mechanism

The concept of AMP as an amplification signal for changes in ATP was first proposed by H. A. Krebs in 1964; this was developed when it was realized that not only was muscle phosphofructokinase affected by AMP, but that the enzyme fructose diphosphatase in liver, which catalyses the reversal of the phosphofructokinase reaction in this tissue, was inhibited by AMP. This finding emphasized the role of AMP as a regulatory molecule and demanded an explanation as to its metabolic significance; the previous experience of the Krebs' group with adenylate kinase (Eggleston and Hems, 1952) provided the background information for Krebs to develop this most important concept. This concept provided some of the impetus for Underwood and Newsholme (1965; 1967a) to study the properties of the phosphofructokinases from rat liver and kidney cortex to ascertain if AMP affected these enzymes in a similar manner to the muscle enzyme. This was found to be the case and from discussions of this dual effect of AMP on liver and kidney cortex phosphofructokinases and fructose diphosphatases, and from experiments with kidney cortex slices, the possibility that apparently energetically wasteful cycles may be operative in tissues was proposed (Underwood and Newsholme, 1967b). The significance of such cycles was first considered by Newsholme and Gevers (1967); they increase the ability of the control reactions in metabolic pathways to respond significantly to small changes in metabolic signals. In other words, such cycles provide inherent amplification for metabolic signals and minimize the change in concentration that a metabolic regulator must undergo to provide satisfactory regulation (as discussed above). The energy that is utilized in such cycles, which is released as heat, is expended in order to provide this amplification, and it cannot therefore be described as a waste of energy (for full discussion see Newsholme and Gevers, 1967). This is another example of how energy is expended in biological systems to provide for metabolic regulation.

4. Evidence for theory of regulation of glycolysis

The theory of metabolic control of glycolysis in muscle at the phosphofructokinase reaction can be summarized as follows: the initiation of muscular contraction increases the utilization of ATP so that there is a decrease in the concentration of ATP, which, through the adenylate kinase reaction, produces an increase in the concentration of AMP. However, the percentage decrease in ATP concentration is small while that of AMP is large, and this latter change increases the activity of phosphofructokinase;

this increased activity will lower the concentration of G-6-P and this will stimulate hexokinase activity. Therefore, provided that the activity of membrane transport of glucose into the cell is higher than that of hexokinase, or that muscular contraction produces (by some unknown mechanism) a stimulation of glucose transport, this stimulation of the two enzymes will increase the rate of glucose degradation so that more ATP is synthesized. Moreover the increased concentration of AMP (and possibly P_i) and the decreased concentration of G-6-P will increase the activity of phosphorylase b, and thus glycogen will be broken down for energy production.

Evidence in support of the above theory is obtained from two sources: firstly from direct measurement of changes in these regulator molecules when the glycolytic rate is changed, and secondly from the fact that the theory can be used to explain a number of biochemical and physiological observations which were previously either not explained or explained inadequately.

(a) *Direct evidence.* Most of the experiments are well documented in the literature and so will be only briefly referred to in this essay. In experiments with the isolated perfused rat heart, the concentration of the regulator molecules are found to change in the expected direction when glycolysis is increased by anoxia, respiratory poisons or uncoupling agents (Newsholme and Randle, 1961, 1964; Regen, Davis, Morgan and Park, 1964); moreover the concentrations of ATP and ADP were found to change very little whereas that of AMP was increased several-fold. Perhaps more physiologically meaningful experiments were performed with the perfused isolated working heart preparation of Neely, Liebermeister, Battersby and Morgan (1967); in this preparation the ventricles of the heart are made to perform varying amounts of mechanical work, and it has been shown that increasing the work output stimulates glycolysis at the reactions catalysed by phosphorylase, hexokinase and phosphofructokinase, and membrane transport is also increased. The changes in the metabolic regulator molecules (AMP, G-6-P, P_i) are consistent with the above theory (Morgan, 1969). The experiments of Sacktor and Wormser-Shavit (1966) and Sacktor and Hurlbut (1966) with the flight muscles of the blowfly are somewhat similar to the experiments of Morgan (1969) in that the flight muscles are made to do mechanical work (i.e. the insect flies) and as a consequence the rate of glycolysis is increased. In particular with the flight muscle of the insect the change from rest to flight results in a very large increase in the rate of ATP utilization and therefore in the rate of metabolism. The stimulation of glycolysis induced by flight was due to an activation of the enzymes phosphorylase, hexokinase and phosphofructokinase (and trehalase), and the changes in the regulator molecules were consistent with the above theory.

It should be noted that this direct evidence is to some extent indirect, and it does not prove that this theory of glycolytic control is substantially correct; it is only consistent with the theory. In order to do this it would be necessary to measure the concentration of the regulator molecules (e.g. ATP, AMP, F-6-P) within the immediate environment of phosphofructokinase in the cell, and to have some information on the properties of this enzyme either *in situ* or in conditions which reflect the probable *in situ* environment of phosphofructokinase. Such investigations are at present technically impossible. It is interesting therefore that perhaps the strongest support for the above theory comes from indirect evidence.

(*b*) *Indirect evidence.* (i) AMP is known to modify the activity of a number of enzymes in a manner that suggests that it may be of regulatory significance, for example phosphorylase, phosphofructokinase, fructose diphosphatase, isocitrate dehydrogenase (see Newsholme and Gevers, 1967, for review). However, other than this proposed regulatory role for AMP, it does not appear to have any other function in the cell, apart from its involvement in the biosynthetic pathway of the adenine nucleotides from IMP; but the rate of this process must be extremely small in comparison with the turnover of the terminal phosphate of ATP, and would not require the very high activity of adenylate kinase, or the maintenance of equilibrium of the reaction catalysed by this enzyme.

(ii) The effect of the inhibitory action of ATP on phosphofructokinase is to raise the K_m of the enzyme for the second substrate, F-6-P. Therefore if the F-6-P concentration in the cell was increased this could overcome the ATP–AMP control of glycolysis. Hence the significance of the fact that the inhibition of hexokinase by G-6-P is non-competitive with respect to glucose; excess glucose in the cell cannot influence the concentration of hexosemonophosphate because of this inhibition. Moreover the concentration of G-6-P is controlled by the activity of phosphofructokinase, which therefore controls the activity of hexokinase non-competitively. Thus the control of glucose utilization is by a concerted control system of hexokinase and phosphofructokinase. The significance of such a system is that it affords flexibility in control; glucose can still be converted to glycogen in the muscle even though phosphofructokinase is inhibited, as a stimulation of the enzyme regulating glycogen synthesis (UDP-glucosyltransferase) will lower the G-6-P concentration and favour phosphorylation of glucose which will be converted to glycogen. Thus glycogen can still be synthesized although the flux through glycolysis is inhibited at the phosphofructokinase reaction. Similarly a hormonal stimulation of glycogen breakdown (this does not involve AMP, G-6-P, etc., see later) will produce an increase in the G-6-P and F-6-P concentrations and therefore stimulate, indirectly, the activity of phosphofructokinase.

This control system of hexokinase and phosphofructokinase is to some extent bypassed in the liver because it contains another specific enzyme for phosphorylating glucose, glucokinase. This enzyme is not inhibited by G-6-P and it has a high K_m for glucose (approximately 10 mM) so that it responds to changes in the concentration of glucose in the hepatic portal vein (approximately 10 mM after a carbohydrate meal). Thus excess glucose entering the portal vein from the gut is removed by the liver and converted to G-6-P by glucokinase; this increases the concentration of G-6-P and F-6-P and therefore stimulates phosphofructokinase and glycolysis. The reason that such a bypass can operate in liver and not muscle is that in liver the end product of glycolysis, pyruvate, can be utilized in the biosynthesis of fatty acid (see Newsholme and Gevers, 1967 for full discussion). It is interesting that the control mechanism of glycolysis in muscles provides the basis for an explanation of the ability of liver to control the blood glucose level.

(iii) It is possible to pose the question as to why phosphofructokinase is inhibited by ATP if changes in the concentration of ATP are not significant in regard to changes in the activity of the enzyme. In view of the suggested role of AMP it might have been expected that phospho-fructokinase would be directly activated by AMP, rather than AMP causing de-inhibition of the ATP effect. The explanation for this has been alluded to above: the most primitive form of feedback control of this enzyme may have been the ATP inhibition mechanism, but this suffers from the disadvantage of inefficiency in energy transfer as discussed above. However, it is a general biological axiom that nature, when evolving new mechanisms, simply adapts or modifies mechanisms already in existence rather than introducing completely new mechanisms. Therefore ATP inhibition represents an evolutionary primitive control mechanism and the enzyme has adapted by providing the de-inhibitory response to AMP, which now appears to play the major role in regulation of activity of phosphofructokinase in many organisms.

(iv) So far little has been said about the fact that the ATP inhibition of phosphofructokinase is relieved by FDP, which is the product of this enzymatic reaction. A possible function for this effect is to provide further amplification in the response of phosphofructokinase to changes in regulatory molecules. Thus, whenever the activity of phosphofructokinase is stimulated (e.g. by AMP) this should lead to an increase in the concentration of FDP which would cause further de-inhibition of the enzyme and therefore increased activity in a positive feedback manner. However an increase in concentration of FDP consequent upon stimulation of phosphofructokinase will depend on whether enzymes of the latter half of glycolysis (e.g. glyceraldehyde-3-phosphate dehydrogenase, pyruvate kinase) are also stimulated. If these enzymes are stimulated by specific regulatory molecules (but not by an increase in substrate) the stimulation of phosphofructokinase would not necessarily lead to an increase in the concentration of FDP; it would depend on the extent of stimulation of each enzyme.

However, perhaps the most interesting aspect of the de-inhibition of phosphofructokinase by FDP, and the most important from the point of view of support for the theory of control described above, is that it can account for oscillations in glycolysis. Direct observation on the reduction of pyridine nucleotides by yeast cells has been made by reflectance fluorimetry; these observations showed that when a certain concentration of glucose was supplied to the yeast cells (under anaerobic conditions) damped oscillations in the state of reduction of the pyridine nucleotides were observed (Chance, Estabrook and Ghosh, 1964). Further work on measurement of the concentrations of glycolytic intermediates in the yeast has shown that the oscillations in the redox state of the pyridine nucleotides reflect oscillations of the glycolytic intermediates. Similar oscillations have now been observed in extracts of mammalian tissues (under anaerobic conditions), and also in the perfused rat heart (Chance, 1965). The basis for these oscillations is considered to be the inhibition of phosphofructokinase by ATP (and de-inhibition by AMP) and the positive feedback effect of FDP. In the initial reactions of glycolysis ATP is hydrolysed and therefore its concentration decreases, and, through changes in AMP, phosphofructokinase activity is stimulated. Therefore the concentration of FDP increases which further stimulates phospho-fructokinase, but it also acts as substrate to increase the rate of the latter half of glycolysis; this process continues until the rate of flux through the latter half of glycolysis is greater than the first half of glycolysis (which is limited by the activity of hexokinase); consequently the concentration of FDP begins to decrease (it is being used faster than it is formed) and that of ATP is increased as it is being produced at a faster rate than it is used. Therefore phosphofructokinase activity is inhibited and the concentration of FDP continues to decrease; this reduces the rate of the latter half of glycolysis so that the rate of ATP production falls below the rate of utilization by the first half of glycolysis, and concentration of ATP begins to decrease; this initiates another period of increased activity of phospho-fructokinase, and maintains the oscillatory cycle.

This represents an oversimplified account of oscillations in glycolysis. The explanation should perhaps take into account the properties of other enzymes of glycolysis (e.g. glyceraldehyde-3-phosphate dehydrogenase, pyruvate kinase); nonetheless the important point is that the properties of phosphofructokinase form the basis for an explanation of such oscillations.

At this point in the essay it is perhaps pertinent to re-emphasize the major weakness in the experimental approach to metabolic control, that of extrapolation from properties of an isolated enzyme in an artificial system to the behaviour of that enzyme in the living cell. The ability of the properties of phosphofructokinase to explain the oscillations in glycolysis lend support to the validity of this extrapolation, at least for phosphofructokinase.

(v) So far I have discussed how this theory of control of glycolysis is able to explain a number of related biochemical or physiological phenomena. From the knowledge of the factors that may regulate these enzymes it is now possible to propose a completely new role for a biological compound whose role has been unquestioningly accepted since 1934. The Lohmann reaction was discovered by Lohmann in 1934 and this indicated that creatine phosphate (CP) is a store of energy rich phosphate for transference to ADP when the cell required energy. The following reaction summarizes this role of creatine phosphate

$$
\begin{aligned}
ATP &\rightarrow ADP + P_i \qquad &\text{(energy utilization)} \\
CP + ADP &\rightleftharpoons ATP + C \qquad &\text{(Lohmann reaction)} \\
\hline
CP &\rightarrow C + P_i \qquad &\text{(overall reaction)}
\end{aligned}
$$

It is generally accepted that creatine phosphokinase catalyses an equilibrium reaction in the cell, and that on muscular contraction, or under anaerobic conditions, CP is broken down; but, in this case, it is difficult to understand the reason for the creatine phosphate breakdown (which is almost total) as it has already been shown that there is very little change in ATP or ADP under these conditions. An alternative idea is that the creatine phosphokinase is only involved in the cell in the resynthesis of CP; and that on initiation of rapid ATP hydrolysis, CP is hydrolysed directly to creatine (C) and P_i (possibly a creatine phosphate phosphatase). The significance of CP might be, therefore, not so much a store of energy-rich phosphate, but a store of P_i, which is released under these specific conditions as it is a regulatory molecule for hexokinase, phosphorylase and phosphofructokinase (and in aerobic tissues for oxidative phosphorylation). There is, of course, no evidence whatsoever to support this new role for creatine phosphate, except that it would account for the breakdown of creatine phosphate in the absence of changes in ATP or ADP, and it provides CP with a rather similar role to AMP.

D. Another mechanism for the regulation of glycolysis in muscle

The theory of the regulation of glycolysis described in Section III(A) explains how the rate of glycolysis is increased when a muscle fibre contracts; the increased rate depends on the stimulation of myofibrillar ATPase and the subsequent decrease, albeit a small decrease, in the ATP concentration in the muscle fibre; this initiates the various amplification procedures of regulation that result in an increased rate of glycolysis from both glucose and glycogen. It could be argued on teleological grounds that advantage might be gained in employing the same regulatory mechanism for the stimulation of both the myofibrillar ATPase and the regulatory enzymes of glycolysis.

The action potential along the sarcolemma is carried towards the centre of the muscle fibre by a system of transverse tubules (T system) and this produces (probably indirectly) a release of Ca^{2+} from the terminal cisternae of the sarcoplasmic reticulum. The increased concentration of Ca^{2+} in the sarcoplasm activates the myofibrillar ATPase which leads to muscular contraction; relaxation is brought about by removal of Ca^{2+} by the sarcoplasmic reticulum (see Weber, 1966, for review).

It has been suggested, therefore, that Ca^{2+} might form a link between nervous stimulation of muscle and the activation of glycolysis. Indeed ever since Ca^{2+} was found to activate phosphorylase b kinase in muscle (see later), it has been suggested that this is the means by which glycogen is broken down during electrical stimulation of muscle (see E. G. Krebs and Fischer, 1962). Further indirect evidence supported this; *in vitro* electrical stimulation of frog sartorius muscle was shown to activate phosphorylase b kinase, which leads to a conversion of phosphorylase b to a, but no change was observed in the concentration of cyclic $3 \cdot 5$ AMP, a known activator of b kinase. Therefore it was suggested that Ca^{2+} was responsible for the activation of this enzyme. There are however three experimental observations against such a role for Ca^{2+} in muscle: firstly, the concentration of Ca^{2+} required to activate myofibrillar ATPase (and therefore present in the sarcoplasm during contraction) is 10^{-5} M, whereas a concentration of 10^{-3} M Ca^{2+} is required to activate phosphorylase b kinase; secondly, the Ca^{2+} activation of b kinase is not easily reversible and therefore of doubtful physiological significance (Meyer, Fischer and E. G. Krebs, 1964); and thirdly, the protein factor required along with Ca^{2+} to activate b kinase may be a proteolytic enzyme and therefore of little physiological significance (see Belocopitow, Fernandez,

Birnbaumer and Torres, 1967). In a preliminary report, Ozawa, Hosoi and Ebashi (1967) claim that phosphorylase b kinase from rabbit muscle was stimulated by very low concentrations of Ca^{2+}: 3×10^{-7} M Ca^{2+} had a very marked effect. They also state that the Ca^{2+} effect was 'fairly reversible'. In view of the above discussion this finding is of obvious importance but it is unfortunate that there is, as yet, no further detailed account of this work.

Recently Margreth, Catani and Schiaffino (1967) investigated the properties of phosphofructokinase from frog skeletal muscle and found that it was inhibited by Ca^{2+}. These workers also found that a proportion of the enzyme sedimented during centrifugation with the sarcoplasmic reticulum fraction. From these findings they suggested that in skeletal muscle phosphofructokinase is present within the sarcoplasmic reticulum, where normally the concentration of Ca^{2+} would be sufficient (10^{-3} M) to inhibit the enzyme. On stimulation of the muscle, Ca^{2+} would be released from the reticulum, so that the Ca^{2+} concentration inside the reticulum would be decreased and this would therefore activate phosphofructokinase. The major problem with this work is lack of satisfactory evidence that phosphofructokinase is normally located within the sarcoplasmic reticulum: thus phosphofructokinase is an enzyme which is known to polymerize very readily (see Mansour, 1965), so that in a concentrated extract of muscle aggregates of the enzyme may be formed which are sufficiently large that they sediment in the fraction containing the reticulum. In other words much more detailed work is required before it can be asserted that this enzyme is located within the reticulum.

Helmreich, Danforth, Karpatkin and Cori (1965) have suggested from work on the control of glycolysis in frog sartorius that changes in adenine nucleotides could not account for the increased glycolytic flux produced by electrical stimulation. The latter increased the activity of hexokinase, phosphorylase and phosphofructokinase but did not affect the concentrations of the adenine nucleotides. They concluded that the enzymes must be controlled by some other factor, and suggested that this might be Ca^{2+}. Unfortunately the value for the AMP concentration in resting muscle quoted by these workers is exceptionally high ($0\cdot4$ μmoles/g), in comparison to concentrations reported by other workers; with such a high resting concentration of AMP it is perhaps not surprising that there was no observed change in this compound on electrical stimulation.

Other problems in the attempt to link the control of Ca^{2+} concentration within the muscle to the control of glycolysis are the possible variation in the systems for removal of Ca^{2+} from the sarcoplasm and/or the variation in sensitivity of myofibrillar ATPases to Ca^{2+}. Thus in heart and red skeletal muscle it is possible that the mitochondria may play a complementary role to the reticulum in removal of Ca^{2+} from the sarcoplasm (see Weber, 1966). In certain insects the frequency of contraction of the flight muscles is not related to the frequency of nervous stimulation, and these are termed fibrillar muscles. The latter respond to lower concentrations of Ca^{2+} than non-fibrillar muscle, and the extent of activation of myofibrillar ATPase of fibrillar muscle by Ca^{2+} is much less than with non-fibrillar muscle (Maruyama, Pringle and Tregear, 1968).

A systematic study of the properties of three important enzymes of glycolysis (hexokinase, phosphofructokinase and fructose diphosphatase) in relation to possible control by Ca^{2+} has been carried out by Vaughan and Newsholme (1969). We have studied effects of Ca^{2+} on these enzymes from red and white vertebrate muscle and from insect fibrillar and non-fibrillar muscle; these four types of muscle were chosen for this investigation as it seemed possible that any Ca^{2+} control mechanism of the glycolytic enzymes could be different in these various muscles.

The results of this investigation have shown that increasing the Ca^{2+} concentration from 10^{-9} to 10^{-5} M (the concentration range which activates myofibrillar ATPase) has no effect on the activities of any of the enzymes tested, nor does it change the inhibition of hexokinase by glucose-6-phosphate, nor the inhibition of phosphofructokinase by ATP, nor inhibition of fructose diphosphatase by AMP. Higher concentrations of Ca^{2+} (10^{-3} M which is about the concentration expected in the sarcoplasmic reticulum) have been found to inhibit hexokinase, phosphofructokinase and fructose diphosphatase, but there was no effect of these higher Ca^{2+} concentrations on the ability of regulatory molecules (e.g. ATP, G-6-P, AMP) to modify the activities of these enzymes.

In summary, the evidence to date does not support the hypothesis that Ca^{2+} controls the activities of the glycolytic enzymes in muscle. In retrospect, this is perhaps not surprising because energy is required by muscles not only for musclar contraction, but also for processes of biosynthesis, ion transport, etc.; particularly in growth and development of muscle, ATP would be required primarily for biosynthesis and there would be obvious disadvantages in coupling the regulation of glycolysis and therefore energy production to the regulation of contraction.

E. How hormones can modify the regulation of glycolysis

Although it is probable that a large number of hormones may effect carbohydrate metabolism in muscle and that a number of different reactions may be affected, I will concentrate in this essay on the action of adrenaline (and glucagon) on phosphorylase, and the hormonal control at the phosphofructokinase reaction. Hormones are present in higher organisms in order to modify the metabolism of the individual target tissue for the benefit of the organism as a whole. But the metabolic process that the hormone affects is undoubtedly regulated by the fundamental control system of the cell, which is operative in the absence of hormones, or indeed any external stimuli. This poses the problem of how a hormone can impose changes on the activity of a process that is already under cellular control; we have discussed the control of glycolysis in muscle and this provides a useful fundamental control mechanism to attempt to understand hormonal action at a molecular level.

In Section II the explanation of a closed loop system of control of a metabolic pathway was explained as a regulatory factor which measures the rate of the metabolic pathway, and modifies the activity of the regulatory enzyme of this pathway. If this represents the fundamental control mechanism of the cell, the hormone could influence this control in two ways; firstly, it could change the concentration of the regulator by a mechanism independent of the normal means of modifying the regulator concentration, and secondly, the sensitivity of the regulatory enzyme to the regulator could be changed by the hormone. Examples to illustrate how these mechanisms may operate in the control of breakdown of glycogen, and the control of the phosphofructokinase reaction, will be discussed.

1. *The significance of citrate in the control of phosphofructokinase in muscle*

As discussed in Section III(C)(1) the concentration of ATP in the muscle fibre must be maintained fairly constant in order to provide efficient transfer of chemical energy; because of the adenylate kinase system it would not be possible for hormones to modify the concentration of AMP (an important regulator of the activity of phosphofructokinase) as this would lead to changes in the concentrations of ATP and ADP. Nonetheless it can be shown that the activity of phosphofructokinase in rat heart is inhibited *in vivo* by hormones that cause mobilization of fatty acids from adipose tissue, and that it can be inhibited in the isolated perfused rat heart by perfusing with a medium containing fatty acids or ketone bodies (see Randle and coworkers, 1966, for review); as anticipated there is no change in the intracellular concentration of the adenine nucleotides under these conditions. The properties of phosphofructokinase (Section III(B)) show that citrate potentiates the ATP inhibition of phosphofructokinase. Therefore a theory was proposed that the fatty acids inhibit the activity of phosphofructokinase by raising the intracellular concentration of citrate, and evidence has been obtained to support it.

H

Thus the concentration of citrate in rat heart is increased either under conditions of fatty acid mobilization *in vivo*, or in the isolated heart when it is perfused with medium containing fatty acids, and under these conditions it is known that the activity of phosphofructokinase is inhibited and the rate of glycolysis is decreased.

The raised concentration of citrate is dependent upon the β-oxidation of the fatty acids and the oxidation of acetyl-CoA by the TCA cycle; the possible mechanism for the increase in citrate concentration has been discussed by Randle, Denton and England (1968). Thus, although hormones cannot modify the ATP concentration, for the reasons given above, they can influence the effectiveness of the inhibitory action of ATP by changes in the citrate concentration; viewed from the aspect of phosphofructokinase activity, an increase in citrate concentration is equivalent to an increase in the concentration of ATP. However, this is not always the case, as the properties of phosphofructokinase show that citrate only inhibits by potentiation of the ATP inhibition, so that if the latter is removed (e.g. increases in AMP, FDP or F-6-P) citrate (at any concentration) will exert no effect on phosphofructokinase. This property ensures that control of this enzyme by the primitive cellular mechanism is always dominant whenever there is an excessive demand for energy; under these conditions glycogen and/or glucose will be broken down to provide extra energy from glycolysis irrespective of the citrate concentration.

The physiological significance of this hormonal control of glycolysis is the ability of the animal to dictate the type of fuel the muscle should use during starvation. As there is only a limited reserve of carbohydrate which, in addition to that produced by gluconeogenesis from non-carbohydrate sources, is required for the nervous system and the red cells, glucose must be conserved for these tissues during starvation. The main fuel reserve for starvation is triglyceride in the adipose tissue and this is mobilized chiefly as fatty acid. The ability of the fatty acids (and ketone bodies) to inhibit phosphofructokinase (via the elevated concentration of citrate) ensures that fatty acid oxidation provides most of the fuel for energy production of the muscle so that glucose is conserved for the other tissues. This is, therefore, the physiological significance of the citrate effect on phosphofructokinase.

2. *Interconvertible forms of enzymes and hormonal control*

The detailed properties of the enzymes phosphorylase *a* and *b* of muscle and the properties of the enzymes which cause interconversion of these two forms have provided an understanding of how hormones can modify fundamental control mechanisms. The basic information for the control of the various enzymes involved in glycogenolysis can be found in the following papers (E. G. Krebs and Fischer, 1962; Sutherland, 1962; Morgan and Parmeggiani, 1964); and the description of the hormonal action causing a conversion between the form of phosphorylase controlled by cellular metabolism and that which is independent of such control has been provided by Newsholme (1965) and Newsholme and Gevers (1967).

The properties of phosphorylase b have already been described (Section III(B)): it is activated by AMP and P_i, and these effects are removed by ATP and G-6-P. However, phosphorylase a is affected only to a small extent by these compounds, and is catalytically active in the absence of AMP.

In resting muscle almost all the phosphorylase exists in the b form, which is inhibited by low AMP and high ATP and G-6-P concentrations; therefore glycogen is not broken down. Adrenaline causes an increase in the intracellular concentration of $3',5'$ AMP, and this activates phosphorylase b kinase, which is the enzyme that converts phosphorylase b to a. However, phosphorylase a is active despite the low concentration of AMP, etc., and therefore, even in resting muscle, glycogen is broken down. If adrenaline is removed the b kinase activity is decreased and phosphorylase a is converted back to phosphorylase b by the enzyme phosphorylase a phosphatase. This represents the mechanism by which the hormone can bypass, at least transiently, the fundamental control mechanism of the cell. The physiological significance is related to the anticipatory role of adrenaline; the reserve fuel of the muscle is mobilized for energy production before the muscle actually contracts, so that for the 'fight or flight' muscular activity the rate of energy supply will not be limiting. In this particular case it is perhaps not so much the total amount of mechanical work done, but that a maximum amount of work is done in a minimum time which is important from the point of view of energy production and from the point of view of the animal's survival. The cellular control of phosphorylase b is probably too slow to be adequate for this sort of energy demand.

This particular mechanism of hormonal control, enzymatic interconversion of two forms of a regulatory enzyme, one of which is controlled by cellular metabolism, also occurs with the enzyme controlling glycogen synthesis, UDP-glucosyl transferase. At the present time there is not sufficient information about the properties of other regulatory enzymes to know if such a mechanism of hormonal control is possible. Therefore it remains to be seen how far this concept of hormonal control can provide a precedent for the mechanism of action of other hormones.

IV. THE SIGNIFICANCE OF SOME VARIATIONS IN ENZYME ACTIVITIES IN MUSCLE

The elucidation of the intermediate stages of glycolysis, TCA cycle, etc., was important for understanding the means by which chemical energy of food stuff was converted into the specific chemical energy used in biological systems (i.e. ATP). Such pathways constitute the basic biochemical structure of the cell so that they are present in almost every cell and organism despite differences in metabolism and physiological function. Recent studies in intermediary metabolism are probing into the more intimate details and interrelationships of metabolism and these studies may provide a basis for understanding how metabolism is associated with different physiological function, and whether the latter can be explained by variations in metabolic processes. As discussed above such studies are providing information on how some physiological phenomena are controlled at the biochemical or molecular level.

Muscle itself provides a range of physiological function from the very high frequency of contraction found in the flight muscles of small insects to the continuous contraction of the anterior byssus retractor muscle of the mussel.

At the present time in my laboratory we are using the variations in muscle metabolism in order to understand more about the control of carbohydrate degradation in muscle in relation to energy provision for contraction. This work involves the measurement of maximum catalytic activities of some of the more important enzymes of glycolysis and the TCA cycle from a variety of muscles from different animals. Some of the results provide information on the type of fuels which might be used by the muscle to support energy formation, while other results question the significance of the glycerophosphate cycle (or similar cycles) in vertebrate muscle.

A. Glycogen and glucose as fuels for energy production in muscle

It has been known for a long time that carbohydrate can function as a fuel for energy production, particularly in white muscle of vertebrates. The results reported in Table 4 (see Crabtree and Newsholme, 1970) show that in this muscle hexokinase activity is very low, whereas phosphorylase activity is very high. This supports the view that for a rapid short burst of exercise, which is performed by white muscle, energy is obtained by breakdown of glycogen and not glucose. The role of hexokinase would appear to be to restore the glycogen levels from blood glucose during the prolonged rest period after exercise. Such a result might be expected, as

Table 4. The activities of some glycolytic enzymes from various muscles of various animals. These results are taken from Crabtree and Newsholme (1970). Activities of all enzymes were measured at 25°

Animal	Muscle	Enzyme activities (μmole/min/g fresh wt of muscle)					
		Hexo-kinase	Phospho-rylase	Phospho-fructokinase	Glycero-phosphate dehydrogenase	Lactate dehydro-genase	Glycero-phosphate oxidase
Insecta:							
Locust (*Locusta migratoria*)	flight	8·0	8·0	13	124	1·6	33
	femoral hind leg	2·3	20	16	33	20	18
(*Schistocerca gregaria*)	flight	12	8·0	—	141	2·9	43
Cockroach (*Periplaneta americana*)	flight	18	30	19	216	1·5	48
Honey bee (*Apis mellifera*)	flight	29	4·0	—	257	—	44
Bumble bee (*Bombus hortorum*)	flight	26	8·0	12	513	1·8	50
Blowfly (*Sarcophaga barbata*)	flight	17	57	31	270	2·5	97
(*Caliphora erythrocephala*)	flight	35	55	—	—	—	90
Pisces:							
Dogfish	red	1·9	12	—	3·6	61	0·1
	white	0·1	62	—	6·2	344	0·6
Amphibia:							
Frog (*Rana temporaria*)	sartorius	1·3	29	—	—	319	0·4
Aves:							
Pigeon	pectoral	1·0	18	24	50	314	0·2
Domestic fowl	pectoral	0·5	83	97	76	870	0·6
Mammalia:							
Rabbit	adductor magnus (white)	0·1	30	31	85	372	0·8
	semitendinosus (red)	0·6	8	8	22	60	0·2
Rat	heart	2·5	12	10	30	311	0·2

the blood supply to these vertebrate muscles is exceptionally poor and the amount of glucose available to the muscle at any instant of time would be very low; the significance of large amounts of glycogen in these muscles is therefore apparent. The deficiency of blood supply necessitates that this muscle relies almost exclusively on anaerobic glycolysis for energy production (see later).

The rate of oxygen uptake by perfused rat heart is 13 μmoles/minute/ gram fresh weight (Neely and coworkers, 1967) and this represents a rate of utilization of glucose of approximately $2 \cdot 5$ μmoles/minute/gram. The hexokinase activity in rat heart is $2 \cdot 5$ μmoles at 25° (Table 4) and therefore is approximately $5 \cdot 0$ at 37°, and this activity could therefore account for all the oxygen uptake of the perfused heart. This is consonant with the findings of Williamson and Krebs (1961) that in the insulinized perfused heart glucose oxidation could account for about 60% of the oxygen uptake. The activity of hexokinase from other red muscles is of the same order of magnitude, which suggests that in these muscles, also, glucose oxidation could play an important quantitative role in energy formation. However, it is known that red muscle can oxidize fat to support muscular activity and it seems likely, therefore, that it can use either glucose or fat for energy production. In the extreme condition of long distance flights in both migratory birds and insects it is known that fat is used as the main source of fuel for the flight muscle. Indeed the energy/weight ratio of fat compared to carbohydrate demands that fat is used (see Weis-Fogh, 1967). However, in less extreme conditions it is possible that fat or carbohydrate can be used by these muscles. The choice of fuel may well depend upon the availability of fatty acids, as it is known that the rate of oxidation is proportional to the concentration in the blood. Thus under conditions of starvation, fatty acids will be oxidized in preference to glucose, as the concentration of fatty acids is increased.

It should be noted that this fatty acid effect can only apply to red muscles and not to white muscles (as there is little or no TCA cycle and no fat oxidation). As glycolysis is the only means of supplying energy for these muscles it would be disadvantageous if it was inhibited by fatty acids, or any other factor apart from ATP and the energy control mechanism. Thus it would be interesting to know if, *in vitro*, phosphofructokinase from white muscles was inhibited by citrate.

B. The problem of re-oxidation of NADH$_2$ produced during glycolysis

The conversion of glyceraldehyde-3-phosphate dehydrogenase to 1,3-diphosphoglycerate in glycolysis requires the conversion of NAD to NADH$_2$, and in order to maintain glycolysis this NADH$_2$ must be continually oxidized to NAD. In white (anaerobic) muscle this is achieved by lactate dehydrogenase: the end product of glycolysis, pyruvate, is converted to lactate and this involves the conversion of $NADH_2$ to NAD. Thus glycogen is converted to lactate, ATP is produced, and no oxygen requiring process is involved; however much less ATP is produced from the degradation of glucose (or glycogen) compared to the complete oxidation of this compound.

The major problem of re-oxidation of glycolytically produced $NADH_2$ in aerobic muscle is that the mitochondria cannot oxidize external $NADH_2$. In insect muscle this problem has been overcome by the glycerophosphate cycle (see Klingenberg and Bücher, 1960; Sacktor, 1961). In the extra mitochondrial compartment the $NADH_2$ is re-oxidized by the enzyme glycerophosphate dehydrogenase, which converts dihydroxyacetone phosphate to L-3-glycerophosphate; the latter enters the mitochondria where the enzyme glycerophosphate oxidase catalyses the conversion of L-3-glycerophosphate to dihydroxyacetone phosphate, which diffuses back into the cytoplasm to maintain the operation of the cycle. The hydrogens, which are removed by the mitochondrial oxidase, enter the respiratory chain (probably as electrons) at the flavoprotein level. This oxidase catalyses a non-equilibrium reaction so that the cycle can operate only in one direction.

This cycle is extremely important in those insect flight muscles that depend on carbohydrate for energy production; in these muscles the activities of the enzymes of both glycolysis and the glycerophosphate cycle are very high (see Table 4).

The activities of glycerophosphate oxidase in vertebrate white and red muscles are very low in comparison to those of the enzymes that may regulate glycolysis (i.e. phosphofructokinase, phosphorylase). Thus in white muscle the maximum activity of the oxidase is only about 1% of the maximum activity of the glycolytic enzymes. It has been suggested that the importance of the oxidase in white muscle is in the operation of the glycerophosphate cycle (Pette, 1966). However the very low activities of the oxidase in both red and white vertebrate muscles strongly suggest that the cycle can play only a very minor role in re-oxidation of glycolytic $NADH_2$ in either muscle. This poses no problem for white muscle in which $NADH_2$ oxidation is achieved by conversion of pyruvate to lactate. However in red (aerobic) muscle a large proportion of the pyruvate is oxidized by the mitochondria, and some other means of re-oxidation of $NADH_2$ is required. Another possibility is a malate–oxaloacetate cycle which involves formation of malate in the cytoplasm, re-oxidation to oxaloacetate within the mitochondria and transfer of oxaloacetate into the cytoplasm. However Haslam and H. A. Krebs (1968) have measured the rate of entry of malate into isolated rat heart mitochondria *in vitro* and found that this rate can account for only 4% of that required for the operation of a cycle when glucose is the main respiratory fuel. Thus, at the present time, there is no satisfactory explanation for the mechanism of re-oxidation of glycolytic $NADH_2$ in vertebrate red muscle.

Indeed in red vertebrate muscle, in which pyruvate enters the mitochondria for oxidation, there is the converse problem to that described above. The activity of lactate dehydrogenase in this muscle is very high (Table 4) in comparison to the rate of pyruvate formation, and it seems surprising that a large proportion of the pyruvate produced by glycolysis is not converted to lactate, and this would prevent it from entering the mitochondria for oxidation. There are two forms of lactate dehydrogenase (isoenzymes), the M and H form, and the H form predominates in red while the M form is found in white muscle. The H form is inhibited by its substrate, pyruvate, whereas the M form is much less inhibited. This has led Kaplan and Goodfriend (1964) to suggest that in aerobic muscle pyruvate is not converted to lactate because pyruvate inhibits lactate dehydrogenase, so that a concentration of pyruvate is maintained for oxidation by the TCA cycle; this does not happen in anaerobic muscle as the M type of lactate dehydrogenase is much less sensitive to pyruvate, so that pyruvate is converted to lactate. This explanation is however unsatisfactory. Firstly, very high (unphysiological) concentrations of pyruvate are required to inhibit the enzyme (10–20 mM); and in the perfused heart addition of pyruvate to the perfusion medium causes the formation of large amounts of lactate (Garland, Newsholme and Randle, 1964), despite the fact that the intracellular pyruvate concentration must have increased. Secondly, the very high activities of lactate dehydrogenase in the various red muscles (in comparison to the glycolytic rate) suggests that very high concentrations of pyruvate would be required to inhibit the enzyme to such an extent as to restrict the flux of pyruvate to lactate (i.e. convert the reaction from equilibrium to non-equilibrium).

It seems possible that the control of lactate dehydrogenase activity in red muscle and the mechanism for re-oxidation of glycolytic $NADH_2$ may be closely related. It is an interesting point that insect flight muscle has solved the problem of controlling lactate dehydrogenase by lack of this enzyme in the muscle; this may be explained by the fact that this muscle re-oxidizes its glycolytic $NADH_2$ by the glycerophosphate cycle, and this depends upon the activity of cytoplasmic glycerophosphate dehydrogenase; the latter catalyses an equilibrium reaction between the NAD, $NADH_2$, L-3-glycerophosphate and dihydroxyacetone phosphate.

Thus the absence of lactate dehydrogenase in insect flight muscle is essential, otherwise a lactate dehydrogenase equilibrium reaction would be established and therefore pyruvate would continually be converted to lactate (while glycolysis proceeded), and this would represent a loss of substrate for the oxidative processes of the muscle. Thus the possession of the glycerophosphate cycle must preclude the presence of lactate dehydrogenase in the same muscle.

From the standpoint of metabolic symmetry the converse situation exists in heart and red vertebrate muscle. The activities of lactate dehydrogenases are high in these muscles, and therefore they cannot possess active glycerophosphate or other similar cycles for the removal of glycolytic $NADH_2$. The low activities of the glycerophosphate oxidases in these muscles (Table 4) are predicted by this argument. A further prediction is that some other means of re-oxidation of glycolytic $NADH_2$ must exist in vertebrates red muscle. Moreover, if this process of $NADH_2$ oxidation maintained the extramitochondrial concentration of $NADH_2$ at a low level, it would explain why pyruvate was not converted to lactate under aerobic conditions, despite the presence of a very active lactate dehydrogenase. Thus it is extremely interesting that Rasmussen (1969) has recently reported evidence for an $NADH_2$ oxidase from pigeon heart mitochondria, which is located outside the normal permeability barrier to $NADH_2$. Although the oxidation appeared to require the usual electron carriers, there was no concomitant phosphorylation of ADP. Furthermore the K_m of the oxidase for $NADH_2$ was very low, approximately $1 \cdot 8$ μM, and this would be expected to maintain the extramitochondrial $NADH_2$ concentration very low. It will indeed be of interest to ascertain if this oxidase is absent from the mitochondria of insect flight muscle.

The significance of the lactate dehydrogenase in red muscle, and the advantage in evolving a new process for glycolytic $NADH_2$ re-oxidation, may be that it permits the tissue to function in excess of its aerobic energy producing capacity for a short period of time. The extra energy would be produced from glycolysis and particularly from the glycogen stored in this tissue, and this would explain the relatively high activities of phosphorylase in red muscle despite the fact that it can use glucose and/or fat for energy supply. This ability to produce extra energy by anaerobic glycolysis would be of little value in insect flight muscle because, with the tracheal system of respiration, it is unlikely that oxygen availability is ever limiting for energy formation. In this case substrate availability is probably the limiting factor because substrates for respiration have to diffuse from the haemolymph to the muscle without the aid of a capillary circulation, and therefore it is important that the flight muscle uses its fuel with the utmost efficiency.

References

Belocopitow, E., Fernandez, M., Birnbaumer, L., and Torres, H. N. (1967). *J. Biol. Chem.*, **242**, 1227.
Bücher, Th. (1965). In *Control of Energy Metabolism*, p. 55. Ed. Chance, B., Estabrook, R. W., and Williamson, J. R. London: Academic Press.
Bücher, Th., and Rüssmann W. (1964). *Angew. Chem. Internat. Edit.*, **3**, 426.
Burk, D. (1939). *Cold Spring Harbor Symp. Quant. Biol.*, **7**, 420.
Chance, B. (1965). In *Control of Energy Metabolism*, p. 415. Ed. Chance, B., Estabrook, R. W., and Williamson, J. R. London: Academic Press.
Chance, B., Holmes, W., Higgins, J., and Connelly, C. M. (1958). *Nature*, **182**, 1190.
Chance, B., Estabrook, R. W., and Ghosh, A. (1964). *Proc. Nat. Acad. Sci.*, **51**, 1244.
Crabtree, B., and Newsholme, E. A. (1970). *Biochem. J.* In preparation.
Eggleston, L. V., and Hems, R. (1952). *Biochem. J.*, **52**, 156.
England, P. J., and Randle, P. J. (1967). *Biochem. J.*, **105**, 907.
Garland, P. B. (1968). In *Metabolic Roles of Citrate*, p. 41. Ed. Goodwin, T. W. London: Academic Press.
Garland, P. B., Newsholme, E. A., and Randle, P. J. (1964). *Biochem. J.*, **93**, 665.
Haslam, J. M., and Krebs, H. A. (1968). *Biochem. J.*, **107**, 659.
Helmreich, E., Danforth, W. H., Karpatkin, S., and Cori, G. F. (1965). In *Control of Energy Metabolism*, p. 299. Ed. Chance, B., Estabrook, R. W., and Williamson, J. R. London: Academic Press.
Kaplan, N. O., and Goodfriend, T. G. (1964). In *Adv. Enzyme Reguln.*, **2**, 203. Ed. Weber, G. London: Pergamon Press.
Klingenberg, M. (1964). *Angew. Chem. Internat. Edit.*, **3**, 54.
Klingenberg, M., and Bücher, Th. (1960). *Ann. Rev. Biochem.*, **29**, 669.
Krebs, E. G., and Fischer, E. H. (1962). *Adv. Enzymol.*, **24**, 263.
Krebs, H. A. (1946). *Enzymologia*, **12**, 88.
Krebs, H. A. (1957). *Endeavour*, **16**, 125.
Krebs, H. A. (1964). *Proc. Roy. Soc. B.*, **159**, 545.
Lohmann, K. (1934). *Biochem. Z.*, **271**, 264.
Mansour, T. E. (1963). *J. Biol. Chem.*, **238**, 2285.
Mansour, T. E. (1965). *J. Biol. Chem.*, **240**, 2165.
Margreth, A., Catani, C., and Schiaffino, S. (1967). *Biochem. J.*, **102**, 35C.
Maruyama, K., Pringle, J. W. S., and Tregear, R. T. (1968). *Proc. Roy. Soc. B.*, **169**, 229.
Meyer, W. L., Fischer, E. H., and Krebs, E. G. (1964). *Biochemistry*, **3**, 1033.
Meyerhof, O. S., and Fiala, S. (1950). *Biochem. Biophys. Acta*, **6**, 1.
Monod, J., Wyman, J., and Changeux, J. -P. (1965). *J. Mol. Biol.*, **12**, 88.
Morgan, H. E., and Parmeggiani, J. A. (1964). *J. Biol. Chem.*, **239**, 2440.
Morgan, H. E. (1969). Personal communication.
Neely, J. R., Liebermeister, H., Battersby, E. J., and Morgan, H. E. (1967). *J. Biol. Chem.*, **236**, 262.

Newsholme, E. A. (1965). *Sci. Progr. (London)*, **53**, 237.

Newsholme, E. A., and Randle, P. J. (1961). *Biochem. J.*, **80**, 655.

Newsholme, E. A., and Randle, P. J. (1964). *Biochem. J.*, **93**, 641.

Newsholme, E. A., and Gevers, W. (1967). *Vitam. & Horm.*, **25**, 1.

Ozawa, E., Hosoi, K., and Ebashi, S. (1967). *J. Biochem. (Japan)*, **61**, 531.

Passonneau, J. V., and Lowry, O. N. (1962). *Biochem. Biophys. Research Commun.*, **7**, 10.

Pasteur, L. (1876). In *Etudes sur la Biere*. Paris: Gauthier-Villars.

Pette, D. (1966). In *Regulation of Metabolic Processes in Mitochondria*, p. 28. Ed. Tager, J. M., Papa, S., Quagliariello, E., and Slater, E. C. Amsterdam: Elsevier.

Randle, P. J. (1963). *Ann. Rev. Physiol.*, **25**, 291.

Randle, P. J., Garland, P. B., Hales, C. N., Newsholme, E. A., Denton, R. M., and Pogson, C. I. (1966). *Recent Progr. Hormone Res.*, **22**, 1.

Randle, P. J., Denton, R. M., and England, P. J. (1968). In *Metabolic Roles of Citrate*, p. 87. Ed. Goodwin, T. W. London: Academic Press.

Rasmussen, U. F. (1969). *FEBS Letters*, **2**, 157.

Regen, D. M., Davis, W. W., Morgan, H. E., and Park, C. R. (1964). *J. Biol. Chem.*, **239**, 43.

Rolleston, F. S., and Newsholme, E. A. (1967). *Biochem. J.*, **104**, 524.

Sacktor, B. (1961). *Ann. Rev. Ent.*, **6**, 103.

Sacktor, B., and Hurlbut, E. C. (1966). *J. Biol. Chem.*, **241**, 632.

Sacktor, B., and Wormser-Shavit, E. (1966). *J. Biol. Chem.*, **241**, 624.

Sutherland, E. W. (1962). *Harvey Lectures*, **57**, 17.

Underwood, A. H., and Newsholme, E. A. (1965). *Biochem. J.*, **95**, 868.

Underwood, A. H., and Newsholme, E. A. (1967a). *Biochem. J.*, **104**, 296.

Underwood, A. H., and Newsholme, E. A. (1967b). *Biochem. J.*, **104**, 300.

Vaughan, H., and Newsholme, E. A. (1969). *Biochem. J.*, **114**, 818.

Weber, A. (1966). In *Current Topics in Bioenergetics*, p. 203. Ed. Sanadi, D. R. London: Academic Press.

Weis-Fogh, T. (1967). In *Insects and Physiology*, p. 143. Ed. Beament, J. W. L., and Treherne, J. E. Edinburgh and London: Oliver & Boyd.

Wilkins, B. R. (1966). In *Regulation and Control in Living Systems*, p. 12. Ed. Kalmus, H. London: John Wiley.

Williamson, J. R. (1965). *J. Biol. Chem.*, **240**, 2308.

Williamson, J. R., and Krebs, H. A. (1961). *Biochem. J.*, **80**, 540.

METABOLISM OF SPERMATOZOA, PAST, PRESENT AND FUTURE

Charles Terner

Department of Biology, Biological Science Center, Boston University, Boston, Massachusetts, U.S.A.

When I saw Sir Hans in Boston recently, he told me that he was becoming interested in sperm metabolism and asked me what spermatozoa can do and what aspects I had found most interesting in them. This essay gives me an opportunity to tell Sir Hans how I became involved in the study of spermatozoa after I had left Sheffield to take up my first research appointment in Reading. In the following pages I shall try not only to remind him of our brief conversation and to include some additional factual information, but also to express some thoughts on the consequences to the process of human reproduction of our ability to manipulate these unique motile cells, the study of which has occupied many of my waking and sleeping hours on both sides of the Atlantic, from the metabolic point of view, of course.

Twenty years ago, visitors calling on Professor Krebs, then head of the Department of Biochemistry and director of the M.R.C. Unit for Research in Cell Metabolism in the University of Sheffield, were often surprised to find him sitting in front of a Warburg apparatus which was shaking rather violently, or to see him standing by a sink washing his glassware. The Warburg apparatus would appear antiquated to our present-day students, accustomed to expensive automatic equipment. The largest room was equipped with batteries of Warburg baths, three tanks per bench sharing one electric motor which drove the stirring paddles and the shaking mechanism by means of belts and pulleys which allowed a fairly wide choice of shaking speeds. When the motor broke down or the master belt broke, three baths stopped shaking, but all was not lost since the operators could still turn the pulleys by hand and continue the shaking until the end of the experiment. In the meantime the bath could be stirred by a friend who agitated the paddles or used his bare hands. Each tank had a separate heating system, consisting of a gas ring and a small Bunsen burner placed underneath. With a little practice it was possible to maintain a temperature of 40°C by watching the thermometer and adjusting the flame of the Bunsen burner. When refrigeration was needed, ice was dropped into the water. Incredible as it may seem, it all worked very well indeed and in addition had the distinction of being copied from Professor Warburg's original design.

A letterhead was on display on the blackboard in which the Unit for Research in Cell Metabolism appeared as 'Unfit for Research in Cell Metabolism', a printer's error which was corrected in subsequent printings. Since paper was still in short supply, these sheets were kept as scrap note paper and distributed among the students, for economy rather than as a reminder.

When I came to Sheffield as a graduate student in the late 40's, the work that was to win Professor Krebs the Nobel Prize had already been done and had brought him world-wide recognition. Yet the 'cycle' was rarely discussed in the laboratory and no student was ever asked questions on it in examinations. Thus some of us may have passed through Sheffield with merely a nodding acquaintance with the cycle, but it caught up with us later on when, on our first professional assignments, we were expected to be experts. When I joined Professor Folley's laboratory at the National Institute for Research in Dairying, Shinfield, near Reading, he immediately confronted me with the question whether the Krebs' cycle was functioning in the mammary gland. Armed with a set of reprints of Professor Krebs' papers that I had had the foresight to request before leaving Sheffield, I struggled through the classical experiments, using mammary gland slices. On reading and re-reading the reprints, the surprising fact dawned on me that the cycle had been accepted on the basis of Professor Krebs' experiments with only two preparations, minced pigeon breast muscle and *E. coli* suspensions. That confirmation in other tissues was slow in coming testifies to the complete acceptance of the cycle as a fundamental and universal principle. Perhaps this is comparable to the practice in molecular biology today of accepting general rules from experiments with subcellular fractions of *E. coli* or rat liver. In Professor Krebs' laboratory there was no such restriction on the type of material used. I first worked on gastric secretion as a graduate student assigned to R. E. Davies, himself then still a graduate student and whose theory of ion secretion in gastric mucosa (his Ph.D. thesis) foreshadowed the proton translocation theory of Mitchell (1967). My postdoctoral period working directly with Professor Krebs on ion transport in brain, kidney and retina reinforced my interest in the function of organs other than liver.

There was an atmosphere of tireless activity in the laboratory; the traditional morning coffee break was not wasted in idle gossip, but spent in discussion of the most recent scientific and rarely of political developments. Mao's forces were in the process of gaining control of China;

Lysenko was being demoted; the Berlin airlift sent a slight jitter through the degree candidates, barely out of the Second World War, but the Prof. said there was still enough time to do a few good experiments.

The Prof.'s personal assistants, Len and Reg, were members of the permanent staff then and are still working with him. Although fully occupied with their own work, they were always willing to help and over the years they must have earned the gratitude of generations of graduate students. Reg Hems had a fine voice and would sing cowboy songs Bing Crosby style with a Yorkshire accent, all too rarely since his devotion to his work did not lend itself to such idleness. I did not know Len's surname until, in response to a telephone call for Mr. Eggleston, I saw Len rush into the office. My surprised remark: 'So you are the great Eggleston!' kept him amused for some time. Everybody except the Prof. was addressed by his or her first name. Nevertheless, this caused some confusion, as in the case of an undergraduate student, Hans Kornberg, who was spending a summer vacation working in the laboratory. He was overheard answering the telephone: 'No, no, this is *Little* Hans speaking'.

We students felt that we had come to the laboratory at an auspicious moment and there was a feeling of excitement and expectation. The field was wide open; the Krebs' cycle and Lipmann's concept of the high-energy bond had opened up a clear path for future research. The problem of the terminal oxidation of carbohydrate, which had been a stumbling block in the way of further progress, had been solved and with an understanding of intermediary metabolism and expertise in the Warburg manometric technique we felt well equipped to attack most biochemical problems.

In the laboratory of Professor Folley the effect of insulin on the biosynthesis of fatty acids in mammary tissue was being studied by the Warburg respirometer technique. Professor Folley preferred the ingenious Dickens–Šimer vessels which measured the R.Q. by a chemical reaction introduced by Professor Krebs while he was still in Professor Warburg's laboratory. When radioactive isotopes became available, Professor Folley was quick to adopt the technique of measuring the incorporation of precursors such as ^{14}C-labelled acetate into fatty acids. At Shinfield I met and made friends with D. R. Melrose who was then on the staff of the Reading Cattle Breeding Centre. Through him I became acquainted with the problems of artificial insemination of cattle. As a side-line to my main duty to work on mammary gland metabolism we engaged on a collaborative study of the metabolism of bull spermatozoa with the purpose of searching for a biochemical method of assessing semen quality. Since that time the study of spermatozoa has remained with me as a permanent research activity.

Although bull spermatozoa had long been known to respire, in the early 50's the field of sperm metabolism was dominated by anaerobic glycolysis. Following the demonstration that fructose is the main sugar in bull and ram semen (Mann, 1945) the rate of fructolysis by bull spermatozoa was studied in many laboratories in a search for a correlation between fertility and glycolytic power. Such excessive preoccupation with anaerobic metabolism was not for 'Krebs cyclists'. Melrose and I carefully washed bull spermatozoa free from seminal plasma, added various substrates and measured the rate of their oxidative utilization by chemical analysis. We then elaborated a manometric test of 'sperm quality' based on incubating washed spermatozoa with fluoride to reduce the endogenous respiration, and adding pyruvate as a substrate, ($\pm$)-2,4-dinitrophenol as an uncoupling agent. We found that bull spermatozoa of 'high quality' (i.e. from bulls of high fertility) responded to the addition of pyruvate with a small increase in respiration which was greatly stimulated by the addition of dinitrophenol. On the other hand, spermatozoa from bulls of low fertility responded to the addition of pyruvate with a larger increase in respiration, but without further increase on addition of dinitrophenol. The biochemical response which was later confirmed by Graves and coworkers (1964) suggested to us that there is in good spermatozoa a tight coupling of phosphorylation and respiration which can be uncoupled by dinitrophenol, and that in 'poor spermatozoa' phosphorylation and respiration are spontaneously uncoupled. We concluded that the tight coupling of good spermatozoa indicated a production by oxidative phosphorylation of metabolic energy far in excess of the energy produced by glycolytic reactions which alone were known to satisfy the energy needs for sperm motility. This was strengthened by our observation of a Pasteur effect in spermatozoa. We suspected that the energy might be used to drive biosynthetic reactions (Melrose and Terner, 1953). This conclusion was coolly received at the time, since not much purpose was seen in biosynthetic reactions in mature spermatozoa whose supposedly sole biochemical function was to generate enough ATP to support motility for their sole physiological function, fertilization. Nevertheless, Lord Rothschild, then chairman of the Agricultural Research Council, saw our paper and offered us a grant in support of a field test. Characteristically, the grant was made to Professor Kay, the director of the Institute, who in turn delegated it to Professor Folley, the head of the Department, who then put Melrose and I in charge of a young graduate, George Glew, whom we engaged upon recommendation of the University of Sheffield. In looking back, this bureaucratic way of running a simple procedure through the hierarchy was in marked contrast with our later experience in the United States in which granting agencies would support young investigators directly and on a much more generous scale. On the other hand, Lord Rothschild departed from the rules by coming into my laboratory to have my 'theory' explained to him personally. His habit of getting through to junior staff members directly had made him very popular with the rank and file, but was known each time to send a shudder through the higher ranks of the academic establishment. Despite the apparent abundance of red tape, the system worked smoothly and was fair to everyone concerned. Glew set out to tour the cattle breeding centres of England with the Institute's mobile laboratory, equipped with an electric Warburg bath of 'modern' design, especially bought for the purpose. Although the results of the field test turned out as we had anticipated, it was not taken up by cattle breeding centres which seemed reluctant to invest in a Warburg apparatus and find an assistant trained to run it.

My move to the Worcester Foundation in 1955 to join Dr. Gregory Pincus interrupted the work on sperm metabolism only temporarily. Although Dr. Pincus had 'hired' me with another research project in mind, he let me pursue my interest in biosynthetic reactions in spermatozoa and helped me to obtain a research grant from the National Institutes of Health. Now that funds were available for the purchase of what appeared to me a luxurious supply, compared to my previous experience of cautious rationing of ^{14}C-labelled precursors, the incorporation of glucose, glycerol, acetate and pyruvate into the various classes of lipids, first of bull spermatozoa and later also of rabbit, human and fish spermatozoa was soon demonstrated (Terner and Korsh, 1962, 1963b; Terner, 1965; Minassian and Terner, 1966). It was confirmed by Scott and coworkers (1967) in ram spermatozoa. We also helped to correct the impression, then prevalent, that the metabolism of human spermatozoa was purely glycolytic, by showing that they are able to oxidize ^{14}C-labelled glucose, pyruvate and acetate to $^{14}CO_2$ (Terner, 1960). It was difficult while at the Worcester Foundation to obtain human semen locally, but after moving to Boston we had the help of Dr. Rock, who placed the donors of his Reproductive Study Centre at our disposal. A graduate student not only did the experimental studies, but she also took care of the accounts for the payment of the fees by keeping a list of the donors; we were soon able to recognize them by name from the sperm count and semen volume without ever meeting them.

Perhaps it is now time to return to Sir Hans' question: 'What can spermatozoa do?'. It seems to me that spermatozoa behave much like any other normal cells. Motility has fascinated the observer since the days of Leeuwenhoek, but this is by no means a unique phenomenon since there are many other motile unicellular organisms. Spermatozoa are, of course, of special interest because of their role in fertilization. Since motility can be so easily observed, it has long been used as a qualitative and quantitative measure of the viability and fertilizing capacity of spermatozoa. During storage in the mammalian epididymis the spermatozoa are non-motile and acquire motility on ejaculation following dilution with secretions of the male accessory glands. Poor motility at this stage correlates well with poor fertilizing capacity. Mammalian spermatozoa, once activated, can remain motile for several days, both in the female reproductive tract and *in vitro* when diluted with certain media. They also undergo a maturation process, capacitation, in the uterus or the Fallopian tubes before they are capable of fertilizing an egg (Austin, 1951; Chang, 1951). Trout spermatozoa are immotile in the milt recovered from the male, but become intensely motile on dilution with ovarian fluid or $0 \cdot 7\%$ NaCl, but rapidly lose their motility again within a minute or two.* Thus, trout spermatozoa washed by centrifuging and re-suspending in saline are long past the stage of activation by the time they are placed into the reaction vessels, yet they will respire for several hours and will incorporate acetate and glucose into lipids (Terner and Korsh, 1963a and b).

Having demonstrated the ability of spermatozoa of a number of species to synthesize lipids from various precursors, we have come back full circle to our early hypothesis in which we assumed a correlation between biosynthetic capacity and fertilizing power. If nothing else, the biosynthetic capacity of spermatozoa may be considered a normal property common to many cell types. It may, however, be of special importance in prolonged survival of spermatozoa in the female reproductive tract. Because of their limited lipid reserves, the spermatozoa may depend on their ability to re-synthesize their reserves from precursors taken up from secretions of the female environment. It is doubtful whether carbohydrate is available to spermatozoa during their ascent of the female reproductive tract. But we have observed the ability of human and rabbit spermatozoa to metabolize glucosamine in both oxidative and biosynthetic reactions in the absence of glucose, and it is possible that glucosamine may become available by hydrolysis of mucopolysaccharides of the female tract (Terner, 1965). We are in the process of investigating the effects of uterine secretions on the metabolism of mammalian spermatozoa.

Researchers engaged in the study of reproductive cells, even at the basic level, cannot avoid being concerned, at least in thought, with wider problems. The threat of overpopulation and widespread poverty and starvation has made the dissemination of information on methods of

* Spermatozoa of other species of fish remain active for much longer periods of time.

birth control a question of national survival to rich and poor countries alike. Despite the success of progestational steroids in suppressing ovulation, there is now also an increasing interest in male anti-fertility agents. Such agents, in order to be acceptable, must of course be fully compatible with the selfish nature of the male: they must allow fertility to return promptly upon cessation of medication, and they must at no stage interfere with male sexual capacity. It is fair to say that such interference would make them unacceptable to both sexes. Steroidal agents may be expected to interfere with spermatogenesis at an early stage, but might have undesirable side effects. Non-steroidal agents may selectively inhibit a vital metabolic function of the sperm, but such agents must have no effect on other organs or tissues. Agents acting at a later stage, such as on the mature spermatozoon, may be relatively inefficient and unreliable in abolishing the fertilizing capacity of very large numbers of spermatozoa. It may be possible to abolish the fertilizing capacity of spermatozoa while they are traversing the female reproductive passages, perhaps by inhibiting the process of capacitation, the exact nature of which is still unknown. Although a decapacitation factor has been found in seminal plasma (Chang, 1957; Williams and coworkers, 1967), it is known that rabbits can be inseminated with epididymal spermatozoa (which do not carry the factor) and that these will fertilize ova after undergoing a maturation process in the female tract. It seems possible to us that agents interfering specifically with biosynthetic processes of spermatozoa might prevent their maturation, and a search for agents acting on the spermatozoa preferably while still in the male reproductive tract may be indicated, so as to distribute the burden of taking pills more evenly between the sexes.

Experience gained by veterinarians and clinicians in the handling of semen and its use for artificial insemination of a number of species of domestic animals and also man, followed by the development of techniques of storing semen in the deep-frozen state (Polge and coworkers, 1949), has suggested some unorthodox applications. Muller (1961) pointed out that it is now possible to upgrade the human species by the use of semen donated to couples of more modest genetic endowments by men who have had the opportunity of proving their 'truly exceptional genetic quality'. He recommended the storage of the semen for several decades, perhaps until after the death of the donors, to prevent the young women to be inseminated from developing some wrong ideas of personal involvement.

Frozen semen also offers a possibility to cope with the disastrous effects of a nuclear war in which the few surviving males may have suffered sterilization by radiation damage. Underground storage of frozen semen, collected before the nuclear explosion, may make it possible to repopulate the devastated country provided enough normal women have survived. Immigration from areas remote from the stricken targets seems less acceptable. The thought that after the greater powers have destroyed each other's populations, their previous 'Lebensraum' might be taken over by other races, less productive materially, but more prolific by virtue of their primordial reproductive power, seems unthinkable and intolerable to the technologically superior nations. But it has happened before and other races inhabit vast areas of lands once the domain of highly civilized populations which, if not extinct, have been decimated and reduced to the status of underprivileged minorities in their native lands. At a time of racial consciousness, it would be interesting to see what ethnic groups the governments of countries with mixed populations would select for genetic survival. It may be suspected that the prejudice against minorities will express itself in the selection of semen from males of the predominant race. In ensuring the preservation of only the ethnic majority, uniformity may be achieved, the dream of absolute rulers, ever afraid of non-conformity of thought and suspicious of the disloyalty of the underprivileged minorities. Yet it may be remembered that their presence has served as a crutch to unpopular regimes who cleverly diverted the hostility of the discontented population from the ruling clique to the oppressed and despised minority. Although religious and political persecution has been practised with great success, the stirring up of animosity against ethnic groups is unsurpassed as a political weapon; a man may pretend to have changed his political and religious beliefs, but he cannot change his race. Therefore, for political regimes of the oppressive type, and no doubt these will be the major ones to emerge after a nuclear disaster, the survival of an ethnic minority is indispensable and the planners looking ahead to the era of reconstruction would serve their own selfish interests well by including in their human semen banks germ cells from well defined minority groups whose descendants will be sufficiently marked genetically to be easily recognizable. The planners would have to hope that an unforeseen twist of fate should not upset the expected balance and place the present majority group into the unfortunate position of a minority.

The case for making procreation a minor clinical procedure, after careful shopping for semen, rather than the result of an impulse of the moment, can be carried further to include the choice of germ cells from truly superior women. Such women can be found easily enough, but it may be difficult to persuade them to allow themselves to be inseminated with semen from donors even of the most attractive physical and intellectual characteristics, since they may be unwilling to interrupt their professional and social activities to undergo the ordeals of pregnancy and childbirth. There is a way out of this dilemma. Although *in vitro* fertilization of human ova and embryonic development in tissue culture may be a thing of the more distant future, it will soon be possible to transfer a fertilized human egg from its genetic mother to a foster mother prior to implantation. The foster mother will agree, for a fee which may vary with the degree of social and technological development of her country and in accordance with a carefully written contract, to bear the child to full term or such time as may be deemed appropriate by recognized medical authorities, to give birth to it and to deliver it to its genetic mother and her husband who may or may not be the genetic father, but who would agree to become the child's legal guardian. Thus the process of reproduction in the human species which heretofore has had its foundation in sexual love, and until quite recently was in the shadow of the fear of pregnancy and its complications, including death in childbirth, will be reduced to an aseptic manufacturing process, like the breeding of pedigree cattle by artificial insemination. The relationship between the genetic mother and father of the most advanced species of this planet may become as impersonal and remote as it is between the male and female flowers of pollen bearing plants. Progress? Perhaps.

It used to be the custom to support one's thesis by lifting a passage from the scriptures and quoting it, even though out of context. I found one that seems to suit the foregoing remarks in the preface of *Essays in Biochemistry* (Greville and Campbell, 1966) in which the editors quoted Isaiah, ch. 9, v. 3: 'Thou hast multiplied the nation, and not increased the joy'. Although I suspect that the editors had in mind the thankless nature of their task of compiling their volume, it seems possible that the prophecy may be fulfilled at last. What the prophet had really meant is open to individual interpretation, especially since in the new translation published by The Jewish Publication Society of America, Isaiah, ch. 9, v. 2 (sc.) reads: 'Thou hast multiplied the nation, thou hast increased their joy', thus displaying a less puritanical spirit. We can only guess what future archaeologists will find when the radioactivity of the debris over our cities has decayed and the remnants of our civilization have been dug up. Perhaps there will be enough evidence left for them to conclude that the scientist–priest class of the twentieth century had had some elementary knowledge of science, but that the people of our days, even more so than those of the much older Mesopotamian civilizations, had been excessively preoccupied with sex.

References

Austin, C. R. (1951). *Aust. J. Sci. Res.*, B, **4**, 581.

Chang, M. C. (1951). *Nature, Lond.*, **168**, 697.

Chang, M. C. (1957). *Nature, Lond.*, **179**, 258.

Graves, C. N., Lodge, J. R., and Salisbury, G. W. (1964). *J. Dairy Sci.*, **47**, 1407.

Greville, G. D., and Campbell, P. N. (1966). In *Essays in Biochemistry*, vol. 2, p. vii. Ed. by Campbell, P. N., and Greville, G. D. London and New York: Academic Press.

Mann, T. (1945). *Biochem. J.*, **39**, 458.

Melrose, D. R., and Terner, C. (1953). *Biochem. J.*, **53**, 296.

Minassian, E. S., and Terner, C. (1966). *Am. J. Physiol.*, **210**, 615.

Mitchell, P. (1967). *Fed. Proc.*, **26**, 1370.

Muller, H. J. (1961). *Science*, **134**, 643.

Polge, C., Smith, A. U., and Parkes, A. S. (1949). *Nature, Lond.*, **164**, 666.

Scott, T. W., Voglmayr, J. K., and Setchell, B. P. (1967). *Biochem. J.*, **102**, 456.

Terner, C. (1960). *Am. J. Physiol.*, **198**, 48.

Terner, C. (1965). *Nature, Lond.*, **208**, 1115.

Terner, C., and Korsh, G. (1962). *Biochemistry*, **1**, 367.

Terner, C., and Korsh, G. (1963a). *J. Cell. Comp. Physiol.*, **62**, 243.

Terner, C., and Korsh, G. (1963b). *J. Cell. Comp. Physiol.*, **62**, 251.

Williams, W. L., Abney, T. O., Chernoff, H. N., Dukelow, W. R., and Pinsker, M. C. (1967). *J. Reprod. Fertil.*, Suppl. 2, 11.

ENZYMIC AND ENERGETIC ASPECTS OF THE SODIUM PUMP

R. Whittam

Department of Physiology, University of Leicester

Introduction

It was realized about 30 years ago that there was still a problem in explaining the distribution of ions across cell membranes. Before the Second World War it had been widely believed that concentration gradients of ions between different compartments of the body were maintained by the selective permeability of cell membranes and the presence inside cells of non-diffusible anions mainly in the form of protein. An adequate account of the distribution of sodium, potassium and chloride stemmed from this concept. With the development of tracer studies, however, pioneer work showed that ions in most tissues are exchangeable with those in plasma. Explanations were no longer possible solely in terms of equilibria based on classical thermodynamics of the kind discussed by Donnan (1911, 1924). Another view was developed based upon the notion, first suggested among others by Hill (1931), that apparent equilibria in biology are really steady states which require for their maintenance a continuous supply of energy from cell metabolism. Living cells are not in thermodynamic equilibrium in the classical sense but represent an open system in the steady state.

How does the living cell accomplish its remarkable transformation of energy without the temperature gradient that a machine needs? It is one of the great achievements of the last 30 years that the details of energy production in catabolism are now understood in straightforward chemical terms (Krebs and Kornberg, 1957), and a start is being made in explaining the energy utilization involved in processes like muscular contraction and the active transport of ions (see Davies, this volume for work on muscle). When I started research I was fascinated by energetics and the way in which living matter accomplishes energy transformation. I jumped at the chance to work on one aspect of this problem in Sheffield. The intellectual stimulation and vision emanating from Professor Krebs helped me tremendously in my hesitant first steps in research. His insight is shown in the way he discussed the problem of active transport. In 1951 Professor Krebs wrote 'A "steady state system" is a mixture of chemical substances which continuously enter chemical reactions, or, (if the mixture is heterogeneous) are transported from one part of the system to another, and yet do not change their concentrations because the rates of removal are equal to the rates of replacement. Steady state systems are not in equilibrium and therefore never constitute a complete or "closed" system.' These ideas are similar to those of Gowland Hopkins (1913) who, in discussing the cell, said, 'Its life is the expression of a particular dynamic equilibrium which obtains in a polyphasic system'.

This kind of notion has been put on a sound theoretical basis through the work of physical chemists. They applied the classical work of Lars Onsager on irreversible thermodynamics to the problem of active transport (see Katchalsky and Kedem, 1962). An important point relevant to mechanism is that a chemical reaction coupled to a vectorial flow of matter must itself show spatial asymmetry.

Krogh (1946) gave a good account of work up to the time when active and passive transport largely replaced permeability as the description of this field of research. It had become clear that there must be a special mechanism for the transport of ions, the term 'sodium pump' having been first used by Dean (1941) to account for sodium extrusion from muscle. The selectivity of cell membranes towards such similar ions as sodium and potassium shows that chemically indiscriminate physical forces cannot account for the observed ion movements.

The problem of how molecules in a membrane direct the passage of ions against concentration gradients is different in kind from much traditional biochemistry which has been concerned with the purification and characterization of enzymes. This problem is concerned, in contrast, with how a functional unit in the membrane selectively takes up the ion to be transported in the face of a higher concentration of another similar ion. Thus, sodium is in a much lower concentration than potassium inside cells and yet is transported outwards. A similar consideration applies to extracellular potassium. After the selection of the ion, there is then movement against a concentration gradient and energy transduction is involved. Energy is needed to pump sodium ions from the intracellular fluid with a low concentration to the extracellular fluid with a high concentration. Pirie (1964) has aptly commented 'the basic problem of contemporary biochemistry is not how a reaction is carried out, nor how its specificity is controlled, but how energy derived from one process is used to drive another'. Directionality has also to be considered in studying enzyme action in a transport system. In discussing the sodium pump, I am limiting myself to two aspects. First there is the problem of the form in which energy from the degradation of foodstuffs is made available for the endergonic process of active transport, and secondly, what is the nature of the enzymes involved in active transport?

Nature of the energy supply for the sodium pump

It is hard to realize in 1968 the controversies there were in the early 1950's regarding a possible direct coupling of electron transport in the cytochrome system with ion transport across cell membranes. Conway (1953) had a mechanism—conveniently called a 'redox pump'—which connected the transference of electrons from hydrogen atoms with the active transport of sodium ions from cells. According to this view there would be a direct stoichiometric relationship between electron transport in the cytochrome system and sodium ions transported across the cell membrane. This theory has been extended and developed by Robertson (1960), and was also discussed and independently suggested, particularly in relation to acid secretion by the gastric mucosa, by Davies (1948) and Davies and Krebs (1952). According to Davies and Krebs (1952) and Davies and Ogston (1950) there was also a possibility that energy from ATP could be utilized for transport processes. Thus, an alternative to a cytochrome–redox system as a link between metabolism and ion transport is a mechanism which depends directly on ATP. A redox reaction independent of the cytochrome system, yet depending on ATP, is still an open possibility (see Whittam and Wiley, 1967).

The attraction of a mechanism depending on ATP follows from its ubiquitous supply in living matter. The early evidence supporting this view was based largely on the effects of inhibitors such as 2,4-dinitrophenol, cyanide, iodoacetate and fluoride, as well as anoxia (see Whittam, 1960). This kind of work was in keeping with a requirement for ATP but did not prove it. Somewhat stronger evidence was the parallelism between the rate of ATP hydrolysis and the rate of potassium transport in human red blood cells (Whittam, 1958). Similar work with giant nerve axons showed a dependence of sodium efflux on arginine phosphate which is known to give rise to ATP (Caldwell, Hodgkin, Keynes and Shaw, 1960). ATP itself was not as effective as arginine phosphate and it seemed that a high ratio of ATP/ADP might be necessary (see de Weer, 1968).

Enzymic evidence for a role of ATP

By far the most compelling evidence showing that ATP hydrolysis is related to sodium transport has come from work on the enzymic hydrolysis of ATP. Skou (1957) demonstrated a synergistic stimulation by sodium and potassium of ATPase activity in a homogenate of crab nerve. The only previous instance of stimulation of enzymic action by sodium was Utter's (1950) finding with a brain homogenate. In retrospect, Utter's work finds an explanation in the presence in brain of the same enzymic activity that Skou described. Skou's discovery has opened the way to a large amount of work on the mechanism of ATP hydrolysis. There are two ways of tackling the problem. There is first the approach in which the ATPase activity is characterized in fragmented membranes which have not been particularly purified.

Perhaps the main discovery from work of this kind is the finding that the reaction can be split into two steps which have different requirements for sodium and potassium. In the course of ATP hydrolysis there appears first to be a reaction requiring sodium which causes a transfer of the terminal phosphate of ATP to an acyl group of the enzyme (Albers, Fahn and Koval, 1963; Whittam, Wheeler and Blake, 1964; Hokin, Sastry, Galsworthy and Yoda, 1965; Post, Sen and Rosenthal, 1965). This transphosphorylation does not involve a loss of the high energy character of the terminal phosphate bond. In the absence of potassium the reaction does not proceed further and there is no breakdown of phosphorylated protein. However, when sodium and potassium are present together the phosphate intermediate cannot be detected, indicating that it must have been broken down by the action of potassium. Moreover, simultaneous addition of the inhibitors, ouabain or oligomycin, prevents the action of potassium. The intermediate is not then hydrolysed. The sequence of reactions can be written as follows:

$$Activated\ by\ Na^+$$
$$ATP + PROTEIN \rightarrow PROTEIN\text{-}PHOSPHATE + ADP$$
$$inhibited\ by\ Ca^{2+}$$

$$Activated\ by\ K^+$$
$$PROTEIN\text{-}PHOSPHATE \rightarrow PROTEIN + P_i$$
$$inhibited\ by$$
$$ouabain\ and\ oligomycin$$

Overall reaction: $ATP \rightarrow ADP + P_i$

This kind of work with membranes of various tissues (kidney and brain cortex, electric organ of *Electrophorus electricus*) suggests that the first step of the reaction involves the formation of a complex between Mg-ATP, sodium ions and the enzyme. The phosphate intermediate is then produced and subsequently broken down by the action of potassium.

Complex chemical nature of the sodium-activated ATPase

In pursuing this line of work it seems essential that the enzyme should be purified and so far this has proved to be intractable. Ways have been described involving the use of hypertonic sodium iodide—by an adaption of the method for the extraction of myosin—which markedly raised the enzymic activity (Nakao, Tashima, Nagano and Nakao, 1965). Similarly, the use of surface active agents, like digitonin, also causes some degree of refinement of the preparation. In spite of great efforts the enzyme has not yet been obtained in a crystalline form. There is indeed some doubt whether this is possible. For example, Tanaka and Strickland (1965), working with microsomes from ox brain, found that a protein could be obtained which did not possess ATPase activity depending on sodium and potassium—although it possessed ATPase activity independent of these ions. Their striking finding was that addition of unsaturated lecithin caused ATPase activity to appear which was sensitive to sodium and potassium. Their work suggests that the enzyme activity is not so much the simple catalysis by a protein but catalysis by a functional unit of the membrane in which lipid as well as protein is needed. The requirement for lipid suggests that the protein alone perhaps lacks the conformation it gets when lecithin is added and upon which the sensitivity to alkali metals depends.

Influence of structure on enzymic activity

The importance of structure regarding the activity of enzymes generally is a relatively neglected area of research, but there are two other examples where enzyme activity is stimulated in a comparable way. Sekuzu, Jurtshuk and Green (1963) showed that the enzyme 3-hydroxybutyrate dehydrogenase becomes inactive on purification, yet the activity can be restored by lecithin. Kagawa and Racker (1966) have also shown that ATPase activity in a purified preparation from mitochondria is insensitive to oligomycin yet addition of a factor derived from mitochondria (which contains lipid) can restore sensitivity to oligomycin in the soluble ATPase preparation. These instances point to the influence on enzymic activity of lipids that form complex structures with proteins. Again, polymers of amino acids with either predominantly positive or negative charges can be attached to enzymes and markedly affect activity because of changes in charge in the immediate milieu of the enzyme. A systematic approach studying enzymes rendered insoluble by attachment to artificial structures of various kinds has shown the great effect of the electrical charges surrounding the protein (see Silman and Katchalski, 1966). Work on changes occurring when a soluble enzyme is made insoluble by attachment to an artificial membrane is only beginning (Whittam, Wheeler and Edwards, 1968).

Since the ATPase involved in the sodium pump is part of a functional unit, it is not surprizing that lecithin appears to be necessary for its activity. Another indication of the importance of lipid is that lecithinase acts on erythrocyte membranes causing them to lose their response to sodium and potassium (Schatzmann, 1962).

The sodium pump considered as a chemical reaction

A quite different approach to the mechanism of action of the ATPase derives from considering its functional role. In some way the hydrolysis of ATP brings about a movement of sodium outwards and potassium inwards. In order to measure the ion movements associated with ATPase activity it is obviously necessary to work with intact membranes which are able to separate two aqueous solutions with different ionic compositions. The enzyme action is accompanied by a movement of cofactors (sodium and potassium) to opposite sides of the membrane. ATP, ADP and P_i remain inside the cell but there is a simultaneous migration of sodium outwards and potassium inwards. The ATPase activity is not stimulated unless these movements can occur. It is not meaningful to talk of the chemical reaction driving the transport process, because as the enzyme only acts when the ion movements can occur. The two events— chemical reaction and flow of ions—are inextricably coupled.

Activation by internal sodium and external potassium

It is clearly important to establish the stoichiometry for the number of ions (m and n for potassium and sodium, respectively) transported for the hydrolysis of one molecule of ATP in accordance with the following reaction:

$$m K_e + n Na_i + ATP + H_2O \rightarrow m K_i + n Na_e + ADP + P_i$$

This equation brings out the spatial asymmetry of the ATPase and the fact that ion movements are as much a part of the reaction as is the splitting of ATP. The subscripts, e and i, refer to external and internal ions. The equation implies that associated with ATP hydrolysis there is a flow of sodium and potassium ions in opposite directions, but it does not say that the flow is against a concentration gradient; that is the thermodynamic aspect of transport. The view of active transport as a movement against a concentration (or electrochemical potential) gradient was based on sound thermodynamic reasoning (Ussing, 1949), but it has no bearing on mechanism. A later approach based on irreversible thermodynamics has somewhat more relevance to mechanism insofar as there is a requirement that the chemical reaction concerned with the flow of matter should itself be spatially asymmetric. Is this important theoretical requirement met with the ATPase system of the sodium pump? Do the ions activate from the sides of the membrane from which they are transported? Sodium efflux is stimulated by external potassium and vice versa in a way sensitive to ouabain (Glynn, 1957; Post and Jolly, 1957; Whittam and Ager, 1965), thus leading to the question whether ATPase activity is stimulated in the same synergistic way and from the same locations. Are the rates of transport and ATPase activity determined just by the concentrations of internal sodium and external potassium, or do the size of the concentration gradients exert an influence? These questions all have a bearing on mechanism. How are they studied experimentally?

In the work with fragmented membranes the activation by sodium and potassium could not be attributed to one side or the other of the membrane because both sides were equally exposed to the same bathing solution. A test of the question of the site of activation of the ions was made with ghosts of human red cells which were prepared so that the internal fluid could be varied in composition (Hoffman, Tosteson and Whittam, 1960). By incubating ghosts containing ATP which were rich and poor in internal sodium in Ringer solutions, which were either potassium-free or contained various amounts of potassium, it was clearly shown that the ATPase activity is indeed asymmetrical in nature. The presence or absence of external sodium did not affect ATPase activity; it was only internal sodium and external potassium which cooperatively stimulated the reaction (Glynn, 1962; Whittam, 1962).

Active transport as a pace-maker of metabolism

In approaching the question of the stoichiometry of ion movements in relation to ATP hydrolysis an experimental drawback is that it is not as satisfactory to measure ion movements in ghosts as in cells. The permeability of ghosts is somewhat raised by the treatment required to change their ionic composition. However, a new method of changing the cells' ionic composition opportunely became available in the work of Bolingbroke and Maizels (1959). They showed that red cells can be loaded with different alkali metals during treatment with non-electrolytes. When red cells are placed in lactose solution they become reversibly permeable to alkali metals without losing their haemoglobin. This method was used to obtain cells with a wide range of internal sodium and potassium, and the rates of movement of these ions were measured (Whittam and Ager, 1965).

An indirect way of measuring ATPase activity had to be used because ATP itself could not be introduced into the lactose-treated cells in the same way that it can be introduced into ghosts. Thus, although cells are better from the point of view of the kinetics of active transport, they are less satisfactory than ghosts in measuring the ATPase activity.

Lactate production regulated by the activity of the sodium pump

Nevertheless, because of the relatively simple glycolytic metabolic pathway in human red cells an assessment can be made of the contribution of lactate production in supplying energy for the sodium pump. When the sodium pump was inhibited with ouabain, or was inactive in the absence of external potassium, lactate production was lower than the value under optimum conditions when the sodium pump was functioning. The fall in lactate production was the same with ouabain as with deprivation of external potassium. The effect of ouabain was not directly on an enzyme of glycolysis because it had no effect in the absence of external potassium. These observations show that the effect of ouabain on lactate production was elicited only when the sodium pump was functioning. If, now, the amount of lactate production affected by external potassium and ouabain is taken as the amount which would otherwise supply ATP for the sodium pump, this amount of ATP can be calculated, since there is a net synthesis of one molecule of ATP associated with the formation of one molecule of lactate in the glycolytic pathway. There is, therefore, a basal rate of metabolism which is independent of the sodium pump, and, in addition, there is a variable rate controlled by active transport. The transport-controlled part can be varied from 25–75% of the basal rate (Whittam and Ager, 1965). Active transport acts as a pacemaker of metabolism in glycolysing red blood cells just as it does in respiring tissues like liver, brain and kidney (see Whittam, 1964). The feedback control is mediated by ADP acting, in red cells, as a substrate for phosphoglycerate kinase (Parker and Hoffman, 1967).

Stoichiometry of the sodium pump

The finding that a part of energy production is regulated by energy utilization for the sodium pump allows a comparison to be made to see if the two cellular activities change in step together. Further, it became possible to measure the stoichiometry (ions transported/ATP hydrolysed) for different rates of transport. The transport rates of sodium and potassium and their associated lactate production were varied in three ways, which depended on direct modification of the rate of the sodium pump and not alteration of transport arising from non-specific inhibition of the energy supply such as is found with iodoacetate or glucose deprivation (Whittam, 1958). The changes were made:

(a) By altering external potassium;
(b) By altering internal sodium;
(c) By partial inhibition with ouabain.

There was always a parallel change in metabolism (indicated by lactate production and the appearance of inorganic phosphate) and the rate of transport. It is worth emphasizing that it is only in red cells and red cell ghosts that this correlation has been established. The evidence for the sodium-activated ATPase being part of the sodium pump in other tissues is still circumstantial and less direct than with red cells.

Schatzmann and Rüss (1965) made a valuable study with red cell ghosts and showed an exact parallelism in the percentage inhibition by ouabain of ATPase activity, and of sodium and potassium transport. The same correlation between ATPase activity and transport was found when the transport rate was also varied by changing the internal sodium and external potassium concentrations (Whittam and Ager, 1965). With each procedure a comparison was made of the number of ions transported per molecule of ATP. The ratio was the same with each experimental procedure. The potassium:ATP ratio was about 2·4, and the sodium:ATP ratio was about 3·2. The stoichiometry was constant for cells in which the transport was either downhill, on the level, or uphill. These values (Whittam and Ager, 1965) agree with other assessments of the stoichiometry (Glynn, 1962; Sen and Post, 1964; Garrahan and Glynn, 1967a).

The energetics of sodium and potassium transport

The details of the ATPase reaction have yet to be worked out. However, from the functional point of view it is worthwhile considering some energetic aspects of the reaction. The first point is whether the energy available from a given rate of ATP hydrolysis is sufficient for the osmotic work performed. As mentioned earlier in connection with enzymes attached to a solid matrix, different properties can arise with solid-state enzymes compared with enzymes in dilute solution. Many enzymes in nature are of this form, and certainly most of those involved in energy transformation. Green (1959) and Lehninger (1960) have drawn attention to the fact that the non-aqueous nature of solid structures in cells might allow stabilization of otherwise unstable intermediates. Moreover, there is the further point that reactions catalysed by enzymes in an environment which is rich in lipid do so in a region where the chemical potential of water is low. No investigations have yet been made of the influence of the water concentration on the ATPase reaction. It is not easy to determine the free energy change in a chemical reaction which takes place in the lipid environment of the cell membrane. Since an allowance cannot be made for this factor the next best thing is to calculate the free energy change as if the reaction took place in aqueous solution. In calculating the free energy change the following equation has been used.

$$\Delta G' = \Delta G^\circ - 2 \cdot 3\, RT \left[\mathrm{pH} - 7 \cdot 5 - \log_{10}\left(\frac{[\mathrm{ADP}][\mathrm{P_i}]}{[\mathrm{ATP}]} \right) \right]$$

Determinations were made of the concentrations of ATP, ADP and P_i in red cells so that the free energy change ($\Delta G'$) could be calculated making use of the standard free energy (ΔG°) of ATP hydrolysis of $-8 \cdot 5$ kcal/mole (see Burton, 1958). The value comes to -13 kcal/mole under the conditions pertaining to intact red cells which were transporting sodium and potassium. In order to calculate the work done, the appropriate equation is as follows:

$$\Delta G = 2 \cdot 3\, RT \left[n \log_{10}\left(\frac{140}{[\mathrm{Na^+}]_i} \right) + m \log_{10}\left(\frac{[\mathrm{K^+}]_i}{10} \right) \right] + (n - m)EF$$

The concentrations in the Ringer solution were: Na, 140 mM; K, 10 mM. R is the gas constant, T the absolute temperature, F the faraday, E the membrane potential (about $0 \cdot 01$ v), and $[\mathrm{Na^+}]_i$ and $[\mathrm{K^+}]_i$ are the intracellular $\mathrm{Na^+}$ and $\mathrm{K^+}$ concentrations in μequiv/ml of cell water. $n = 3 \cdot 2$ and $m = 2 \cdot 4$. ΔG represents the minimum energy utilized for the transport for sodium and potassium during the hydrolysis of one mole of ATP in a way sensitive to ouabain. Within the range of the physiological internal sodium concentrations it was calculated that the energy requirement did not exceed 9 kcal. The results, therefore, show that the energy available (13 kcal) exceeded the energy requirement for the active transport, and that the efficiency was about 70%.

Independence of activity of the sodium pump on concentration gradients

The fact that the stoichiometry was the same for downhill as for uphill movements raises an important point regarding the concept of active transport. The outward movement of sodium ions appears to be determined only by the internal sodium concentration and is not affected by the external sodium concentration. This means that an outward downhill movement of sodium ions into a sodium-free Ringer solution can occur through the sodium pump in the same way that uphill transport is brought about. The results show that transport coupled to ATPase activity may be either with or against a concentration gradient. It is the connection between the chemical reaction and the flow of matter which is the main characteristic of the sodium pump. Movement against a concentration gradient is not an essential feature of it. It is obvious that in order to achieve a vectorial flow of ions a spatially oriented chemical reaction must be involved, since there cannot be a coupling between a scalar chemical reaction and vectorial flow of matter. From the chemical point of view it is easier to investigate a mechanism where only internal sodium determines the rate of the reaction and not a combination of internal and external sodium. The same consideration applies with regard to activation of external potassium.

A useful way of regarding the sodium pump is, therefore, as a chemical reaction linked to the flow of matter—irrespective of whether or not the ion movement is against a concentration gradient. It seems that over a wide range of activity the sodium pump functions like a bicycle with a fixed gear in which the ratio of the revolutions per minute of the pedals and the distance moved by the bicycle is constant whatever the gradient.

The question could be raised: what happens to the stoichiometry when the cells contain a very low sodium concentration and a very high potassium concentration? The stoichiometry seems to decrease under these conditions and a possible explanation derives from a general consideration about the physiological regulation of the sodium and potassium content of cells. Why do cells not pump out all their sodium? The reason is that as internal sodium reaches a low level, internal potassium then reaches a high level and starts to inhibit activation of the pump by sodium. There would be fewer sodium ions transported outwards per ATP if potassium ions took their place on the pump mechanism—as appears likely. Similarly, fewer potassium ions would enter if external sodium entered the cell on the potassium mechanism. It is known from our work discussed below on the competition between these two ions that activation by potassium is subject to competition by sodium. With fragmented membranes there are dual effects of each ion, such that at low concentrations there is activation whereas at high concentrations the same ion begins to inhibit because of competition with the companion ion (Priestland and Whittam, 1968). It seems, therefore, that the internal sodium and potassium concentrations of cells are regulated by the activity of the sodium pump. A stage is reached where net transport no longer occurs because internal potassium has become so high as to inhibit effectively the activation of internal sodium.

I

Mechanism of action of the sodium-activated ATPase

The mechanism of action of the sodium-activated ATPase can be usefully considered in the light of general knowledge of the behaviour of enzymes. This knowledge largely stems from work with purified enzymes, and there are two salient features of the activity. There is the attachment of substrate to the active centre forming an enzyme–substrate complex which breaks down to give the products of the reaction. Indeed, the attachment of substrate to the active centre may involve an induced fit of substrate with the enzyme in a way that depends on the whole conformation of the enzyme and not just on the kinds of amino acids in the region of the active centre (Koshland, Yankeelov and Thoma, 1962). Many inhibitors act directly on the active centre. However, there are other agents which influence enzymic activity whose action cannot be attributed to an effect on the active centre. There are sites in enzymes—called allosteric—that are distant from the active centre but which, nevertheless, determine the rate of catalysis (Monod, Changeux and Jacob, 1963). This concept has led to much work with purified enzymes that has fulfilled the predictions of Monod and coworkers (1963).

A case can be made out from the general features of the sodium transport system that protein conformational changes and an allosteric mechanism are likely to be involved. Thus, the hydrolysis of ATP occurs exclusively within the cell, and the products are liberated with the cell (Schatzmann, 1964; Whittam and Ager, 1964). In spite of the enzyme action occurring at the inner surface of the cell membrane, the activity is nonetheless stimulated by external potassium. Perhaps the simplest explanation is that potassium acts on a distant site of the protein that is responsible for the hydrolysis, and as such the mechanism would fall into the category of allosteric. Similarly, the reaction of ATP with the enzyme requires internal sodium, yet the splitting of ATP allows sodium to be liberated to the outside of the cell. Again, a reasonable explanation is that owing to different conformations of the enzyme, which is in combination with lipid, the changing molecular architecture permits sodium to move only in one direction, namely outwards.

Allosteric and cooperative effects

Several discussions of this aspect of the sodium pump have been made (see Tosteson, 1963; Skou and Hilberg, 1965; Whittam, 1967). Indeed, detailed speculations as to the molecular mechanism of possible allosteric effects have been made by some authors on the basis of the general features of the sodium pump which were outlined above (e.g. Opit and Charnock, 1965; Jardetzky, 1966). These hypothetical schemes have great intellectual fascination and are highly plausible as mechanisms for the sodium pump. The difficulty is that evidence in favour of such mechanisms, or indeed of any other mechanisms at the molecular level, is almost completely lacking. For the experimentalist the tendency is perhaps to denigrate schemes of this kind, mainly for the reason that they do not suggest critical experiments with which they can be tested. Professor Krebs has at times halted eloquent but somewhat tendentious arguments by simply asking 'and what is your first experiment?'. As an example of theoretical schemes which cannot be tested, it is salutary to remember that in 1952 Danielli put forward six different explanations for the observed kinetics of sugar transport and pointed out that there was no experimental way of distinguishing between them. In the case of possible allosteric mechanisms for the sodium pump great ingenuity and subtlety has been brought to bear in the theoretical proposals but greater ingenuity is needed to devise experimental tests of the possible systems.

Sigmoid kinetics for activation by sodium and potassium

One observation cited in favour of an allosteric mechanism is that activation by one ion (sodium or potassium) shows sigmoid kinetics in the presence of an excess of the other ion when the ATPase activity of fragmented membranes is measured. This finding was one of the first to be made in the enzymic work on ATPase activity and has recently been emphasized in work by Robinson (1967) and Squires (1965), who suggest that this deviation from a rectangular hyperbola implies an allosteric mechanism. This effect is certainly consistent with an allosteric mechanism, but also with other interpretations which ought to be considered. A sigmoid response can be obtained without an allosteric mechanism as, for example, in work with succinic dehydrogenase (Gawron, Mahajan, Limetti, Kananen and Glaid, 1966). If a reaction involves a number of steps there can be cooperative effects in which more than one molecule of substrate is required to initiate the reaction, and this requirement leads to sigmoid kinetics. The theoretical treatment of enzyme kinetics, with particular reference to effects of this kind, has been given by Ferdinand (1966) and by Rabin (1967). It seems clear that deviation from Michaelis–Menten kinetics is not sufficient ground in support of an allosteric mechanism unless there is also evidence relating to the nature of sub-units or conformational changes during enzymic activity. The best evidence for allosteric effects is where sub-units of the enzyme have been demonstrated that separately possess effector and catalytic sites (Gerhart and Schachmann, 1965), and where direct evidence of a conformational change arising from attachment of an allosteric effector with the enzyme has also been found (Dratz and Calvin, 1966). These are necessary conditions before an allosteric property can be justifiably attributed to an enzyme.

Competition between ions gives sigmoid kinetics

It is therefore necessary critically to examine the ATPase evidence further. In work with fragmented membranes, in which these features can be found, it is inevitable that sodium and potassium are accessible to all points of the surface of the fragments which are catalysing ATP hydrolysis. This means that activation by sodium takes place in the presence of potassium at what would have been the inner surface of the membrane in the intact cell. Similarly activation by potassium must occur in the presence of sodium. When sodium is in low concentration and potassium in high concentration, or vice versa, one ion is subject to competition by the other ion, although, at the same time, both ions must be present in order to elicit the co-operative stimulation characteristic of the ATPase. It is clear that in such a suspension of particles, competition between ions may not be readily recognizable as a separate event from the cooperative stimulation of activity. The kinetics of activation need to be studied with intact membranes so that activation is not complicated by simultaneous interfering effects of the other ion.

When ATPase activity of intact membranes was compared with ATPase activity of fragmented membranes there was a striking difference in the kinetics of activation by sodium and potassium (Priestland and Whittam, 1968). Experiments were made with red cell ghosts in which activating effects of sodium (from inside) can be distinguished from inhibitory effects (from outside). The sigmoid curve was found with ghosts incubated in Ringer solution containing sodium but not in the absence of external sodium. Thus, the stimulation by external potassium with intact membranes shows a sigmoid curve, just as is found with fragmented membranes, but not in the absence of external sodium. External sodium is not required for ATPase activity and in its absence a rectangular hyperbola could be fitted to the experimental points. The simplest explanation seems to be that there is a decrease in the response to low concentrations of potassium ($0 \cdot 1$–$0 \cdot 3$ mM) and that external sodium is able to compete with potassium. If a sigmoid curve does exist in the absence of external sodium it might still be found by a more refined examination of activation by external potassium at very low concentrations. Baker and Stone (1966) and Stone (1968), in a theoretical analysis of results of human red cells, predicted that a sigmoid response due to an allosteric mechanism might occur with an external potassium concentration in the region of $0 \cdot 05$ mM. This concentration is difficult to achieve experimentally and the possibility is still open that a sigmoid response at this level of external potassium might be present. Nevertheless, since the large sigmoid response can be abolished by incubating cells in the absence of external sodium, clearly this effect is not valid positive evidence for an allosteric effect.

Cooperative effects between ions of the same element

In spite of the note of caution prominent in the above paragraph it is not implied that cooperative effects are absent in the operation of the sodium pump. There clearly must be cooperation between internal sodium and external potassium. Furthermore, there is some evidence for a requirement for two potassium ions at an external site in order for the system to operate. In the measurement of stoichiometry, it turned out that about three sodium and two potassium ions were transported per molecule of ATP hydrolysed. It is, therefore, interesting that Sachs and Welt (1967) fitted kinetic data on potassium influx to a model which involved the cooperative action of two potassium ions on the external surface of the membrane. In frog muscle also there is evidence for the involvement of more than one sodium ion in the sodium pump, inasmuch as sodium efflux is proportional to the third power of the internal sodium concentration (Keynes and Swan, 1959). This result is consistent with the view that more than one sodium ion is needed for the sodium pump to operate. Again, this conclusion is consistent with the stoichiometry found with red cells. Cooperative action of more than one sodium ion at the internal surface and of more than one potassium ion at the external surface is a reasonable conclusion about mechanism from experimental results.

There is a dilemma in future work on this problem because the chemical purification which is needed for enzymic studies leads to loss of the characteristic property of the sodium pump, and yet retention of these properties with some degree of intact membrane means that application of the techniques used with isolated enzymes is not possible. Indications of possible future developments are given in the last paragraph of this essay.

Reversal of the direction of action of the sodium pump

In studying an ATPase reaction its reversal would not normally be expected unless the reaction was coupled to another which had a large positive free energy change. Experiments with fragmented cell membranes under several conditions showed only little labelling of ATP with tracer P_i, evidently because there was no source of energy for the reaction (Skou, 1960; Fahn, Koval and Albers, 1966). However, with the intact membranes of red cell ghosts it is possible to test whether ATP within the ghosts becomes labelled with P_i depending on the direction of sodium and potassium movements. Instead of a chemical reaction being coupled to ATP synthesis, the question arises whether the exergonic dissipation of ionic concentration gradients might reverse the ATPase reaction through reversal of the direction of operation of the sodium pump. Garrahan and Glynn (1967b) tested this question with ghosts rich in potassium and poor in sodium incubated in a potassium-free sodium Ringer solution. The sodium pump could not operate because there was no external potassium, and the concentration gradients favoured downhill movements of sodium inwards and of potassium outwards. Labelling of ATP was shown which depended on the ionic gradients, and was largely abolished by ouabain and partly abolished by oligomycin. Both these compounds inhibit the sodium pump. Incorporation was very much lower in potassium Ringer compared with sodium Ringer. It seemed safe to conclude that running the sodium pump backwards led to a net synthesis of ATP at the expense of energy derived from ionic concentration gradients (Garrahan and Glynn, 1967b).

Requirement for both sodium and potassium

One of the salient features of the normal operation of the sodium pump is the requirement for both sodium and potassium ions to be transported simultaneously. This means that sodium is not transported outwards without potassium going inwards and vice versa. It is, therefore, relevant to the mechanism of the apparent reversal of the ATPase reaction to enquire whether reverse movements of both ions (i.e. of sodium inwards and potassium outwards) are also required. This is important, as it appeared that the second step of the ATPase reaction catalysed by potassium might be reversible on its own (Garrahan and Glynn, 1967c).

Reconstituted ghosts of human red cells were prepared containing tracer P_i, small amounts of ATP and ADP, and different concentrations of sodium and potassium. The ghosts were incubated in Ringer solutions of various compositions designed to allow normal operation of the sodium pump, inhibition of the sodium pump (when ouabain was added) or non-activation of the sodium pump (when potassium was omitted). As found by Garrahan and Glynn (1967b), there was always some labelling of ATP from P_i whatever the distribution of ions across the cell membranes, but the incorporation was increased when potassium-rich ghosts were incubated in sodium Ringer. When potassium-rich ghosts were incubated in a sodium-free Ringer, in which the cations were choline, the extra incorporation was not observed, neither was there inhibition by ouabain. Furthermore, when the ghosts were rich in sodium, so that there was no driving force for the downhill movement of sodium inwards, there was again no extra labelling in a way that was related to the distribution of ions. The extra incorporation of P_i into ATP was only found when there were downhill movements of *both* sodium and potassium (Lant and Whittam, 1968). This extra labelling was also abolished by adding to the Ringer solution sufficient potassium to facilitate normal operation of the sodium pump. The optimum conditions for labelling were therefore high internal potassium, low internal sodium and a potassium-free medium containing sodium.

It is reasonable to equate the labelling of ATP by tracer phosphate with the net synthesis of ATP. It has not been possible to demonstrate net synthesis by chemical means because of the fact that the incorporation occurs at only about 2% of the reaction causing hydrolysis of ATP (Garrahan and Glynn, 1967b; Lant and Whittam, 1968). The main outcome of the work on the ionic requirement for labelling is that it has to be possible for downhill movements of both sodium and potassium to occur. If only the movement of one of these ions is possible then the labelling is not found. Moreover, even if downhill movements do occur but the pathway through the sodium pump is inhibited by ouabain, again the labelling is not found. The third way of stopping the labelling is to include sufficient potassium in the Ringer solution so that the normal operation of the sodium pump can proceed. Taken together, these results indicate that the labelling of ATP depends upon conditions under which downhill movements of sodium and potassium can occur—apparently by the system which normally brings about their uphill movement.

Coupling of sodium influx and potassium efflux through the sodium pump pathway

The above results on the backwards running of the sodium pump lead to the question whether there might also be a coupling of downhill ion movements in view of the points of similarity between the forwards and backwards reaction. In order to test whether potassium efflux is coupled to sodium influx, measurements were made of the unidirectional fluxes with radioactive tracers (Lant, Priestland and Whittam, 1970). Potassium efflux from cells was decreased about 25% when ouabain was added to potassium-free sodium Ringer. This means that just as ouabain inhibited labelling of ATP under these same conditions, so it also inhibited a small part of the downhill potassium movement. When ouabain was added to a choline chloride solution lacking both sodium and potassium, it had no effect on potassium efflux. This result shows that inhibition by ouabain depended on external sodium. The implication is clearly that the potassium efflux might be accompanied by an entry of sodium which is also sensitive to ouabain. When sodium influx was measured from a potassium-free sodium Ringer solution it was inhibited by ouabain. The inhibition was greater than the ouabain-sensitive potassium efflux, almost certainly due to the exchange diffusion of sodium which has been described by Garrahan and Glynn (1967d) under similar conditions. However, it appears that besides exchange diffusion of sodium there is a component of sodium influx which balances the potassium efflux, both of these components being sensitive to ouabain. The ouabain-sensitive sodium influx was greater than the comparable efflux by an amount in the same region as the ouabain-sensitive potassium efflux.

These experiments are not entirely satisfactory since it would really be necessary to make simultaneous measurements of sodium influx and efflux, and of potassium efflux on the same batch of cells. Instead of making these somewhat complex measurements, the net changes in sodium and potassium were determined instead. The net gain of sodium and the net loss of potassium from cells were in accord with the findings on unidirectional fluxes in showing that a small fraction of both sodium entry and potassium loss was inhibited by ouabain. It thus appears that there is an interdependence, or coupling, of ouabain-sensitive downhill sodium and potassium movements which parallel the requirements for incorporation of phosphate into ATP (Lant, Priestland and Whittam, 1970).

Future prospects

I have not attempted in this essay to cover the transport of ions across the membranes of mitochondria, bacteria and plant cells, because these different systems do not have the sodium pump which is the principal transport system in the plasma membrane of animal cells. What are the likely lines of development during the next few years? Undoubtedly, there will be great interest in the concept that energy transformation may be reversible in the sense that energy in chemical bonds may be derived from the energy liberated by the dissipation of ionic gradients. Equally important, events at the molecular level of organization allow conformational changes in macromolecules such that the membrane is spatially asymmetrical in the way sodium and potassium ions are selected and transported across it. This is perhaps the least experimentally accessible question in the whole field, for the physiological function arises from the operation of a complex assembly of molecules. In contrast, the methods of investigation at present available for characterizing macromolecules inevitably involve their separation from the membrane and consequent purification. A hopeful indication of a new approach in this direction is the recent work of Cohen, Keynes and Hille (1968) on changes in birefringence during conduction in nerve axons. With very sensitive methods, they have shown changes in light scattering and birefringence which can be most simply explained on the basis of a conformational change in a molecule or molecules of the membrane. This work might be extended to the situation in the membranes of cells in which it is possible to vary at will the operation of the sodium pump. Another powerful indication of structure is optical rotatory dispersion or circular dichroism, and Mommaerts (1966) has made interesting observations on the circular dichroism of visual pigments. These physical methods are showing effects related to the structure of macromolecules associated with physiological function. Further understanding of the function and mechanism of the sodium pump seems likely to depend upon work at two levels of organization. One, with intact cells, in which the sodium pump is seen as an integral part of cellular activity with controlling effects on other activities such as metabolism and cell volume; and the other, where the mechanism is investigated at the molecular level with physicochemical techniques.

References

Albers, R. W., Fahn, S., and Koval, G. J. (1963). *Proc. Natl. Acad. Sci. U.S.*, **50**, 474.

Baker, P. F., and Stone, A. J. (1966). *Biochim. Biophys. Acta*, **126**, 321.

Bolingbroke, V., and Maizels, M. (1959). *J. Physiol.*, **149**, 563.

Burton, K. (1958). *Nature, Lond.*, **181**, 1594.

Caldwell, P. C., Hodgkin, A. L., Keynes, R. D., and Shaw, T. I. (1960). *J. Physiol.* **152**, 561.

Cohen, L. B., Keynes, R. D., and Hille, B. (1968). *Nature, Lond.*, **218**, 438.

Conway, E. J. (1953). *Int. Rev. Cytol.*, **2**, 419.

Danielli, J. F. (1952). *Symp. Soc. Exp. Biol.*, **8**,

Davies, R. E. (1948). *Biochem. J.*, **42**, 609.

Davies, R. E., and Krebs, H, A. (1952). *Symp. Biochem. Soc.*, **8**, 77.

Davies, R. E., and Ogston, A. G. (1950). *Biochem. J.*, **46**, 324.

Dean, R. B. (1941). *Biol. Symposia*, **3**, 331.

Donnan, F. G. (1911). *Z. Elektrochem.*, **17**, 572.

Donnan, F. G. (1924). *Chem. Rev.*, **1**, 73.

Dratz, E. A., and Calvin, M. (1966). *Nature, Lond.*, **211**, 497.

Fahn, S., Koval, G. J., and Albers, R. W. (1966). *J. Biol. Chem.*, **241**, 1882.

Ferdinand, W. (1966). *Biochem. J.*, **99**, 278.

Garrahan, P. J., and Glynn, I. M. (1967a). *J. Physiol.*, **192**, 217.

Garrahan, P. J., and Glynn, I. M. (1967b). *J. Physiol.*, **192**, 237.

Garrahan, P. J., and Glynn, I. M. (1967c). *J. Physiol.*, **192**, 189.

Garrahan, P. J., and Glynn, I. M. (1967d). *J. Physiol.*, **192**, 159.
Gawron, O., Mahajan, K. P., Limetti, M., Kananen, G., and Glaid, A. J. (1966). *Biochemistry*, **5**, 4111.
Gerhart, J. C., and Schachmann, H. K. (1965). *Biochemistry*, **4**, 1054.
Glynn, I. M. (1957). *J. Physiol.*, **136**, 148.
Glynn, I. M. (1962). *J. Physiol.*, **160**, 18P.
Green, D. E. (1959). *Advances in Enzymology*, **21**, 73.
Hill, A. V. (1931). *Adventures in Biophysics*, Oxford University Press.
Hoffman, J. F., Tosteson, D. C., and Whittam, R. (1960). *Nature, Lond.*, **185**, 186.
Hokin, L. E., Sastry, P. S., Galsworthy, P. R., and Yoda, A. (1965). *Proc. Nat. Acad. Sci. U.S.A.*, **54**, 177.
Hopkins, F. G. (1913). *Rep. Brit. Ass.*, p. 652.
Jardetzky, O. (1966). *Nature, Lond.*, **211**, 969.
Kagawa, Y., and Racker, E. (1966). *J. Biol. Chem.*, **241**, 2461.
Katchalsky, A., and Kedem, O. (1962). *Biophys. J.*, **2**, Suppl., 53.
Keynes, R. D., and Swan, R. C. (1959). *J. Physiol.*, **147**, 591.
Koshland, D. E., Yankeelov, J. A., and Thoma, J. A. (1962). *Fed. Proc.*, **21**, 1031.
Krebs, H. A. (1951). In *Radioisotope Techniques*, **1**, 1. H.M.S.O.
Krebs, H. A., and Kornberg, H. L. (1957). *Ergebn. Physiol.*, **49**, 212.
Krogh, A. (1946). *Proc. Roy. Soc., B*, **133**, 140.
Lant, A. F., and Whittam, R. (1968). *J. Physiol.*, **199**, 457.
Lant, A. F., Priestland, R. N., and Whittam, R. (1970). *J. Physiol.*, **207**, 291.
Lehninger, A. L. (1960). *Fed. Proc.*, **19**, 952.
Mommaerts, W. F. H. M. (1966). *J. Mol. Biol.*, **15**, 377.
Monod, J., Changeux, J. P., and Jacob, F. (1963). *J. Mol. Biol.*, **6**, 306.
Nakao, T., Tashina, Y., Nagano, K., and Nakao, M. (1965). *Biochem. Biophys. Res. Commun.*, **19**, 755.
Opit, L. J., and Charnock, J. S. (1965). *Nature, Lond.*, **208**, 471.
Parker, J. C., and Hoffman, J. F. (1967). *J. Gen. Physiol.*, **50**, 893.
Pirie, N. W. (1964). *Proc. Roy. Soc., B*, **160**, 149.
Post, R. L., and Jolly, P. C. (1957). *Biochim. Biophys. Acta.*, **25**, 118.
Post, R. L., Sen, A. K., and Rosenthal, A. S. (1965). *J. Biol. Chem.*, **240**, 1437.
Priestland, R. N., and Whittam, R. (1968). *Biochem. J.*, **109**, 369.
Rabin, B. R. (1967). *Biochem. J.*, **102**, 22c.
Robertson, R. N. (1960). *Biol. Rev.*, **35**, 231.
Robinson, J. D. (1967). *Biochemistry*, **6**, 3250.
Sachs, J. R., and Welt, L. G. (1967). *J. Clin. Invest.*, **46**, 65.
Schatzmann, H. J. (1962). *Nature, Lond.*, **196**, 677.
Schatzmann, H. J. (1964). *Experientia*, **20**, 551.
Schatzmann, H. J., and Rüss, B. (1965). *Helv. Physiol. Pharm. Acta.*, **23**, C47.
Sekuzu, I., Jurtshuk, I., and Green, D. E. (1963). *J. Biol. Chem.*, **238**, 975.
Sen, A. K., and Post, R. L. (1964). *J. Biol. Chem.*, **239**, 345.
Silman, I. H., and Katchalski, E. (1966). *Ann. Rev. Biochem.*, **35**, 873.
Skou, J. C. (1957). *Biochim. Biophys. Acta.*, **23**, 394.
Skou, J. C. (1960). *Biochim. Biophys. Acta.*, **42**, 6.
Skou, J. C., and Hilberg, C. (1965). *Biochim. Biophys. Acta.*, **110**, 359.
Squires, R. F. (1965). *Biochem. Biophys. Res. Commun.*, **19**, 27.
Stone, A. J. (1968). *Biochim. Biophys. Acta.*, **150**, 578.

Tanaka, R., and Strickland, K. P. (1965). *Arch. Biochem. Biophys.*, **111**, 583.
Tosteson, D. C. (1963). *Fed. Proc.*, **22**, 19.
Ussing, H. H. (1949). *Physiol. Rev.*, **29**, 127.
Utter, M. F. (1950). *J. Biol. Chem.*, **185**, 499.
Weer, R. de (1968). *Nature, Lond.*, **218**, 730.
Whittam, R. (1958). *J. Physiol.*, **140**, 479.
Whittam, R. (1960). *Ann. Rep. Chem. Soc.*, **57**, 379.
Whittam, R. (1962). *Biochem. J.*, **84**, 110.
Whittam, R. (1964). In *The Cellular Functions of Membrane Transport.* Ed. J. F. Hoffman, p. 139. New Jersey: Prentice-Hall.
Whittam, R. (1967). In *The Neurosciences: An Intensive Study Program.* p. 313. New York: Rockefeller Press.
Whittam, R., and Ager, M. E. (1964). *Biochem. J.*, **93**, 337.
Whittam, R., and Ager, M. E. (1965). *Biochem. J.*, **97**, 214.
Whittam, R., Wheeler, K. P., and Blake, A. (1964), *Nature, Lond.*, **203**, 720.
Whittam, R., Wheeler, K. P., and Edwards, B. A. (1968). *Biochem. J.*, **107**, 3P.
Whittam, R., and Wiley, J. S. (1967). *J. Physiol.*, **191**, 633.

METABOLISM AND FUNCTION OF KETONE BODIES

D. H. Williamson and R. Hems

*External Staff of the Medical Research Council, Metabolic Research Laboratory,
Nuffield Department of Clinical Medicine, Radcliffe Infirmary, Oxford*

'The finding that ketone bodies are ready substrates of respiration suggests that their presence in the circulating blood serves to supply tissues with a fuel of respiration; that their function is analogous to that of glucose and the non-esterified fatty acids.'

Krebs (1961)

I. INTRODUCTION

It is perhaps unfortunate that ketone bodies were discovered in the urine of diabetics (Gerhardt, 1865; Jakasch, 1882; Minkowski, 1884), because this led to the natural conclusion that they were useless products of metabolism, a view which is still held by a number of biochemists and clinicians. The object of this essay is to correct this false impression and to emphasize the physiological role of ketone bodies rather than their contribution to the pathological situation of diabetic ketoacidosis. It is our intention to give a brief account of the current state of the field of ketone body metabolism and to omit any detailed historical description of its development which can be obtained from the reviews listed at the end of the essay.

II. PHYSIOLOGICAL AND PATHOLOGICAL KETOSIS

It is well-established that the only organ of the rat or man which contributes significant amounts of ketone bodies to the circulating blood is the liver (for a review see Campbell and Best, 1956) and that this organ, unlike peripheral tissues, is unable to utilize ketone bodies to any appreciable extent. The two main ketone bodies, acetoacetate and D-3-hydroxybutyrate),* can be interconverted in liver and then diffuse into

---

* The third ketone body, acetone, will not be considered here, since it is usually a minor component and is not utilized to any great extent by animals.

the blood to supply the extrahepatic tissues (Figure 1). If the rates of ketone body formation and utilization were always equal there obviously would be no rise in blood ketone bodies in any situation. As this is not the case there must be an 'imbalance', however slight, between the rates of production by the liver and utilization by the extrahepatic tissues in order to obtain an increase in blood ketone body concentration (i.e. ketosis). This has led to the general assumption that an increase in the

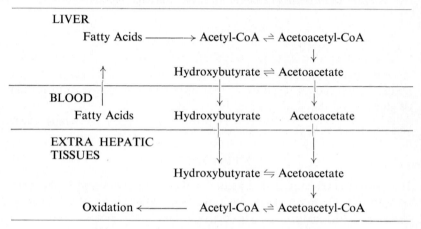

Figure 1: Outline of ketone body metabolism

circulating concentration of ketone bodies is indicative of increased synthesis by the liver. Experimental data to support this, at least in the starved and alloxan-diabetic rat, has recently been obtained by measurements of ketone body turnover with [14C]-labelled hydroxybutyrate (Bates, Krebs and Williamson, 1968). However, this assumption is not necessarily always valid as illustrated by the rise in blood ketone body concentrations in starved rats treated with cyclopropanecarboxylate, which has been shown to be due to reduced utilization of acetoacetate by kidney and other tissues (Williamson and Wilson, 1965).

In the last decade it has become widely accepted that glucose and free fatty acids are the two major respiratory fuels of rat and man, and that alterations in the proportions of these fuels in the blood contribute to the maintenance of 'caloric homeostasis' (Fredrickson and Gordon, 1958). Thus the plasma non-esterified fatty acid concentration rises whenever the blood glucose level is low, as in starvation or on a low-carbohydrate diet, or when glucose is not readily available to the tissues, as in diabetes. The increase in free fatty acids in these situations is accompanied by parallel increases in the concentrations of ketone bodies. Extrahepatic tissues can utilize ketone bodies and consequently the moderate rise in ketone body concentration when the availability of glucose is restricted can be viewed as a 'physiological ketosis' which contributes to the maintenance of a relatively constant energy supply (Krebs, 1966). To illustrate this point the relative proportions of glucose, free fatty acids and ketone bodies (acetoacetate plus hydroxybutyrate) in the blood of fed and starved human subjects and rats are shown in Table 1. The fairly constant concentrations of ketone bodies in blood with minimal excretion in the urine throughout a prolonged period of starvation suggests their formation and utilization are finely regulated. In contrast, the 'pathological ketosis' of the untreated diabetic, resulting in ketoacidosis, with concomitant excretion of large amounts of ketone bodies (wasted energy) and alkali via the urine, is the result of the breakdown of normal control mechanisms.

This raises the question of the advantages to the organism of a fuel whose production in excessive amounts can have disastrous and even fatal consequences. A partial answer is that the supply of free fatty acid is limited by two factors: their relatively low solubility and their toxicity at high concentrations, and therefore ketone bodies can be considered as a supplementary means of transporting the energy contained in the free fatty acids (McKay, 1943; Krebs, 1966). Transport of lipid fuels in more than one form has the added advantage that it allows the direction of a particular fuel to specific organs. The apparent ability of ketone bodies to assist in the regulation of the release of free fatty acids and glycerol from adipose tissue and thus control their own formation is another point in their favour.

Knowledge of the enzyme reactions concerned in the synthesis and utilization of ketone bodies and the ways in which these processes are regulated is necessary before any clear understanding can be reached of the physiological role of ketone bodies or the reasons for the failure of control mechanisms in 'pathological ketosis'.

III. SYNTHESIS OF KETONE BODIES

The liver is the main site of acetoacetate formation in non-ruminants. This organ is thought not to oxidize acetoacetate because of the absence of a key enzyme, 3-oxoacid-CoA transferase involved in ketone body utilization (Mahler, 1953). However, experiments on rat liver perfused with acetoacetate and no other added substrate indicate that the keto acid is slowly removed (Söling, 1967; Wieland, 1968).

Table 1. Concentrations of metabolic fuels in blood of man and rat.

Species	State	Glucose (mM)	Acetoacetate (mM)	Hydroxy-butyrate (mM)	Total ketone bodies (mM)	Free fatty acids (μEqv/ml)	O$_2$ Equivalents for complete combustion (mM)	Contribution of ketone bodies (%)
Man	Starvation (16 h)	4·7	0·013	0·016	0·029	0·42	39·2	0·25
	Starvation (40 h)	3·6	0·65	2·24	2·89	1·15	64·2	19·6
	Starvation (7 days)	3·5	0·95	3·58	4·53	1·19	71·9	27·7
Rat	Fed	6·1	0·064	0·072	0·136	0·15	41·0	1·2
	Starvation (24 h)	3·9	0·52	1·72	2·24	0·48	45·7	21·4
	Starvation (48 h)	4·1	0·47	1·62	2·09	0·50	46·8	19·6

The data on man have been taken from the work of Cahill, Herrera, Morgan, Soeldner, Steinke, Levy, Reichard and Kipnis (1966) and are for plasma. The values for whole rat blood have been compiled from Berry, Williamson and Wilson (1965), and unpublished experiments in this laboratory

A. Enzymes concerned in Hepatic Ketogenesis

Ketone bodies were originally considered to be intermediates in the β-oxidation of fatty acids. This view proved to be untenable when Lynen and Ochoa (1953) showed that the normal intermediates of fatty acid degradation are all CoA derivatives, and when Lehninger and Greville (1953) discovered that L-3-hydroxybutyryl-CoA is the intermediate formed during the oxidation of fatty acids, whereas the free hydroxy-butyrate appearing in body fluids has the D-configuration. These findings stimulated work on the intermediate stages in the formation of ketone bodies from acetyl-CoA and led to their elucidation during the late 1950's.

The first step is the condensation of two molecules of acetyl-CoA to give acetoacetyl-CoA in a reaction catalysed by the enzyme, acetoacetyl-CoA thiolase (E.C. 2.3.1.9.; Lynen, 1953):

$$2 \text{ Acetyl-CoA} \rightleftharpoons \text{Acetoacetyl-CoA} + \text{CoA} \qquad (1)$$

Other, less specific enzymes (e.g. 3-ketoacyl-CoA thiolase, E.C. 2.31.16) can also catalyse this reaction. The conversion of acetoacetyl-CoA to acetoacetate in liver can occur in two ways:

(*a*) Direct deacylation (Stern and Miller, 1959):

$$\text{Acetoacetyl-CoA} \rightarrow \text{Acetoacetate} + \text{CoA} \qquad (2)$$

(*b*) Hydroxymethylglutaryl-CoA (HMG-CoA) pathway (Lynen, Henning, Bublitz, Sorbo and Kröplin-Rueff, 1958):

$$\text{Acetoacetyl-CoA} + \text{Acetyl-CoA} \rightarrow \text{HMG-CoA} + \text{CoA} \qquad (3)$$
$$\text{HMG-CoA} \rightarrow \text{Acetoacetate} + \text{Acetyl-CoA} \qquad (4)$$

The enzymes catalysing reactions (3) and (4) are HMG-CoA synthase (E.C. 4.1.3.5) and HMG-CoA lyase (E.C. 4.1.3.4) respectively. In the combined thiolase–HMG-CoA pathway acetyl-CoA is not only the precursor of acetoacetate but also plays a catalytic role. The equilibrium of the acetoacetyl-CoA thiolase reaction (1) lies far to the left (Goldman, 1954) and acetoacetate synthesis only proceeds because the HMG-CoA synthase and lyase reactions (3 and 4) are not reversible (Decker, 1962).

There has been considerable controversy as to which of these two pathways plays the major role in hepatic ketogenesis (for a review see Bressler, 1963). This seems to have been resolved by more recent experiments. Sauer and Erfle (1966) found that a considerable proportion of the activity previously ascribed to acetoacetyl-CoA deacylase in guinea pig liver was in reality due to hydrolysis of acetoacetyl glutathione, a contaminant of acetoacetyl-CoA synthesized from commercial preparations of glutathione. Measurements of the activities of the individual enzymes of the two pathways in rat liver (Williamson, Bates and Krebs, 1968) indicate that the activity of the deacylase pathway can only account for about 20% of the maximal rates of ketogenesis observed with perfused rat liver (Krebs, Wallace, Hems and Freedland, 1969), whereas the capacity of the HMG-CoA pathway is in excess of these rates.

The interconversion of acetoacetate and hydroxybutyrate is catalysed by D-3-hydroxybutyrate dehydrogenase (E.C. 1.1.1.30):

$$\text{Acetoacetate} + \text{NADH} + \text{H}^+ \rightleftharpoons \text{D-3-Hydroxybutyrate} + \text{NAD}^+ \quad (5)$$

This enzyme is located on the inner membrane of rat liver mitochondria (Norum, Farstad and Bremer, 1966) and can only be solubilized with great difficulty.

Acetone is formed from acetoacetate by non-enzymic decarboxylation:

$$\text{Acetoacetate} \rightarrow \text{Acetone} + \text{CO}_2 \quad (6)$$

Although the pathway of hepatic ketogenesis has been delineated, relatively little is known of the properties of the individual enzymes from mammalian liver, and this is one area where future work should be directed.

B. Control of Hepatic Ketogenesis

Knowledge of the intermediary metabolism of acetoacetate and hydroxybutyrate has prepared the ground for the study of the mechanisms which control the rate of ketone body production by the liver. Current views on these mechanisms are based on studies of the metabolism of precursors of ketone bodies both *in vivo* and in isolated tissue preparations. Information on the concentrations of direct precursors, and on the inhibition of key enzymes by metabolic intermediates has also been of importance in formulating theories about the nature of these control mechanisms. Possible sites for the control of hepatic ketogenesis are outlined in Figure 2 and are discussed in greater detail below.

Concentration of free fatty acids

The major precursors of ketone bodies are the plasma free fatty acids and their concentrations are increased in all conditions (starvation, severe exercise, high-fat diet and insulin deficiency or insensitivity) associated with a raised blood ketone body concentration. Ample evidence exists that the uptake of fatty acids from the plasma by tissues is proportional to the fatty acid concentration (Fritz, Davis, Heltrop and Dundee, 1958; Eaton and Steinberg, 1961; Evans, Opie and Shipp, 1963; Aydin

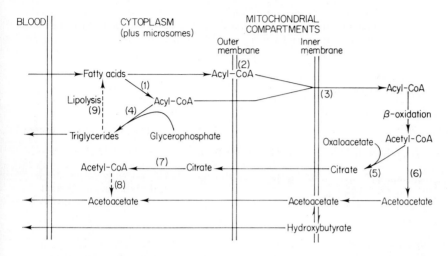

Figure 2. Enzymes concerned: (1) [Acyl-CoA synthetase (microsomal; E.C. 6.2.1.3); (2) Acyl-CoA synthetase (mitochondrial outer membrane; E.C. 6.2.1.3); (3) Carnitine–palmityl transferase (E.C. 2.3.1. . . .); (4) Glycerol-phosphate acyl transferase (E.C. 2.3.1.15); (5) Citrate synthase (E.C. 4.1.3.7); (6) HMG-CoA pathway (mitochondrial); (7) Citrate lyase (E.C. 4.1.3.6); (8) HMG-CoA pathway (cytoplasmic); (9) Lipase (? glucagon-activated)

and Sokal, 1963) and this has led to the suggestion that the rate of ketone body synthesis is to a large extent dependent on the concentration of circulating free fatty acids (Fritz, 1961). Experimental support for this hypothesis has been provided by *in vivo* experiments in which some parallelism between the concentrations of plasma free fatty acids and blood or hepatic ketone bodies was reported (Ontko and Zilversmit, 1966; J. R. Williamson, Wright, Malaisse and Ashmore, 1966; Start and Newsholme, 1968a). In contrast to these experiments is the finding that free fatty acid concentrations do not decrease appreciably in the blood of starved rats after administration of compounds (glycerol or dihydroxy-acetone) which cause a large fall (80%) in the hepatic ketone body concentration (Williamson, Veloso, Ellington and Krebs, 1969). A disassociation of free fatty acid and ketone body levels has also been reported by Foster (1967). Closer study of some of the experiments cited above (Table 2) indicates that the relationship between the concentrations of ketone bodies and their precursors is by no means a strict one, especially when other oxidizable fuels are freely available. Thus it is clear that other

Table 2. Comparison of the concentrations of plasma free fatty acids and blood ketone bodies in various experimental conditions. The values in this table are for rats and have been compiled from the sources indicated

Experimental condition of rats	Plasma free fatty acids (μEq/ml)	Blood ketone bodies (μmoles/ml)	Source of values
Corn oil-fed injected with saline	0·50	0·30	Ontko and Zilversmit (1966)
Corn oil-fed injected with heparin	1·74	0·58	
Normal fed	0·28	0·30	J. R. Williamson, Wright, Malaisse, and Ashmore (1966)
Normal fed injected with anti-insulin serum	0·83	0·53	
Normal fed	0·27	0·26	D. H. Williamson: unpublished experiments
Starved 48 h	0·79	2·63	

factors are involved in the control of ketone body formation. It must, however, be emphasized that there is little doubt that a necessary prerequisite for a sustained increase in hepatic ketogenesis is a rise in the plasma free fatty acid concentration.

β-Oxidation pathway versus triglyceride synthesis

Two major metabolic pathways are available to the free fatty acids entering the liver: catabolism via the β-oxidation pathway or diversion to triglyceride formation. Obviously, the higher the proportion of free fatty acids converted into triglycerides the less there is available for oxidation to acetyl-CoA and possible synthesis of ketone bodies. There is a decreased output of triglycerides by livers of starved rats (Otway and Robinson, 1967) and this lower output means that a higher proportion of the plasma free fatty acids are diverted to the β-oxidation pathway.

Fritz (1961) has proposed that the main factor controlling the intrahepatic fate of free fatty acids is the availability of α-glycerophosphate which is required as an acceptor for the acyl portion of fatty acyl-CoA derivatives during triglyceride synthesis. There is some evidence that the hepatic concentration of glycerophosphate decreases in starvation, although the absolute values reported in the literature vary considerably (Bortz and Lynen, 1963; Tzur, Tal and Shapiro, 1964; Zakim, 1965), but the concentration is not decreased in livers from alloxan-diabetic rats

(Wieland and Loffler, 1963; D. H. Williamson, unpublished work). The glycerophosphate concentration depends to a large extent on the cytoplasmic [free NAD^+]/[free NADH] ratio (Hohorst, Kreutz and Bücher, 1959) and consequently its concentration is not necessarily a good indicator of its availability, since net synthesis depends on the supply of glycerol from the blood or of triose phosphate from the Embden–Meyerhof pathway. The fact that there is a greater flux of glycerol to the liver from the release of adipose tissue triglyceride stores in starved and diabetic subjects (Cahill and coworkers, 1966; Carlson and Orö, 1963) does not seem to have been considered in connection with the 'glycerophosphate availability' hypothesis for the control of triglyceride synthesis.

A decrease in the net conversion of free fatty acids into triglycerides can be brought about by two other mechanisms on which there is little information:

(a) decrease in the activity of glycerolphosphate acyltransferase (E.C. 2.3.1.15) which catalyses the first step in glyceride synthesis, or

(b) increase in the rate of lipolysis of intrahepatic triglycerides.

Rat liver contains a number of lipases which are distinct from lipoprotein lipase (Olson and Alaupovic, 1966; Mahadevan and Tappel, 1968) and at least one can be activated by glucagon (Bewsher and Ashmore, 1966), but it is not known if the activity of these enzymes increase in starvation or alloxan diabetes. Similarly, there have been no reports of changes in the amount of glycerolphosphate acyltransferase in situations associated with increased ketogenesis. The factors controlling the size and turnover of the intrahepatic lipid pool obviously require further study.

Another factor which may be important in deciding the amount of free fatty acid oxidized is the activity of carnitine-palmityl transferase (palmityl-CoA:carnitine-palmityl transferase, E.C. 2.3.1. . . . .), the enzyme responsible for the transfer of fatty acyl-CoA derivatives across the inner mitochondrial membrane to the site of fatty acid oxidation (Yates and Garland, 1966). This enzyme is considered to be the rate-limiting step in the oxidation of long-chain acyl-CoA (Shepherd, Yates and Garland, 1966) and its activity increases about 2-fold in starvation (Norum, 1965).

Activity of citrate synthase

The failure to find detectable amounts of the known intermediates indicates that fatty acid oxidation proceeds to the stage of acetyl-CoA without release of free CoA derivatives (Garland, Shepherd and Yates, 1965) and that the rate of degradation of long-chain acyl-CoA is primarily controlled by respiratory chain phosphorylation. The accumulation of acetyl-CoA in livers from starved, fat-fed and alloxan-diabetic rats (Wieland and Weiss, 1963a; Tubbs and Garland, 1964) suggests that the *in vivo* activity of citrate synthase is diminished or that its capacity is inadequate to deal with the increased rate of acetyl-CoA production in these situations. The V_{max} activity of citrate synthase from rat liver is of the order of 7–10 μmoles/min/g wet wt (Srere and Foster, 1967; Garland, 1968). The K_m for oxaloacetate is $2 \cdot 1$ μM (Garland, 1968) and as the intramitochondrial oxaloacetate concentration is likely to be well below this value (Williamson, Lund and Krebs, 1967) it is possible that the *in vivo* activity of citrate synthase cannot cope with the maximal rate of acetyl-CoA production (2–4 μmoles/min/g). The amount of citrate synthase (as measured *in vitro*) in the liver is not altered in starvation (Srere and Foster, 1967) or alloxan diabetes (Srere, 1968) so that, excluding the possibility that its capacity is insufficient, other explanations for the accumulation of acetyl-CoA must be sought. There are two ways in which the *in vivo* activity of citrate synthase could be decreased:

(a) indirectly by a fall in oxaloacetate concentration, or
(b) direct inhibition by an allosteric effector, and these possibilities will now be considered in more detail.

(a) *Concentration of oxaloacetate.* Wieland and his collaborators (Wieland, Matschinsky, Löffler and Müller, 1961; Wieland, Weiss and Eger-Neufeldt, 1964) have suggested that the severe ketosis associated with alloxan diabetes is partly due to the increased oxidation of fatty acids causing a fall in the $NAD^+/NADH$ ratio which in turn results in a decreased concentration of oxaloacetate. The experimental basis for this hypothesis was the finding of a lower oxaloacetate concentration in livers from alloxan-diabetic rats (Wieland and Löffler, 1963; Hohorst, Kreutz, Reim and Hübener, 1961) and the demonstration that cytoplasmic malate dehydrogenase was in equilibrium with the cytoplasmic [free NAD^+]/[free NADH] (Hohorst, Kreutz and Bücher, 1959). The permeability of liver mitochondria for oxaloacetate is restricted (Haslam and Krebs, 1968), and therefore the overall concentration of oxaloacetate in liver has little bearing on the concentration of the keto acid at the intramitochondrial site of citrate synthase. Thus the probable determinants of the oxaloacetate concentration at this site are the mitochondrial malate concentration and the mitochondrial [free NAD^+]/[free NADH], assuming these are in equilibrium via the mitochondrial malate dehydrogenase (see Williamson and coworkers, 1967). The mitochondrial [free NAD^+]/[free NADH] decreases in starvation compared to the fed state and as there is little change in the malate concentration in the whole liver it can be calculated that the mitochondrial oxaloacetate concentration falls, but this is not true for the severe ketosis of alloxan diabetes where the calculated concentration actually rises (Williamson and coworkers, 1967).

Krebs (1966) has also suggested that oxaloacetate deficiency may be a contributory factor in severe ketosis, but that this deficiency arises from diversion of oxaloacetate towards carbohydrate synthesis via phosphoenol-pyruvate formation. This suggestion stemmed from the realization that the more severe forms of ketosis are always accompanied by increased rates of gluconeogenesis (Van Itallie and Bergen, 1961; Engel and Amatruda, 1963). Supporting evidence for a deficiency of oxaloacetate in these situations is the lower concentrations of its precursors, aspartate and glutamate, in livers of alloxan-diabetic and phlorrhizin-treated rats (Kirsten, Kirsten, Hohorst and Bücher, 1961; Williamson, Lopez-Vieira and Walker, 1967).

(b) *Direct inhibition.* Citrate synthase is inhibited by long-chain acyl-CoA derivatives (Wieland and Weiss, 1963b; Tubbs and Garland, 1964) and these accumulate in liver in starvation and alloxan diabetes (Bortz and Lynen, 1963a; Tubbs and Garland, 1964). This inhibition of citrate synthase increases the K_m for oxaloacetate, can under certain conditions be reversed by incubation with serum albumin and may involve a conformational change in the enzyme (Wieland, Weiss, Eger-Neufeldt, Teinzer and Westermann, 1966). However, there are a number of reservations concerning the physiological significance of this inhibition. A variety of other enzymes, including glucose-6-phosphate dehydrogenase and glutamate dehydrogenase, are inhibited by low concentrations of long-chain acyl-CoA, and this relative non-specificity suggests that the acyl-CoA derivatives may act as protein 'denaturants' by virtue of their detergent properties (Srere, 1965; Taketa and Pogell, 1966).

A more likely candidate as a 'physiological' inhibitor of citrate synthase is ATP (Hathaway and Atkinson, 1965; Shepherd and Garland, 1966). On the basis of elegant studies with rat-liver mitochondria Shepherd and Garland (1966) suggested that control of citrate synthase by ATP can effectively regulate the relative proportions of acetyl-CoA diverted to acetoacetate or citrate. This is an attractive hypothesis because it would link control of the tricarboxylic acid cycle to the energy status of the mitochondria. Thus an excess of mitochondrial ATP would inhibit its further synthesis via tricarboxylic acid cycle oxidations and direct acetyl-CoA to acetoacetate (a non-energy yielding pathway), while a deficiency of ATP would rapidly be made up by relief of the citrate synthase inhibition. There are certain experimental objections to this hypothesis and these have been discussed by Garland (1968) and Wieland (1968).

Role of concentrations of free CoA and acetyl-CoA

Considerable emphasis has been placed on the positive correlation between hepatic acetyl-CoA concentrations and blood or liver ketone body levels (Wieland and Weiss, 1963a; J. R. Williamson, Herczeg, Coles and Danish, 1966). A similar correlation between acetyl-CoA concentrations and acetoacetate synthesis has been reported in experiments on mitochondria from rat liver (Shepherd, Yates and Garland, 1965). Such a relationship would be expected from nature of the initial steps in ketogenesis (equations **1, 3** and **4**). A more sophisticated indicator is the [acetyl-CoA]/[CoA] ratio which is related to the acetoacetyl-CoA concentration via the equilibrium of the thiolase reaction:

$$\frac{[CoA] \times [Acetoacetyl\text{-}CoA]}{[Acetyl\text{-}CoA]^2} = 6 \times 10^{-5} \text{ (Goldman, 1954).}$$

By rearrangement of this expression the *in vivo* acetoacetyl-CoA concentration can be calculated from those of free CoA and acetyl-CoA (assuming that thiolase is at equilibrium and that the measured reactants are available to it). Such calculations give concentrations of $0 \cdot 35 \times 10^{-9}$M and $2 \cdot 7 \times 10^{-9}$M for livers from fed and starved rats respectively (Williamson and coworkers, 1969). Thiolase is present in both the cytoplasm and mitochondria of rat liver (Williamson and coworkers, 1968) and therefore if the permeability of one of the reactants was restricted the concentrations of acetoacetyl-CoA could be different in the two compartments. The failure of total measured acetyl-CoA (and the calculated acetoacetyl-CoA) to fall in concentration during a period when the rate of ketogenesis was decreasing (Williamson and coworkers, 1969; Foster, 1967), suggests that a considerable proportion of the acetyl-CoA may be cytoplasmic or alternatively, if the acetyl-CoA concentration is representative of that in the mitochondria, there is a regulatory site within the HMG-CoA cycle.

A further complication is the recent speculation of Fritz (1967) that there may be two intramitochondrial acetyl-CoA pools. One adjacent to the fatty acid oxidase–ketone body forming system and the other pool available to citrate synthase; acetyl groups being transferred via carnitine acetyltransferase.

Activity of HMG-CoA pathway enzymes

It is generally accepted that the rate-limiting reaction of the HMG-CoA pathway is that catalysed by HMG-CoA synthase and measurement of the activity of the overall reaction is considered to represent synthase activity. A change in the amount of this enzyme could alter the rate of ketogenesis. Wieland, Löffler, Weiss and Neufeld¹ (1960) have reported a 2-fold increase in HMG-CoA synthase activity in livers from alloxan-diabetic rats, but no change in activity in livers from starved rats. The activities reported by these workers were low in comparison to the rates of ketogenesis observed on incubation of fatty acids with isolated rat-liver preparations (Krebs and coworkers, 1969). More recent measurements of the activity of HMG-CoA synthase indicate activities compatible with these reported rates of ketogenesis, with no change of activity (expressed in terms of body weight of rat) on starvation, but 70% and 140% increases in alloxan diabetes and on feeding a high-fat diet, respectively (Williamson and coworkers, 1968) (Table 3). Thus the ketosis of starvation must

Table 3. Activities and intracellular distributions of HMG-CoA synthase and lyase in livers from normal, starved, alloxan-diabetic and fat-fed rats. The values are means $\pm$S.D. with numbers of observations in parentheses, and are expressed in μmoles acetoacetate formed/min at 25°

State of rats	Enzyme	Activity (units/100 g body wt) Whole homogenate	Cytoplasm	Particles	
Normal	HMG-CoA	$10\pm1(5)$	$1\cdot2\pm0\cdot3(5)$	$8\cdot9\pm0\cdot9(5)$	
Starved for 48 h	synthase	$12\pm5(13)$	$2\cdot5\pm1\cdot0(12)^*$	10	±3 (11)
Alloxan-diabetic		$17\pm3(5)^*$	$2\cdot4\pm0\cdot5(5)^*$	15	±2 (5)*
Fat-fed		$24\pm2(5)^*$	$2\cdot0\pm0\cdot3(5)^*$	22	±2 (5)*
Normal	HMG-CoA	$41\pm8(6)$	$3\cdot2\pm0\cdot9(6)$	38	±9 (6)
Starved for 48 h	lyase	$41\pm9(12)$	$7\cdot8\pm2\cdot6(12)^*$	33	±7 (12)
Alloxan-diabetic		$49\pm1(4)$	$7\cdot0\pm1\cdot8(4)^*$	42	±2 (4)
Fat-fed		$56\pm6(5)^*$	$5\cdot7\pm0\cdot5(5)$	50	±7 (5)

* Significantly different from values for normal rats (P<0·01).

result from increased flow through the HMG-CoA pathway without a concomitant change in the amounts of the individual enzymes. On the other hand, the rise in enzyme concentration in alloxan diabetes and on fat feeding may contribute to the increased hepatic ketogenesis in these situations. These conclusions do not exclude the possibility that changes in HMG-CoA synthase activity are also brought about by allosteric modifiers but so far none have been reported.

Extramitochondrial synthesis of acetoacetate

The major site of ketone body production is within the mitochondria, probably in the matrix adjacent to the fatty acid oxidation complex. Low, but significant activity of the HMG-CoA pathway enzymes have been found in the cytoplasm of guinea-pig (Sauer and Erfle, 1966) and rat liver (Williamson and coworkers, 1968) and this activity is increased in starvation and alloxan diabetes (Table 3). On the basis of these findings an extramitochondrial pathway of ketogenesis has been proposed (Sauer and Erfle, 1966; Williamson and coworkers, 1968). Evidence for the physiological significance of this pathway can be obtained from current knowledge of the origin and fate of cytoplasmic acetyl-CoA. Citrate transported from the mitochondria and then cleaved by citrate lyase (E.C. 4.1.3.6) which is exclusively cytoplasmic, is the main source of cytoplasmic acetyl-CoA (Kornacker and Lowenstein, 1965a and b; Bartley, Abraham and Chaikoff, 1965):

$$\text{Citrate} + \text{ATP} + \text{CoA} \rightarrow \text{Acetyl-CoA} + \text{Oxaloacetate} + \text{ADP} + \\ + \text{Orthophosphate} \qquad (7)$$

In the fed animal this acetyl-CoA is required for fatty acid synthesis and to a lesser extent for the synthesis of mevalonic acid (a precursor of cholesterol) which is formed from HMG-CoA by HMG-CoA reductase (E.C. 1.1.1.34):

$$\text{Hydroxymethylglutaryl-CoA} + 2 \text{ NADPH} + 2 \text{ H}^+ \rightleftharpoons \text{Mevalonate} + \\ + 2 \text{ NADP}^+ + \text{CoA} \qquad (8)$$

Starvation and alloxan diabetes are both associated with a greatly depressed rate of lipogenesis (for a review see Masoro, 1962), while in starvation only there is virtual disappearance of the activity of HMG-CoA reductase (Bucher, Overath and Lynen, 1960). Admittedly there may be a decrease in the activity of citrate lyase in these situations (Kornacker and Lowenstein, 1965a and b; but see Srere and Foster, 1967), but only by about two-thirds, while the hepatic concentration of citrate is not greatly decreased, especially in alloxan diabetes (Tarnowski and Seemann, 1967; Start and Newsholme, 1968b; Wieland, 1968). Thus acetyl-CoA may still be formed in the cytoplasm, though at a somewhat diminished rate, and the increased activity of the extramitochondrial HMG-CoA pathway in these situations may play an important role in its disposal. The contribution of this pathway to the overall rate of hepatic ketogenesis is not likely to be large, but nevertheless it is of interest because its regulation depends to a certain extent on the rate of lipogenesis (and cholesterol synthesis) rather than on the rate of fatty acid oxidation.

Conclusions

Of the multiplicity of factors involved in the *in vivo* regulation of hepatic ketogenesis, the most important are the proportion of the available free fatty acids oxidized to acetyl-CoA and the activity of citrate synthase. The exact mechanisms by which control is exerted at these two metabolic 'branching' points is still open.

IV. UTILIZATION OF KETONE BODIES

The evidence that peripheral tissues, in contrast to liver, can readily utilize acetoacetate and hydroxybutyrate as fuels of respiration is well documented. Oxidation of ketone bodies has been shown with tissue slice preparations (McCann, 1957; Krebs, 1961), isolated perfused organs (Snapper and Grünbaum, 1927; J. R. Williamson and Krebs, 1961) eviscerate preparations (Mirsky and Broh-Kahn, 1937; Söling, Garlepp and Creutzfeldt, 1965) and in the whole animal (Wick and Drury, 1941; Nelson, Grayman and Mirsky, 1941). The utilization of acetoacetate is not affected to any extent by glucose or insulin (for reviews see Campbell and Best, 1956; Stadie, 1958). However, relatively little is known about the control of the extrahepatic metabolism of ketone bodies.

A. Enzymes concerned in Extrahepatic Ketone Body Utilization

The first step in the utilization of acetoacetate is its conversion to acetoacetyl-CoA, and two enzymes have been described which can effect this conversion in extrahepatic tissues:

(a) 3-Oxoacid-CoA transferase (succinyl-CoA: 3-oxoacid-CoA transferase, E.C. 2.8.3.5) (Stern, Coon, del Campillo and Schneider, 1956):

$$\text{Acetoacetate} + \text{Succinyl-CoA} \leftrightharpoons \text{Acetoacetyl-CoA} + \text{Succinate} \quad \textbf{(10)}$$

(b) Acetoacetyl-CoA synthetase (Stern, Coon and del Campillo, 1953):

$$\text{Acetoacetate} + \text{ATP} + \text{CoA} \rightarrow \text{Acetoacetyl-CoA} + \text{AMP} + \\ + \text{pyrophosphate} \quad \textbf{(11)}$$

The presence of such a synthetase has never been established in rat tissues and its significance is doubtful. Activity of 3-oxoacid-CoA transferase has been demonstrated in most extrahepatic tissues of the rat (Williamson, Bates, Page and Krebs, 1970). The equilibrium of the transferase reaction (Stern and coworkers, 1956):

$$K = \frac{[\text{Acetoacetyl-CoA}] \times [\text{Succinate}]}{[\text{Succinyl-CoA}] \times [\text{Acetoacetate}]}$$

$$= 4 \cdot 3 \times 10^{-3} \text{ at pH } 8 \cdot 1 \text{ (no Mg}^{2+})$$

lies in favour of acetoacetate formation. Acetoacetyl-CoA is cleaved by thiolysis to two molecules of acetyl-CoA in the thiolase reaction:

$$2 \text{ Acetyl-CoA} \rightleftharpoons \text{Acetoacetyl-CoA} + \text{CoA} \qquad (12)$$

The equilibrium of this reaction is far to the left ($K = 6 \cdot 0 \times 10^{-5}$ at pH $8 \cdot 5$) and it is the coupling of reactions (10) and (12) which overcomes the unfavourable equilibrium of the 3-oxoacid-CoA transferase and allows the conversion of acetoacetate to acetyl-CoA to proceed more readily. The equilibrium of the overall reaction

$$K = \frac{[\text{Acetoacetate}] \times [\text{Succinyl-CoA}] \times [\text{CoA}]}{[\text{Acetyl-CoA}]^2 \times [\text{Succinate}]}$$

$$= \frac{K_{\text{thiolase}}}{K_{\text{transferase}}} = \frac{6 \cdot 0 \times 10^{-5}}{4 \cdot 3 \times 10^{-3}} = 1 \cdot 4 \times 10^{-2}$$

Thus thiolase occupies a central role in hepatic ketogenesis and in extrahepatic acetoacetate oxidation; in the former it sets the acetoacetyl-CoA concentration, while in the latter it displaces the unfavourable equilibrium of the transferase reaction.

D-(−)-3-Hydroxybutyrate must first be converted toaceto acetate via the intramitochondrial D-3-hydroxybutyrate dehydrogenase before it can be oxidized by peripheral tissues. The finding that the L(+)-isomer can be utilized by homogenates of extrahepatic tissues of the rat (McCann, 1957) suggests the presence of either a racemase (Stern, del Campillo and Lehninger, 1955) or a synthetase (Lehninger and Greville, 1953). The L-3-hydroxybutyryl-CoA formed in the synthetase reaction can be oxidized by 3-hydroxyacyl-CoA dehydrogenase and NAD$^+$ to give acetoacetyl-CoA.

B. Control of Ketone Body Utilization

Measurements of the activity of 3-oxoacid-CoA transferase in various tissues of the rat and in different physiological situations indicate that acetoacetate utilization is not controlled by alterations in the concentration of this enzyme (Williamson and coworkers, 1970).

Experiments on the whole animal suggest that over a wide range the utilization of ketone bodies is directly related to their concentration in the blood (Wick and Drury, 1941; Nelson and coworkers, 1941; Bates and coworkers, 1968). Control of utilization via the availability of acetoacetate is to be expected if the transferase and thiolase reactions catalyse an equilibrium in vivo, since an increase in acetoacetate will result in a reciprocal increase in acetyl-CoA. Thus the control of acetoacetate oxidation, like the regulation of hepatic ketogenesis, is ultimately concerned with the rate of removal and formation of acetyl-CoA. A low acetyl-CoA concentration will favour acetoacetate utilization, while a high one will have the opposite effect. In situations where fat is the major fuel of respiration the concentration of acetyl-CoA in extrahepatic tissues is presumably the resultant of its removal by the tricarboxylic acid cycle and its formation by fatty acid oxidation and acetoacetate utilization. Consequently, an important role for acetoacetate might be the provision of C_2 units when the requirements of the tricarboxylic acid cycle cannot be met by fat oxidation.

The succinyl-CoA concentration may also play an important role in the regulation of acetoacetate utilization. Apart from 3-oxoacid-CoA transferase, two other enzymes compete for the available succinyl-CoA, succinyl-CoA hydrolase (E.C. 3.1.2.3):

$$\text{Succinyl-CoA} + H_2O \rightarrow \text{Succinate} + \text{CoA} \tag{13}$$

and succinyl-CoA synthetase (E.C. 6.2.1.4. & 5):

$$\text{Succinyl-CoA} + \text{GDP (ADP)} + \text{Orthophosphate} \leftrightharpoons \text{Succinate} + \text{GTP (ATP)} + \text{CoA} \tag{14}$$

This latter reaction (the so-called substrate level phosphorylation) is freely reversible ($K = 3 \cdot 3$; Kaufman and Alivisatos, 1955) and changes in the concentrations of the other reactants can alter the concentration of succinyl-CoA and thus possibly affect the rate of acetoacetate utilization. This has been shown experimentally with dinitrophenol-treated beef heart mitochondria, where acetoacetate oxidation was inhibited by a high concentration of phosphate and addition of AMP, GDP or ADP enhanced the effect (Hatefi and Fakouhi, 1968).

C. Extrahepatic Ketogenesis

The *in vitro* formation of small quantities of ketone bodies by peripheral tissues of the rat, especially in the presence of added fatty acids (Jowett and Quastel, 1935; Weinhouse and Millington, 1951; Weidemann and Krebs, 1969), raises the question of the mechanism and physiological importance of this extrahepatic ketogenesis. The virtual absence of HMG-CoA synthase from extrahepatic tissues of the rat (Williamson and coworkers, 1970) strongly suggests that this acetoacetate synthesis is mediated via reversal of the transferase–thiolase system. The reversible nature of the first two steps involved in the utilization of acetoacetate by peripheral tissues automatically confers on these tissues the ability to synthesize ketone bodies from acetyl-CoA. The absence of a preceding non-equilibrium step, excluding the diffusion of acetoacetate into the blood stream, means, however, that the process of extrahepatic keto-genesis cannot be as effective as the irreversible HMG-CoA pathway of the liver.

Evidence that peripheral tissues may add ketone bodies to the blood under certain circumstances has recently been obtained in man (Hagenfeldt and Wahren, 1968). By arterial and venous catherization these workers found that resting muscle took up ketone bodies, but that during severe exercise the arterial-venous difference was reduced, and in some cases was positive. Fatty acid oxidation is increased during exercise, and, as already discussed, the resulting high rate of production of acetyl-CoA may well favour the formation of acetoacetate rather than its utilization. However, it is clear that further work is required before any conclusions can be made as to the physiological significance of extrahepatic ketogenesis.

D. Organ-specific Direction of Ketone Bodies and Other Fuels

In the post-absorptive state stored fat is presented to the tissues in four forms. Free fatty acids derived directly from adipose tissue; tri-glycerides formed in the liver from a portion of the free fatty acids taken up by this organ; acetoacetate and hydroxybutyrate, which can be considered as 'predigested' forms of fatty acids. Some possible reasons for the multiple forms in which fat is made available have already been considered, namely the poor solubility of free fatty acids and their toxicity. Another possibility is that it allows direction of particular fuels to specific organs. Each of the above fuels derived from stored fat requires a different enzyme to initiate its utilization: acyl-CoA synthetase for free fatty acids; lipoprotein lipase for triglycerides; 3-hydroxbutyrate dehydrogenase for hydroxybutyrate; 3-oxoacid-CoA transferase for acetoacetate. The potential of any tissue to metabolize these fuels will therefore depend on its content of the necessary enzymes, and this may vary with the physio-logical state of the animal. An example is the direction of triglycerides to adipose tissue in the fed animal when the activity of lipoprotein lipase is high in this organ, and the decreased uptake of triglycerides in the starved animal when the lipoprotein lipase activity is considerably lower (see Robinson, 1967). Insufficient quantitative information is available to fully assess the importance of this type of direction with regard to other fuels, but some preliminary data on the content of relevant enzymes in liver, heart, kidney, brain and skeletal muscle of the fed rat are shown in Table 4. The liver is clearly well equipped to utilize free fatty acids and to interconvert acetoacetate and hydroxybutyrate, but the virtual absence of 3-oxoacid-CoA transferase and lipoprotein lipase means that any signifi-

Table 4. Comparison of the activities in some rat tissues of the key enzymes required for the utilization of ketone bodies, free fatty acids and triglycerides. Where quantitative information is available the data from the cited sources has been recalculated assuming the activity of heart to be 100 in each case

Tissue	3-Oxoacid-CoA transferase[a]	Thiolase[a,b]	3-Hydroxy-butyrate[c] dehydrogenase	Acyl-CoA[d] synthetase	Lipoprotein[e] lipase
Liver	absent	58	1200	585	? absent
Heart	100	100	100	100	+
Kidney	69	68	155	50	+
Brain	7·5	7·5	55	11·5	absent
Skeletal muscle	5	6·5	22	5·5	+

References: [a] Williamson, Bates, Page and Krebs (1970); [b] Wieland, Reinwein and Lynen (1956); [c] Lehninger, Sudduth and Wise (1960); [d] Pande and Mead (1968); [e] D. S. Robinson, personal communication.

cant uptake of ketone bodies and triglycerides is restricted to the extra-hepatic tissues. Heart and kidney contain the necessary enzymes to deal with all four fuels and this may reflect their high metabolic activity. The activities of the four enzymes in skeletal muscle are low, but this is misleading because of the large contribution of muscle to the body mass. Until recently it was widely accepted that the only significant fuel of the brain was glucose. The demonstration by catheterization of cerebral vessels that human brain uses appreciable amounts of ketone bodies during prolonged starvation (Owen and coworkers, 1967) indicates that the brain can adapt its requirements to the fuels supplied. Brain from fed rats contains the necessary enzymes for ketone body utilization (Table 4), which suggests that this adaptation may not necessarily occur via an increase in enzyme concentration, but rather by an increase in substrate concentration.

V. MODIFICATION OF THE SUPPLY OF METABOLIC FUELS BY THE KETONE BODY CONCENTRATION IN BLOOD

The ketone body concentration in blood can increase 10 to 30-fold in physiological situations (severe exercise, fasting; see Table 1) and this range of concentration change far exceeds that of any other blood metabolite. Many workers have studied the effects of hyperketonaemia produced by administration of ketone bodies on the concentrations of other fuels in blood. Although some of the findings are conflicting sufficient evidence is available to indicate that under certain circumstances the circulating concentration of ketone bodies can assist in the regulation of the release of other metabolic fuels into the blood and on this basis a role for ketone bodies as 'metabolic messengers' would seem established.

A. Supply of Free Fatty Acids and Autoregulation of Ketogenesis

The administration of acetoacetate or hydroxybutyrate to fasting man or animals produces a prompt decrease in the concentrations of free fatty acids in the blood (Mebane and Madison, 1964; Björntorp and Schersten, 1967; Jenkins, 1967; Balasse, Couturier and Franckson, 1967; Balasse and Ooms, 1968; Senior and Loridan, 1968). In the dog this fall in free fatty acid concentration has been shown to be the result of increased uptake by peripheral tissues and decreased adipose tissue lipolysis (Balasse and coworkers, 1967). The supply of free fatty acids to the liver is an important factor in the control of hepatic ketogenesis and thus ketone bodies can to some extent regulate their own formation and so avoid the development of a fatal ketoacidosis during prolonged periods of starvation. In diabetic ketoacidosis, ketone bodies either do not exert their 'feedback' action or other factors related to the diabetic state counteract their effectiveness.

Two mechanisms have been proposed for the decreased flux of free fatty acids from adipose tissue on administration of ketone bodies:

(a) direct inhibition of lipolysis brought about by acetoacetate or hydroxybutyrate, (Björntorp, 1966; Björntorp and Schersten, 1967) or (b) stimulation of insulin secretion by ketone bodies with the resultant suppression of the release of free fatty acids (Madison, Mebane, Unger and Lochner, 1964).

There is considerable speculation as to which of these mechanisms is operative *in vivo*. Madison and coworkers (1964) found a marked rise in the insulin concentration of pancreatic venous blood in dogs in response to infusion of either hydroxybutyrate or acetoacetate, whereas no appreciable changes in peripheral blood insulin have been found in man during administration of ketone bodies (Fajans, Floyd, Knopf and Conn, 1964; Balasse and Ooms, 1968; Senior and Loridan, 1968). Inhibition of the adrenaline-activated lipolysis in adipose tissue by high concentrations of hydroxybutyrate and acetoacetate has been demonstrated both *in vitro* with epididymal fat pads of the rat (Björntorp, 1966) and *in vivo* in the pancreatectomized dog (Björntorp and Schersten, 1967). The latter experiment is proof that insulin is not necessarily involved in the inhibition of lipolysis. It is of interest that two other related carboxylic acids which can occur in high concentrations in blood, lactate (after severe exercise) and acetate (after ingestion of ethanol), also inhibit the release of free fatty acids from adipose tissue *in vivo* (Issekutz, Miller and Rodahl, 1966; Crouse, Gersen, DeCarli and Lieber, 1968).

B. Supply of Glucose and Glycerol

The decrease of free fatty acid concentration after administration of ketone bodies is accompanied by a fall in the concentrations of glucose and glycerol in blood (Balasse and Ooms, 1968; Senior and Loridan, 1968; Björntorp and Scherstén, 1967). In the fasting dog the resulting mild hypoglycaemia appears to be due to a decreased hepatic output of glucose rather than increased utilization (Balasse and coworkers, 1967). This is evidence against a direct effect of insulin on blood glucose concentrations in this situation. In starvation glycerol released from the adipose tissue is a major precursor of glucose (Nikkilä and Ojala, 1964) and consequently the decreased flux of glycerol to the liver after infusion of hydroxybutyrate may well explain the fall in hepatic output of glucose. A more direct effect of ketone bodies on the release of glucose from the liver cannot be excluded on present evidence. Further work is required before the relative importance of the modification of the supply of metabolic fuels by ketone bodies can be correctly assessed. Little is known of the effective concentration range of the ketone bodies, of the species specificity of this method of fuel regulation or how acetoacetate and hydroxybutyrate exert their effects on the pancreas or adipose tissue.

VI. CONCLUDING COMMENT

A future student of the historical development of biochemistry might well consider that the contributions of H.A.K. to the area of ketone body metabolism bear no comparison to his contributions to the elucidation of the mechanisms of urea synthesis and of the tricarboxylic acid cycle. Although this view may be strictly correct, his numerous reviews on the subject of ketosis have stimulated others to study the inter-relationships between carbohydrate and fat metabolism. Much of the recent knowledge of ketone body metabolism outlined in this essay is a direct result of this stimulation.

It is difficult to forecast what remains to be uncovered concerning the function and metabolism of ketone bodies but at least one prediction can be made which has a reasonable chance of being correct. The sensitivity of the concentration of ketone bodies in blood to changes in hormonal and nutritional state, and the existence of rapid and specific methods for the estimation of ketone bodies, suggest that a request for determination of blood ketone bodies may become as common as that for blood sugar.

K

Reviews (chronological order)

McKay, E. M. (1943). *J. Clin. Endocrin.*, **3**, 101.
Campbell, I., and Best, C. H. (1965). *Metabolism*, **5**, 95.
Stadie, W. C. (1958). *Diabetes*, **7**, 173.
Langdon, R. G. (1960). In *Lipid Metabolism*. Ed. by Bloch, K. New York: Wiley.
Fritz, I. B. (1961). *Physiol. Rev.*, **41**, 52.
Krebs, H. A. (1961). *Arch. Intern. Med.*, **107**, 51.
Krebs, H. A. (1961). *Biochem. J.*, **80**, 225.
Van Itallie, T. B., and Bergen, S. S. (1961). *Am. J. Med.*, **31**, 909.
Bressler, R. (1963). *Ann. N. Y. Acad. Sci.*, **104**, 735.
Engel, F. L., and Amatruda, T. T. (1963). *Ann. N. Y. Acad. Sci.*, **104**, 753.
Winegrad, A. I. (1964). In *Actions of Hormones on Molecular Processes*. Ed. by Litwack, G., and Kritchevsky, D. New York: Wiley.
Krebs, H. A. (1966). In *Advances in Enzyme Regulation*. **4**, p. 339. Ed. by Weber, G. Oxford: Pergamon Press.
Greville, G. D., and Tubbs, P. K. (1968). In *Essays in Biochemistry*. **4**, p. 155. Ed. by Campbell, P. N., and Greville, G. D. London: Academic Press.
Wieland, O. (1968). In *Advances in Metabolic Disorders*, **3**, p. 1. Ed. by Levine, R., and Luft, R. London: Academic Press.

References

Aydin, A., and Sokal, J. E. (1963). *Amer. J. Physiol.*, **205**, 667.
Balasse, E., Couturier, E., and Franckson, J. R. M. (1967). *Diabetologia*, **3**, 488.
Balasse, E., and Ooms, H. A. (1968). *Diabetologia*, **4**, 133.
Bartley, J., Abraham, S., and Chaikoff, I. L. (1965). *Biochem. Biophys. Res. Commun.*, **19**, 770.
Bates, M. W., Krebs, H. A., and Williamson, D. H. (1968). *Biochem. J.*, **110**, 655.
Berry, M. N., Williamson, D. H., and Wilson, M. B. (1965). *Biochem. J.*, **94**, 17C.
Bewsher, P. D., and Ashmore, J. (1966). *Biochem. Biophys. Res. Commun.*, **24**, 431.
Björntorp, P. (1966). *J. Lipid. Res.*, **7**, 621.
Björntorp, P., and Scherstén, T. (1967). *Amer. J. Physiol.*, **212**, 683.
Bortz, W. M., and Lynen, F. (1963). *Biochem. Z.*, **339**, 77.
Bressler, R. (1963). *Ann. N. Y. Acad. Sci.*, **104**, 735.
Bucher, N. L. R., Overath, P., and Lynen, F. (1960). *Biochim. Biophys. Acta*, **40**, 491.
Cahill, G. F., Herrera, M. G., Morgan, A. P., Soeldner, J. S., Steinke, J., Levy, P. L., Reichard, G. A., and Kipnis, D. M. (1966). *J. Clin. Invest.*, **45**, 1751.
Campbell, I., and Best, C. H. (1956). *Metabolism*, **5**, 95.
Carlson, L. A., and Orö, L. (1963). *Metabolism*, **12**, 132.
Crouse, J. R., Gerson, C. D., DeCarli, L. M., and Lieber, C. S. (1968). *J. Lipid. Res.*, **9**, 509.
Decker, K. (1962). *Deutsch. Med. Wochschr.*, **87**, 2254.
Eaton, P., and Steinberg, D. (1961). *J. Lipid. Res.*, **2**, 376.

Engel, F. L., and Amatruda, T. T. (1963). *Ann. N. Y. Acad. Sci.*, **104**, 753.

Evans, J. R., Opie, L. H., and Shipp, J. C. (1963). *Amer. J. Physiol.*, **205**, 766.

Fajans, S. S., Floyd, J. C., Knopf, R. F., and Conn, J. W. (1964). *J. Clin. Invest.*, **43**, 2003.

Foster, D. W. (1967). *J. Clin. Invest.*, **46**, 1283.

Fredrickson, D. S., and Gordon, R. S. (1958). *Physiol. Rev.*, **38**, 585.

Fritz, I. B. (1961). *Physiol. Rev.*, **41**, 52.

Fritz, I. B. (1967). *Perspect. Biol. Med.*, **10**, 643.

Fritz, I. B., Davis, D. G., Heltrop, R. H., and Dundee, H. (1958). *Amer. J. Physiol.*, **194**, 379.

Garland, P. B. (1968). In *Metabolic Roles of Citrate*, p. 41. Ed. by Goodwin, T. W. New York: Academic Press Inc.

Garland, P. B., Shepherd, D., and Yates, D. W. (1965). *Biochem. J.*, **97**, 587.

Gerhardt, C. (1865). *Wien. Med. Presse*, **6**, 672.

Goldman, D. S. (1954). *J. Biol. Chem.*, **208**, 345.

Hagenfeldt, L., and Wahren, J. (1968). *Scand. J. Clin. Lab. Invest.*, **21**, 314.

Haslam, J. M., and Krebs, H. A. (1968). *Biochem. J.*, **107**, 659.

Hatefi, Y., and Fakouhi, T. (1968). *Arch. Biochem. Biophys.*, **125**, 114.

Hathaway, J. A., and Atkinson, D. E. (1965). *Biochem. Biophys. Res. Commun.*, **20**, 661.

Hohorst, H. J., Kreutz, F. H., and Bücher, Th. (1959). *Biochem. Z.*, **332**, 18.

Hohorst, H. J., Kreutz, F. H., Reim, M., and Hübener, H. J. (1961). *Biochem. Biophys. Res. Commun.*, **4**, 163.

Issekutz, B., Miller, H. I., and Rodahl, K. (1966). *Fed. Proc.*, **25**, 1415.

Jakasch, R. von (1882). *Z. Physiol. Chemie*, **7**, 487.

Jenkins, D. J. A. (1967). *Lancet ii*, 338.

Jowett, M., and Quastel, J. H. (1935). *Biochem. J.*, **29**, 2181.

Kaufman, S., and Alivisatos, S. G. A. (1955). *J. Biol. Chem.*, **216**, 141.

Kirsten, E., Kirsten, R., Hohorst, H. J., and Bücher, Th. (1961). *Biochem. Biophys. Res. Commun.*, **4**, 169.

Kornacker, M. S., and Lowenstein, J. M. (1965a, b). *Biochem. J.*, **94**, 209 and **95**, 832.

Krebs, H. A. (1961). *Biochem. J.*, **80**, 225.

Krebs, H. A. (1966). In *Advances in Enzyme Regulation*, **4**, 339. Ed. by Weber, G. Oxford: Pergamon Press.

Krebs, H. A., Wallace, P. G., Hems, R., and Freedland, R. A. (1969). *Biochem. J.*, **112**, 595.

Lehninger, A. L., and Greville, G. D. (1953). *Biochim. Biophys. Acta*, **12**, 188.

Lehninger, A. L., Sudduth, H. C., and Wise, J. B. (1960). *J. Biol. Chem.*, **235**, 2450.

Lynen, F. (1953). *Fed. Proc.*, **12**, 683.

Lynen, F., and Ochoa, S. (1953). *Biochim. Biophys. Acta*, **12**, 299.

Lynen, F., Henning,V.. Bublitz. C., Sorbo, B., and Kröplin-Reuff, L. (1958). *Biochem. Z.*, **330**, 269.

Madison, L. L., Mebane, D., Unger, R. H., and Lochner, A. (1964). *J. Clin. Invest.*, **43**, 408.

Mahadevan, S., and Tappel, A. L. (1968). *J. Biol. Chem.*, **243**, 2849.

Mahler, H. R. (1953). *Fed. Proc.*, **12**, 694.

Masoro, E. J. (1962). *J. Lipid. Res.*, **3**, 149.

280   D. H. WILLIAMSON AND R. HEMS

McCann, W. P. (1957). *J. Biol. Chem.*, **226**, 15.
McKay, E. M. (1943). *J. Clin. Endocrin.*, **3**, 101.
Mebane, D., and Madison, L. L. (1964). *J. Lab. Clin. Med.*, **63**, 177.
Minkowski, O. (1884). *Arch. Exper. Path. und. Pharmakol.*, **18**, 35.
Mirsky, I. A., and Broh-Kahn, R. H. (1937). *Amer. J. Physiol.*, **119**, 734.
Nelson, N., Grayman, I., and Mirsky, I. A. (1941). *J. Biol. Chem.*, **140**, 361.
Nikkilä, E, A.. and Ojala, K. (1964). *Life Sci.*, **3**, 243.
Norum, K. R. (1965). *Biochim. Biophys. Acta*, **98**, 652.
Norum, K. R., Farstad, M., and Bremer, J. (1966). *Biochem. Biophys. Res. Commun.*, **24**, 797.
Olson, A. C., and Aluapovic, P. (1966). *Biochim. Biophys. Acta*, **125**, 185.
Ontko, J. A., and Zilversmit, D. B. (1966). *Proc. Soc. Expt. Biol. Med.*, **121**, 319.
Otway, S., and Robinson, D. S. (1967). *J. Physiol.*, **190**, 321.
Owen, O. E., Morgan, A. P., Kemp, H. G., Sullivan, J. M., Herrera, M. G., and Cahill, G. F. Jr. (1967). *J. Clin. Invest.*, **46**, 1589.
Pande, S. V., and Mead, J. F. (1968). *Biochim. Biophys. Acta*, **152**, 636.
Robinson, D. S. (1967). In *The Fate of Dietary Lipids*, p. 175. Ed. by Cowgill, G., and Kinsell, L. W. Washington: U.S. Dept. of Public Health.
Sauer, F., and Erfle, J. D. (1966). *J. Biol. Chem.*, **241**, 30.
Senior, B., and Loridan, L. (1968). *Nature (Lond.)*, **219**, 83.
Shepherd, D., and Garland, P. B. (1966). *Biochem. Biophys. Res. Commun.*, **22**, 89.
Shepherd, D., Yates, D. W., and Garland, P. B. (1965). *Biochem. J.*, **97**, 38C.
Shepherd, D., Yates, D. W., and Garland, P. B. (1966). *Biochem. J.*, **98**, 3C.
Snapper, I., and Grünbaum, A. (1927). *Biochem. Z.*, **185**, 223.
Söling, H. D. (1967). In *Die Pathogenese des Diabetes Mellitus.* p. 6. Ed. by Klein, E. Berlin: Springer Verlag.
Söling, H. D., Garlepp, H. J., and Creutzfeldt, W. (1965). *Biochim. Biophys. Acta*, **100**, 530.
Srere, P. A. (1965). *Biochim. Biophys. Acta*, **106**, 445.
Srere, P. A. (1968). In *Metabolic Roles of Citrate.* p. 11. Ed. by Goodwin, T. W. New York: Academic Press Inc.
Srere, P. A., and Foster, D. W. (1967). *Biochem. Biophys. Res. Commun.*, **26**, 556.
Start, C., and Newsholme, E. A. (1968 *a, b*). *Biochem. J.*, **109**, 37P and **107**, 411.
Stadie, W. C. (1958). *Diabetes*, **7**, 173.
Stern, J. R., and Miller, G. E. (1959). *Biochim. Biophys. Acta*, **35**, 576.
Stern, J. R., del Campillo, A., and Lehninger, A. L. (1955). *J. Amer. Chem. Soc.*, **77**, 1073.
Stern, J. R., Coon, M. J., and del Campillo, A. (1953). *J. Amer. Chem. Soc.*, **75**, 1517.
Stern, J. R., Coon, M. J., del Campillo, A., and Schneider, M. C. (1956). *J. Biol. Chem.*, **221**, 15.
Taketa, K., and Pogell, B. M. (1966). *J. Biol. Chem.*, **241**, 720.
Tarnowski, W., and Seemann, M. (1967). *Z. Physiol. Chemie*, **348**, 829.
Tubbs, P. K., and Garland, P. B. (1964). *Biochem. J.*, **93**, 550.
Tzur, R., Tal, E., and Shapiro, B. (1964). *Biochim. Biophys. Acta*, **84**, 18.
Van Itallie, T. B., and Bergen, S. S. (1961). *Amer. J. Med.*, **31**, 909.
Wick, A. N., and Drury, D. R. (1941). *J. Biol. Chem.*, **138**, 129.

Weidemann, M. J., and Krebs, H. A. (1969). *Biochem. J.*, **112**, 149.

Weinhouse, S., and Millington, R. H. (1951). *J. Biol. Chem.*, **193**, 1.

Wieland, O. (1968). In *Advances in Metabolic Disorders*, Ed. by Levine, R., and Luft, R. New York: Academic Press Inc., **3**, 1.

Wieland, O., and Löffler, G. (1963). *Biochem. Z.*, **339**, 204.

Wieland, O., Löffler, G., Weiss, L., and Neufeldt, I. (1960). *Biochem. Z.*, **333**, 10.

Wieland, O., Weiss, L., and Eger-Neufeldt, I. (1964). In *Advances in Enzyme Regulation*, vol. 2, p. 85. Ed. by Weber, G. Oxford: Pergamon Press.

Wieland, O., Matschinsky, F., Löffler, G., and Müller, U. (1961). *Biochim. Biophys. Acta*, **53**, 412.

Wieland, O., Reinwein, D., and Lynen, F. (1956). In *Biochemical Problems of Lipids*. Ed. by Popjak, G., and LeBreton, E. London: Butterworth.

Wieland, O., and Weiss, L. (1963 *a*, *b*). *Biochem. Biophys. Res. Commun.*, **10**, 333 and **13**, 26.

Wieland, O., Weiss, L., Eger-Neufeldt, I., Teinzer, A., and Westerman, B. (1966). *Klin. Woch.*, **43**, 645.

Williamson, D. H., Bates, M. W., and Krebs, H. A. (1968). *Biochem. J.*, **108**, 353.

Williamson, D. H., Bates, M. W., Page, M. A., and Krebs, H. A. (1970). (In preparation).

Williamson, D. H., Lopez-Vieira, O., and Walker, B. (1967). *Biochem. J.*, **104**, 497.

Williamson, D. H., Lund, P., and Krebs, H. A. (1967). *Biochem. J.*, **103**, 514.

Williamson, D. H., Veloso, D., Ellington, E. V., and Krebs, H. A. (1969). *Biochem. J.*, **114**, 575.

Williamson, D. H., and Wilson, M. B. (1965). *Biochem. J.*, **94**, 19C.

Williamson, J. R., Herczeg, B., Coles, H., and Danish, R. (1966). *Biochem. Biophys. Res. Commun.*, **24**, 437.

Williamson, J. R., and Krebs, H. A. (1961). *Biochem. J.*, **80**, 540.

Williamson, J. R., Wright, P. H., Malaisse, W. J., and Ashmore, J. (1966). *Biochem. Biophys. Res. Commun.*, **24**, 765.

Yates, D. W., and Garland, P. B. (1966). *Biochem. Biophys. Res. Commun.*, **23**, 460.

Zakim, D. (1965). *Arch. Biochem. Biophys.*, **111**, 253.

INDEX

Acetate,
  growth on, 131, 132, 146, 148
  oxidation of, 122
Acetate thiokinase, 157, 162
Acetoacetate, 257–277
Acetoacetyl-CoA thiolase, 261, 268, 272
Acetyl-CoA, 261, 266, 268,270, 272
  catalytic role of, 133, 145, 146, 147
  formation of, 122, 125, 126
  reactions of, 125, 126, 131, 132
Acetylcholine depletion, 175
Acetyl-CoA–carnitine acetyl transferase, 157, 162
Aconitase reaction, 154
Active transport, 236
    as a pacemaker of metabolism, 241–242
Acyl-CoA, 267
Adaptation, enzymic, 147
Adenylate kinase, 203, 204, 206, 213
Adrenaline, 212, 215
Allosteric,
  constant, 202
  effectors, 145, 146
  protein, 202
Allulose-6-phosphate, formation of, 137
Amino acids, families of, 130
Ammonia,
  biosynthetic reactions of, 169–170
  concentration gradients, 180
      between liver and blood, 181
  concentration in blood, 168, 179–181
  concentrations in tissues, 179–181
  formation from glutamine in kidney, 177–178
  in urine, 177
  toxic effects on brain, 174–176
Ammonia load, fate in vivo, 172–174
Ammonia metabolism,
  difficulties in study of, 167
  in brain, 174–176
  in kidney, 176–179
  in liver, 168–174

regulation in mammalian tissues, 167–186
Sheffield 1936–54, 181–185
Amplification, 202, 203
  AMP as signal, 202–203
  another mechanism of, 204
Anaplerotic reactions, 130–135, 146, 147, 149
Arthrobacter globiformis,
  growth on glycine, 125, 130
  pyruvate, carboxylase in, 133, 145
ATP, 267
  as energy source for calcium pump, 92
  as energy source of muscle contraction, 88, 89, 90, 91
  depletion, 175
  enzymic evidence for role of, 237–239
  hydrolysis of, 238
  role in glucose oxidation, 88
ATPase,
  activation by external potassium, 240–241
  activation by internal sodium, 240–241
  sigmoid kinetics for activation by sodium and potassium, 247
  sodium activated, complex chemical nature of, 239
  sodium activated, mechanism of action of, 246
ATP:citrate–oxaloacetate lyase, 155
Automated analysis, 102
Autophagosomes, 111
Axenic culture, 103

Bacilli, thermophilic, 145, 147
Bacteria, photosynthetic, 131, 142, 144
Bacterium formooxydans, growth on formate by, 141
Biochemistry, as an independent discipline, 63

Ca^{2+}, 210, 211, 212

283